DIOSCORIDES ON PHARMACY AND MEDICINE

History of Science Series, No. 3

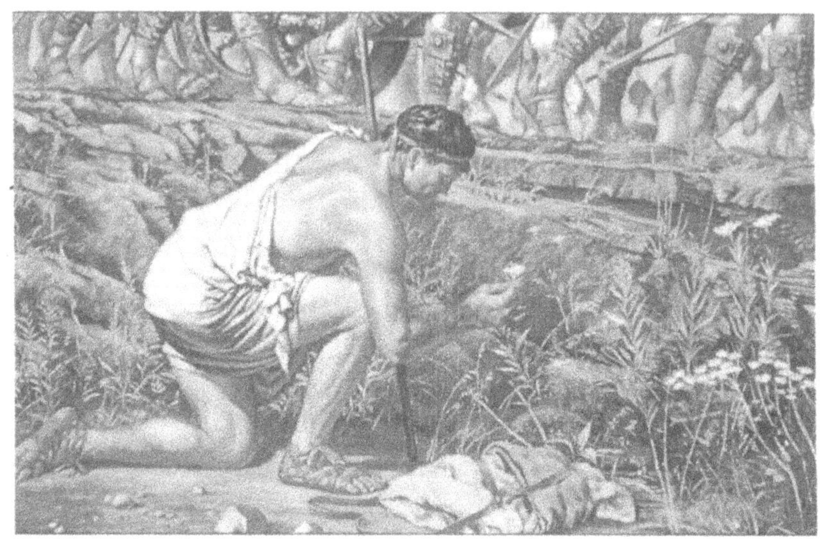

Pedanios Dioscorides, Dioscorides and the Roman legions
(Parke-Davis Great Moments in Pharmacy art series;
courtesy Parke-Davis Division of Warner-Lambert Company).

DIOSCORIDES ON PHARMACY AND MEDICINE

John M. Riddle

FOREWORD BY JOHN SCARBOROUGH

University of Texas Press, Austin

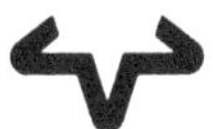

Printed in the United States of America
First paperback edition, 2011

LIBRARY OF CONGRESS CATALOGING IN PUBLICATION DATA

Riddle, John M.
Dioscorides on pharmacy and medicine.

(History of science series ; no. 3)
Bibliography: p.
Includes index.
1. Dioscorides Pedanius, of Anazarbos. De materia medica. 2. Materia medica—Early works to 1800. 3. Medicine, Greek and Roman—Early works to 1800. 4. Medicinal plants—Early works to 1800. I. Title. II. Series: History of science series (Austin, Tex.) ; no. 3. [DNLM: 1. Dioscorides Pedanius, of Anazarbos. 2. History of Medicine, Ancient. 3. Pharmacognosy—history. 4. Pharmacology—history. WZ 100 D594R]
RS79.D563R53 1985 615'.321 85-6220
ISBN 978-0-292-72984-1

To Margie and Erika

CONTENTS

ILLUSTRATIONS

TABLES

FOREWORD

EUDEMUS OF CHIOS was boasting again about his ability to withstand the powers of hellebore. Athenians soon were bored by his constant and loudly proclaimed declarations that only *he* could quaff a drink of this well-known poison and not be purged or be affected in any way. He certainly attracted the attention of the strutting young men of the city, who did not know much about plants, but many of the local farmers laughed at the wide-eyed wonder displayed by the townspeople. Finally, someone got Eudemus very drunk on neat wine at one of the frequently held evening symposia, and the secret—such as it was—became known to all: Eudemus did not have special powers, but carefully drank a cup of vinegar mixed with pumice after he had gulped the seventh measure of his hellebore solution. Perhaps one of the aspiring poets could now compose a good satire on the effrontery of Eudemus, who had exploited the ignorance of city-bred Athenian citizens. Anyone who had relatives in the country—and just about everyone in Athens did—would have known the pumice-and-vinegar antidote, and an ambitious writer of comedy could easily lampoon Eudemus, much as had the great Aristophanes brought howls of laughter with his puns on aphrodisiacs and contraceptive potions a century before.

Eudemus is a "real" historical figure, mentioned by Theophrastus in the *Historia Plantarum* (IX. 17. 2–3), composed about 300 B.C., and the account given above is lightly fictionalized from the bare essentials provided by Theophrastus. Plants and plant lore were a part of the Greeks' life from the beginning of their civilization, and even Homer could take for granted that his listeners would know their weeds, fruits, and herbs. Yet until Theophrastus, there had been little organized attempt to classify the hundreds of plants that surrounded the Greeks in their everyday life, from the crowns of laurel or wild olive leaves awarded to victors at the Pythian and Olympic games to the deadly hemlock that killed the famous Socrates in 399 B.C. How did they "work," these *pharmaka*? How could one tell an "herb" from an ordinary plant? What distinguished a "food plant" from an herb? Since most Greeks were farmers, most Greeks were not overly concerned with such questions, but they were very much interested in the lore that would instruct them in how to plow, when to plant, and when to harvest. Data of the farming year (constellations and seasons) had been recorded in hexameters by Hesiod of Ascra (about 700 B.C.) in the *Works and Days*, but always taken for granted was a common knowledge of plants. Every farm boy and girl grew up knowing them, learning basic properties, leaf shapes, textures of stems, growing seasons, and useful or dangerous fruits and seeds according to the location of the small plots that normally were Greek farms. Greeks cherished the colorful beauty of the numerous flowers of their small peninsula, and one finds references to the cabbage rose as early as Homer; later poets employed the instantly perceived white of the lily, the purples of violets, and the dozens of hues that washed the craggy landscape. Listeners hearing these songs would indeed know exactly which flowers were being referred to. Animals taught much, too: the horses of the wealthy always sought the sweetest clover in the growing greenery of the rainy season, and the pigs in their rooting often pointed out tender shoots and underground tubers.

Pharmacy and herbal lore were parts of a classical Greek common heritage, but Greeks also had an odd manner of asking why and how things were as they were. Over the centuries, thinkers and philosophers had posited a number of theories to explain the world of nature, and by Theophrastus' day, the tripartite concept of elements, qualities, and humors had become quite popular among intellectuals. Elements were the basic blocks of nature's existence, so that a combination of earth, air, fire, and water determined how something "was"; one "knew" something in nature by its qualities, the hot, the cold, the wet, and the dry, and dominance of one element was suggested by its quality (e.g., the "cold, wet earth" or the "hot, dry pepper"). Humors provided an explanation of a balancing (Greek *krasis*) of fundamental liquids in the human body, and a perfect blending gave perfect health; the four humors proposed in the fourth century B.C. by the author of the Hippocratic *Nature of Man* (blood, black bile, yellow bile, and phlegm) nicely matched the four elements and four qualities. One could then assume a drug lore that would promote a restoration of the *krasis* by knowing the dominant element and quality in the administered drug—and thereby treat with its contrary. But this was theory. How could one actually determine if a drug "worked"?

Toxic substances were fairly well understood by the second century B.C., as suggested by the poems of Nicander of Colophon, the *Theriaca* and *Alexipharmaca*. Nicander borrowed heavily from an earlier Greek toxicologist named Apollodorus, who, in turn, may have inherited his notions from Diocles of Carystus, an Athenian contemporary of Aristotle, the teacher of Theophrastus. Again Greek lore of the farm and field shows vividly in Nicander's semiplagiarism of details on the black widow spider, various cobras, wasps, and large centipedes and millipedes, as well as what was to be done if one drank too much of the famous aphrodisiac made from blister beetles. Greek pharmacy had a good botanical morphology from Theophrastus, a rough taxonomy of plants derived in part from folklore, some medical entomology and toxicology as recorded by Nicander, and a mass of details on herbs and herbal concoctions as revealed in the Hippocratic tracts on women's ailments. An organizing principle, however, did not appear in any of these Greek treatises, even though Theophrastus' basic botany had been superb.

Dioscorides lived in one of the most important eras of Western history. The Roman Empire had been created two generations before by the ruthless and brilliant statesmanship of Augustus (27 B.C.–A.D. 14), and Dioscorides of Anazarbus in extreme southeastern Asia Minor would have grown up in a "Greek world" fully under the control of Rome. The traditions suggest that Dioscorides studied botany and pharmacology in Tarsus, a nearby city with a collection of teachers in these specialties, so that when he wrote his fundamental *De materia medica* sometime around A.D. 65, Dioscorides would have inherited a long history of pharmacological data, much as he outlines in the preface to his work. The first century of the new era of Roman peace was also a time of increased trade with far-flung points in the East. New spices and drugs had come into the ken of Greco-Roman pharmacologists, especially after the sailors from Roman Egypt began to re-exploit the knowledge of the monsoons to go to India. Dioscorides could record time-tested remedies using frankincense and myrrh from southern Arabia, but he could also incorporate into his drug listings many of the newer exotica from the East, including Socotrine aloe, cloves, and true cinnamon.

All this is fairly well documented, as one reads through the Greek text of Dioscorides' *Materia medica*. He continually teases clarity from sparse description, reaches precision only after many, many observations of plants, seasons, fruits, seeds, and localities and—this is the cornerstone for Dioscorides—records what drugs "did" in patients.

John Riddle has perceptively and convincingly discerned, for the first time in modern scholarship on ancient pharmacy, that Dioscorides invented a "drug affinity system," and that the classifications in the *Materia medica* are to be explained on this basis, not on morphology or any other traditional manner then known from the pharmacological tradition. Classification by drug affinity meant that the physician had to do two things: know his plants in the field, in all of their seasonal variations, and make precise observations on a number of patients concerning what the herb, mineral, or animal product actually did or did not do. Consequently, Dioscorides' drugs always have "properties" (*dynameis* in Greek), not the vaguely perceived "powers" of earlier Greek tracts on herbs or drug lore. Utterly brilliant as was Dioscorides' innovation, it was generally ignored by almost all later physicians and pharmacologists, including the polymathic and chalcenteric Galen (A.D. 129–after 210). Only with modern pharmacognosy has Dioscorides' methodology come into clear focus, and it is to Riddle's great credit that his *Dioscorides on Pharmacy and Medicine* combines the best of modern analytical biochemistry, pharmacology, and pharmacognosy, with Dioscorides' own words and ideas. This book points the way for the future in the history of pharmacy: Riddle has demonstrated that one must command the ancient texts in their original tongues, and that one must also use the modern pharmacognosy in a judicious association with ancient data. Riddle's Dioscorides emerges as a brilliant observer, careful naturalist, astute botanist, and skilled physician, and it is due to Riddle's own dexterous scholarship that Dioscorides can reclaim his place as one of the great figures in the history of medicine.

JOHN SCARBOROUGH
Department of History and College of Pharmacy
University of Kentucky, Lexington

ACKNOWLEDGMENTS

THE PLEASURE of acknowledging all those who directly assisted me in this study, I confess, fills me with some misgivings. In dealing with the subject of ancient medicine, I encountered specialized subject matter at every turn. In acknowledging all those specialists—friends and colleagues—I risk the suspicion that this study is not so much the product of one person but of an international committee. I must claim responsibility for how I received my colleagues' advice if only to relieve them of a possible burden of error. These people gave me their expertise with indulgent patience. The fact that I am a historian of the classical and medieval periods of Western Europe surely intrigued my colleagues in the physical, biological, and medical sciences when I asked them clumsily phrased questions related to their special fields of inquiry. They saved me from many a blunder and, even when I occasionally and stubbornly did not finally agree with their suggestions, they were never ignored.

Librarians and manuscript curators throughout Europe and the United States assisted me in finding the manuscripts of and commentaries to Dioscorides, but my colleagues in the sciences are the people who enabled me to understand better the genius of Dioscorides. The following specialists assisted me in clarifying Dioscorides' meanings: Gerhard Baader (medical history, Freiuniv., Berlin); Edward Croon, Jr. (pharmacognosy, University of Mississippi); Gerald Elkan (microbiology, North Carolina State University); James W. Hardin (botany, North Carolina State University); Elizabeth Kanof (medicine, Raleigh); Paul Kauffman (ophthalmology, University of Wisconsin); Samuel G. Levin (chemistry, North Carolina State University); Gordon H. Newby (Islamism, North Carolina State University); James Newsome (medicine, University of North Carolina–Chapel Hill); Vivian Nutton (Wellcome Institute, London); Walter E. Stumpf (anatomy and pharmacology, University of North Carolina–Chapel Hill); Samuel B. Tove (biochemistry, North Carolina State University); and Paul Wheatley (social thought, University of Chicago). Sections of the book were read by Samuel Coleman (anthropology, North Carolina State University); Ann Epstein (classics, Duke University); Anthony Lavopa (history, North Carolina State University); James Mulholland (history and mineralogy, North Carolina State University); and Francis Newton (classics, Duke University). The McCormick and Company Research Center Laboratories assisted me in understanding a particularly difficult problem. At an early stage of writing, John Crellin (medical history, Duke University) read a full draft of this work and made helpful suggestions with encouraging and precautionary criticisms. A graduate student in my seminar, Albert Wylie, observed a pattern in the Dioscorides' treatment of minerals that helped me in that section. Barbara Baines and Barbara Namkoong assisted in the editorial work. Two friends, both historians of European history, urged me to relate Dioscorides' achievements to the context of his time. For this encouragement, I am indebted to Stanley Suval and James Banker, whose insight led me to face openly a previously avoided issue.

John Scarborough (University of Kentucky) read the manuscript and made innumerable suggestions. In particular, Professor Scarborough checked my translations and made many corrections, often by making entirely new proposals, which I substituted for mine, making only small alterations to his suggested translations. As a leading scholar in the field of ancient medicine, he combines the highest principles of scholarship with a spirit of generosity and friendship. His contributions are both a support and a challenge to me.

Finally, research for this book was supported by a year's fellowship from the National Endowment for the Humanities, and additional support came from my university.

INTRODUCTION

UNDER THE UMBRAGE of a bewildering variety of medical and magical theories, generations of people took herbs, minerals, and animal substances as medicines when they were sick or injured; when they were fearful of phantoms, bad spirits, or bad germs; when they wanted to preserve good health; or when they wanted to control the reproductive process. Sometimes the medicine was prescribed by a doctor, but more often it was self-prescribed or recommended by friends or relatives. Where did these common folk and their doctors learn what to take for various afflictions or how to prepare the medicine? How did they decide the proper drug amount and how often to take a dose? Did they understand the risks? Most could not read or write, at least not to the extent of comprehending a complex pharmaceutic-medical guide, even if one had existed. The concepts and technical vocabulary of early times did not permit rapid development of medical guides. People acted largely on oral information, as they did when learning manners, cooking, sewing, and the martial arts.

For the sixteen hundred years of the modern era, termed Christian, in the stretch from the Viking north to the Indian Ocean, the knowledge of medicines came more from the prodigious search effort of one man, Dioscorides (fl. ca. A.D. 40–80), than from any other person. While he may not have been the first to discover most of the usages, he industriously collected them from various lands, codified the data, and organized it in a clear, concise, and rational fashion. For this reason he became the chief authority on pharmacy and one of the principal ones on medicine.

Some time around the period A.D. 50–70, Dioscorides published a five-book study, to use his words, "on the preparation, properties, and testing of drugs." The title was περὶ ὕλης ἰατρικῆς or, in Latin, *De materia medica* [*The Materials of Medicine*].[1] Like the vast majority of people born at the beginning of the Christian era, Dioscorides lived and died in relative obscurity. But, like only a few of his generation, through his writings he greatly influenced the lives of those who followed in history. His contributions to medicine were appreciated by almost all generations, but they also were misunderstood by them. This regard for Dioscorides has almost ended in our own twentieth century, however, and now few either appreciate or understand his achievements.

His work is an assemblage of data about the medicinal properties of slightly more than 1,000 natural products drugs, mostly from the plant kingdom. He also included drugs derived from animals and minerals.[2] According to one index compiled in the sixteenth century, Dioscorides related 4,740 medicinal usages for these drugs, involving 360 varieties of medicinal actions, such as stimulants, antiseptics, and anti-inflammatory agents.[3]

Before Dioscorides, medical writers prescribed drugs for the ill and injured, but the scale and thoroughness of Dioscorides' work superseded all previous efforts—this judged both by what is extant of pre-Christian-era works and by what is related by later writers about them. When one considers that the entire Hippocratic corpus listed only about 130 medicinal substances—and the Hippocratic works were by far the largest in volume of the extant medical writings before Dioscorides—then the scale of Dioscorides' work becomes clearer.[4] Dioscorides had predecessors who wrote on drugs—he named many of them—but their works have mostly been lost. Judging by the evidence available to us of the contents of his predecessors' works, Dioscorides' writings were the largest and the most thorough.

The generations who came after him used his work for the data base of their pharmacy and medicine. During periods when the knowledge of Greek was more restricted (as happened in the late Roman Empire and the early Middle Ages), Dioscorides' work was translated into Latin, Arabic, and Armenian. It was read in an area that extended with few interruptions from the Viking North Atlantic to the Islamic parts bordering the Indian and Pacific oceans. Subsequent writers on the materials of medicine contributed their understanding of drugs within the frame, form, and context established by Dioscorides.

With the development of printing and the so-called Renaissance (1450–1600), Dioscorides was not "rediscovered" by the humanists, the way other classical authors supposedly were, because his works had never left circulation. There was, however, a dramatic intensification of interest in him as a medical authority. The Greek text of

Dioscorides was published once in the fifteenth century and five times in the sixteenth. There also were seven Latin and three Arabic translations. One verified edition of a Latin translation was published in the fifteenth century and forty-nine editions in the sixteenth. There were thirty-six different Latin commentaries involving ninety-six separate printings from 1478 to 1600. Forty-three separate printings were produced in modern vernacular translations into Italian, French, German, Czech, Spanish, Dutch, English, and Arabic. Many of these editions are folio volumes with woodcuts of the herbs and animals. They are as impressive in size as they are expressive in medical content. These statistics concern only the editions and commentaries. If we were to include his imitators—those whose contributions were based, at least in part, on Dioscorides' foundation—the numbers increase so substantially as to be unmanageable. The commentators who directly expounded on his text were generally of two types: medical practitioners and university professors who lectured on his work. The intensity of interest and refinement of his part of the educational curriculum in sixteenth-century universities led to a splintering of the study of the materials of medicine into the specialties of pharmacy, botany, and mineralogy.

All of the attention came because he was a resource for information. Dioscorides deliberately stayed away from medical theory and the swirling controversies of his day. This characteristic of his work prevented it from having a debilitating linkage with the transitory theories that succeeded one another down to the modern era. The empirical quality gave his work a timeless position in medical history. No matter what the claims about the cause of disease, the simple remedy for a headache or an upset stomach was readily accommodated to almost any school of thought. As long as people had the simple diagnoses of headaches and upset stomachs, it mattered little in one respect what they thought were their etiologies, as long as the remedies were effective. If one knew the causes, the ailments could be prevented, but once one has the affliction, the cure is paramount.

My own interest in Dioscorides came about more than a score of years ago when, while I was writing my dissertation on an aspect of the history of pharmacy, I found various conflicting citations in Latin and Arabic writings that were attributed to Dioscorides. Some of the quotations could not have come from his original work because, among other reasons, some of the drugs he was quoted as discussing were not known in Greco-Roman times. Various authors were making ingenious use of Dioscorides' authority to support their claims; at least, they thought that Dioscorides had been their authority. There were numerous texts, I discovered, that were erroneously attributed to Dioscorides. I attempted to separate what genuinely belonged to him from what was spurious.

Over the years I became progressively more interested in Dioscorides' influence in medicine. Upon satisfying myself as to his actual writings, I thought that I would write about his influence on Western medicine, through both his own and spurious writings. In repeatedly studying his text, however, I became aware that this person was a highly original medical observer, one whose work could have been explosive to the scientific categories of his and subsequent periods, but, alas, it was not. Instead, his legacy was that of a collector of data and not that of its organizer in an important and meaningful way. I determined two tasks that needed to be performed: an analysis of Dioscorides' work and the tracing of his influence. One study was to understand what Dioscorides proposed and the second was to learn how his work was undone. His own hope was that he would be remembered as an organizer of knowledge, but his successors failed to understand the scheme. Nonetheless, his successors understood the factual data. The latter and not the former provided his place in history.

I shall present the story of Dioscorides in two parts. This volume will deal with the *Materials of Medicine*. In a forthcoming book I shall discuss the influence of that text on later generations. This volume carries part of the story of Dioscorides down to the sixth century because that is when the pictures of herbs in the manuscripts—the best ones, that is—were fitted to Dioscorides' text in place of his original drawings. In writing this volume I found that a study of papyrus and early manuscripts was inextricably connected with a reconstruction of Dioscorides' original arrangement. This volume, therefore, deals with Dioscorides through the sixth century but only to the extent of what light those centuries shed on Dioscorides' work and not in what way Dioscorides' work influenced those six centuries.

Drug Efficacy and History

Many physicians and an embarrassingly large number of historians believe that in older times all physicians were little more than witch doctors who did more harm than good. Images of excessive bloodletting, obnoxious medicines, and incantations come readily to mind. Such views are misleading. Human beings living in former ages were not so unintelligent that they could be fooled if they had received mostly certain and definite harm as a result of their medical care.

Nonetheless, there are serious doubts about the efficacy of early medicine.

Arthur K. Shapiro, an eminent pharmacologist, asserts that the only common link between ancient and modern medicine is the placebo effect.[5] Certainly, as we now know, the placebo effect is very real. When the patient believes that relief has come, it is often because of an unexplained process through which the mind triggers the body's production of endorphins, the body's natural defense against pain. The placebo effect can be psychological, physiological, or psychophysiological.[6] Shapiro's emphasis on the placebo effect in medical history must be taken into account when judging Dioscorides, but, as we shall see in analyzing Dioscorides, he is not correct that placebos are the "only link."

Charles E. Rosenberg believes that, around 1800, patients and physicians shared common beliefs about how the body and drugs worked, and he concludes: "Both physician and educated layman shared a similar view of the manner in which the body functioned, and the nature of available therapeutic modalities reinforced that view."[7] While Rosenberg's point is likely true for the period around 1800, in Dioscorides' time there was absolutely no consensus as to how the body functioned or how drugs reacted on it. On the contrary, it was one of the most virulently controversial periods in medical history. One could argue that, while there was no consensus about human physiology, there could have been trust relationships between patients and physicians who subscribed to the same set of beliefs.

Certainly a critical factor in assessing therapy in any age is the relationship established between the physician and the patient. Since that relationship is important, it should be kept in mind when studying Dioscorides, but only in the back of the mind—to use a modern anatomical metaphor. Patient-physician relations are secondary to the intrinsic question about the efficacy of Dioscorides' remedies. His work was a guide to drugs and not a comprehensive medical therapy text. We have no way of knowing all the uses to which his work was subject. It is certain that some good physicians in every age used Dioscorides' information in treating their trusting and obedient patients. Still there were some poor physicians with suspicious, hardheaded patients who used Dioscorides as well. The question is whether the information in Dioscorides' work largely assisted recovery, relieved pain, and treated diseases, whoever may have employed it.

J. Worth Estes' seminal study of the clinical effectiveness of colonial American drugs led him to conclude: "Neither they nor their doctors could have known the majority would have recovered without any of the 225 preparations then commonly available."[8] Dioscorides would have been, I believe, the first to concede Estes' supposition. Dioscorides' claims for his drugs were usually modest. The gauge for judging the success of most medical therapy, whether in ancient Rome, colonial America, or present Germany, is the recovery of the patient. Some patients, of course, did not recover and some fewer still died. The question remains, could the remedies in Dioscorides' work, if properly administered, have assisted in the recovery or were they largely incidental to the healing processes?

Henry F. Dowling is very emphatic about the efficacy of early drugs. "Less than two dozen effective drugs were known before the year 1700."[9] If no consensus existed about the workings of the body in Dioscorides' time, it is equally true that there exists no consensus today as to the value and effectiveness of early medicines.

In contrast to Dowling's, Rosenberg's, and Shapiro's opinions, and mindful of Estes' point about the healing process exclusive of drug therapy, there are many in today's science communities who see in the study of traditional drugs a means to add to our present knowledge.[10] These people believe that many of the crude drugs from natural sources were pharmaceutically effective. The editorial in the first issue of the *Journal of Ethnopharmacology* (Lausanne, 1979, p. 1) said, "In fact, almost every classical pharmacologic is derived from a classical botanical source originally employed as a native remedy."

Methodology

My central purpose in analyzing Dioscorides' *De materia medica* is not to enter the modern debate about the effectiveness of traditional drugs and medicine. Nonetheless we cannot be disinterested because the issue directly relates to the judgment we shall form about the importance of Dioscorides' contribution. On the one hand, Dioscorides was important because historically his work was influential in science, and this is a fact regardless of any opinions on the part of modern scientists as to the validity of his science. On the other hand, however, we cannot ignore our informed modern perceptions of science when we study a historical work.

For years in studying early medicine, I avoided answering the inevitable question, "Do the remedies work?" When we study early science purely by extrapolating the anticipations of modern science we do little in the way of understanding early science or history. If one searches the historical documents of medicine to find those drugs which appear in our modern medical guides, we distort the record. Such a process only validates modern science by giving its "facts" historical heritage. In the process, it reassures us about our present science by confirming what we already knew and had no particular reason to doubt. Left unexplained in the historical records will be those crude drugs about which modern science is mute, either because the laboratories have yet to examine the plant or animal chemistry or because the chemicals, either as individual compounds or in synergistic relation with other compounds found in the same natural product, have received no clinical testing. The number of instances where modern science studies do not provide adequate testimony to assess the historical data is large enough to be meddlesome.

The task of analyzing Dioscorides' *De materia medica* by identifying the natural substances and translating his Greek to modern terms, then fitting his medicine to modern science, is not easy. Does the effectiveness of a drug rest with the time when it is measured or is its effectiveness somehow absolute? There are drugs given by the Greeks and Romans to relieve particular ailments that modern science has found effective. But, in some instances, modern science has proven the prescribed drugs harmful, as we shall see. Let us suppose that "x" was given for "y" from A.D. 50 through 1350, but in 1650 "x" was in disfavor and no longer given for "y." In 1800 the medical science community re-examined the issue and restored "x" as a therapeutic agent, this time not for "y" but for "w." "W" may or may not have been pathologically similar to "y." But suppose in the most recent pronouncement—laboratory analysis and clinical testing in 1950—"x" was rejected as being pharmaceutically effective for both "y" and "w." This means that the measure of the effectiveness of a drug is dependent on the age in which the measure is made. Accordingly, some ages—to continue with the hypothetical case—judge the science of A.D. 50 as "correct," and other ages as "incorrect." Some people in science today would say that in 1985 one cannot accept as necessarily valid a position based on laboratory and clinical reports of 1950 because of the superseding innovations. The judgment about the effectiveness of "x" tells us something of the age in which the judgment was formed, especially when we study what procedures were used in forming the judgment. It tells us little, however, about this particular piece of medical knowledge for the period we seek to assess. On the basis of a 1950 study, how strongly can we assert the validity of the A.D. 50 assertion of fact? The ancient Roman might well echo the words of the modern poet who said, "Let no age write my epitaph."

The historian of science is familiar with these dilemmas inherent in understanding the past. Even though we eschew judging another age's science (except in a broad interpretation of how people of a period formed their opinions), we cannot escape the prison of our present understanding as we seek to delve into the past. When our sense of nature is violated, we react negatively, even though it may also be with understanding, perhaps even sympathy. Aristotle said that a moved object must be in contact or continuous contact with the thing it moves, but we know that he was *wrong* because motion was the same in Aristotle's day as it is now.[11] We do not, indeed cannot, assume other postulates, for instance, that in Aristotle's day nature was different than today's nature.

While the history of the exact sciences, such as mathematics and physics, poses its own set of problems, the history of medicine is far more complex. In dealing with Dioscorides, the number of variables is so large that we cannot ever be absolutely certain of the historical data. First there is the reading of the manuscripts in order to determine what actually was written. Then we must determine exactly the natural products that Dioscorides was discussing. In the case of plants we must pinpoint the exact species in our Linnaean taxonomy—a precise classification system Dioscorides did not have. We must translate the technical terms, sometimes combining symptoms, to reformulate ancient perceptions in our modern-day terms for diseases and afflictions. Ancient Greek seldom precisely coincides with modern technical English. We need to determine the harvesting and preparation methods, factors we know are vital to proper drug manufacture from natural products. We cannot always know that the plants were the same chemically then as they are now. The modern science of phytochemistry makes us aware of individual variations even among plants of the same species. It is critical in determining the possible effectiveness of any crude, natural drug to know not only the exact species and its environment but also the method of harvesting, the morphology of extraction site (e.g., roots, leaves, etc.), the preparation, and the administration. One modern textbook names thirteen individual patient variable factors affecting drug metabolism, ten variable factors related to drug administration, and thirteen variable factors related to external environmental factors.[12] These variables are operative when we know the pure synthesized drug and not a complex natural product.

Even the most meticulous scholarship in translating Dioscorides' manuscripts and studying their contents is still not going to yield easily the data necessary to evaluate the effectiveness of the drugs or the value of his medicine. Judging Dioscorides' science is fraught with danger. At most points there are paleographical snares, botanical puzzles, medical pitfalls, and semantical traps. We cannot be certain of most of the evidence because we are seldom sure when we have a fact. Even so, the evidence can be accepted as a body through a careful judgment of each particular item. When such evidence is mounted, it appears sufficient to assert reasonable probability. As these cases accumulate, the sheer weight of the evidence allows us to be reasonably certain that Dioscorides was a rational user of drug therapy.

Particular problems in terms and concepts relevant to understanding Dioscorides will be discussed as we encounter them in our analysis. Perhaps this approach is preferable to a long discussion of methodology before one has sampled Dioscorides' writings. One exception to this rule will be the textual problems, but I shall delay that discussion until the second volume. The textual variations in the manuscripts show how scribes in the different periods occasionally made modifications in the text based on their own medical experiences.

Plant Identifications

The identification of Dioscorides' plants requires explanation and special caution. Since modern scientific names for individual plants do not correspond exactly with Dioscorides' "kinds" (εἴδη) of plants and animals, we have to make judgments as to what plants Dioscorides *probably* meant. A number of methods must be combined in making these identifications: (*a*) Dioscorides' description; (*b*) pictures in manuscripts; (*c*) collaborative descriptions made by those closer to Dioscorides in time, for example, Pliny and Theophrastus; (*d*) descriptions and illustrations made since Dioscorides in interpreting his flora; and (*e*) pharmacognosy. Each of these methods will be discussed in context.

When standard authorities seem to agree or nearly agree, the modern binominal identification is given without comment or reference (usually in parenthesis following the Greek term). Sometimes the addition of the scientific name imparts more authority than the evidence merits. One should realize that there are real possibilities for error. Dioscorides may have intended a different plant altogether, or two or more species of the same or different genera, when our tentative identifications are to one specific species. Over the years many botanists have sought to identify Dioscorides' plants. Principal among them are Kaspar Maria von Sternberg, who wrote a study of Matthiolus' commentary to Dioscorides, published in Prague in 1821;[13] Curtius Sprengel, who produced the first modern printed text in Greek of Dioscorides in 1829–1830[14] and who based much of his insight on Janus Saracenus' 1598 commentary;[15] Julius Berendes, who produced a German translation and commentary in 1902;[16] Robert T. Gunther, editor of John Goodyer's 1655 English translation,[17] who added the work of Charles Daubeny;[18] and Otto Stapf, a botanist with Kew Gardens and an expert in Dioscorides' flora. Other important modern references used are A. Carnoy, *Dictionnaire étymologique des noms grecs de plantes* (1959); Jacques André, *Lexique des termes de botanique en latin* (1959); Arthur Hort, *Theophrastus Enquiry into Plants* (1948; plants and nomenclature supplied by William Thiselton-Dyer); and W. H. S. Jones, *Pliny: Natural History*, vols. 6–8 (1951–1963). When there are important differences of opinion, there will be full citations.

I ordinarily give a modern identification to the plant, but sometimes when the plant is very common, such as garden lettuce, radishes, and cabbage, the scientific name is omitted. To include scientific names would, in these cases, needlessly clutter the text and convey an impression that Dioscorides was more precise in a modern way than he was. Normally, once the plant is identified, subsequent references will be only to its common English name.

Another Work By Dioscorides?

Only the *De materia medica* will be reviewed in this volume, but, of all the pseudo-Dioscoridean treatises, there is considerable doubt about the authorship of one treatise, Περὶ ἁπλῶν φαρμάκων, "On Simple Drugs," sometimes called Εὐπόριστα, "Family Medicines." The treatise is assigned to Dioscorides in its various manuscript copies, and through the sixteenth century it was considered by those few who knew it to have been written by Dioscorides. It did not receive wide circulation in the West, at least, until the latter half of the sixteenth century. Sixteenth-century scholars believed that a quotation in the Dioscoridean treatise attributed to Aetius of Amida (sixth century A.D.) was a later interpolation and, therefore, the fact did not shake their confidence in its authorship.[19] In 1795 Ioannes A. Fabricius rejected "On Simple Drugs" as a genuine Dioscorides work.[20] In 1903 Max Wellmann, Dioscorides' modern editor, first said in an encyclopedia article that he thought the work spurious and a product of an anonymous author of the third or fourth century.[21] Later Wellmann changed his mind and reversed himself in a short pamphlet in which he argued for its authenticity (but with many later interpolations).[22]

I confess that I have changed my mind about its authorship, possibly even more often than Wellmann, but I have yet to take a position in print. In this volume, I shall avoid once again an expressed opinion. Instead, a discussion of the treatise will be in the sequel to this volume. Regardless of whether Dioscorides did or did not write "On Simple Drugs," I agree with one part of Wellmann's last opinion on the subject: if authored by Dioscorides, it was earlier in his writing than was *De materia medica.*[23] Whoever wrote "On Simple Drugs," in my opinion, either had not yet seen, or never knew, or did not appreciate the organizational scheme that Dioscorides devised in *De materia medica*. For an analysis of Dioscorides' *major or only* work, it matters little whether or not earlier in his career he wrote "On Simple Drugs." Let us, therefore, postpone a consideration of the piece and turn our attention to *De materia medica*.

Order of Presentation

This study of Dioscorides is presented in five chapters, coincidentally similarly to Dioscorides' five books in his original *De materia medica.* The first part of our study examines what we know of Dioscorides' life—in a word, little—and the state of the medical arts during his time—in a word, controversial. The extent to which Dioscorides relied on other authorities is explored because it is important in judging his originality but less so than one might initially think. Dioscorides' own claim to uniqueness will close the first part.

Dioscorides' five-book *De materia medica* had two organizational schemes, which are examined in Chapters 2 and 3. In the second chapter, the method he chose to relate information about each simple drug will be explored in the same order as he presented for each chapter component: plant name and picture; plant habitats; botanical description; drug properties; medicinal usages; harmful side effects; quantities and dosages; harvesting, preparation, and storage; adulteration; veterinary usages; magical and nonmedical usages; and specific geographical locations. The section on the 4,740 or so medicinal usages is the most complicated because ancient symptoms and diseases do not precisely correspond to our modern ones. Various approaches to their study yield different perceptions, and I shall offer a variety of methods so as to present a multifaceted approach to medical history.

The order of presentation in each chapter was not nearly as important as the order for presenting each chapter. Dioscorides' genius was in the order of arranging chapters in relationship one to another. Therein lay the order he saw in nature. The organization of the chapters on plants constitutes our Chapter 3. The sequel to it postulates that Dioscorides' animal and mineral drugs have the same theoretical affinities as did his plant products.

Chapter 5 concludes this work with the acceptance by the Greco-Roman world of Dioscorides' factual data. Dioscorides' theoretical system was not acceptable either because of competitive, alternative theories or because he completely failed to communicate. The unfolding of these two possibilities is the principal concern of the later study of Dioscorides' influence. Nonetheless, there is involved a pertinent, inseparable problem in the very analysis of Dioscorides' work. Manuscript copyists rearranged Dioscorides' order, thereby producing a different work, one that preserved the information about drugs but destroyed the proposition about drug relationships. Light on this subject is shed by a survey of Galen's pharmaceutical theory, by the early papyrus fragments of both Dioscorides and various herbalists, and by scattered manuscript evidence.

The pictures of plants and animals are the topic in Chapter 5. One who sees the beautiful, illuminated Dioscorides' manuscripts for the first time marvels at the fine colored drawings that begin most chapters. One would expect, therefore, that discussion of the pictures would come at the beginning, not the end, of this book. The reason the pictures are discussed last is that those we have in the manuscripts were the last to be added.

DIOSCORIDES ON PHARMACY AND MEDICINE

The Medical Remedies Discussed in This Book
Are Intended Solely as Historical Analysis.
Any Use of Them for Therapeutic Purposes
Could Be Dangerous.

1. DIOSCORIDES AND THE MATERIALS OF MEDICINE

DIOSCORIDES' HOMETOWN was Anazarbus.[1] The town site is strategically located along a bend in the river Pyramus as it tumbles down from the mountains. At Anazarbus, the river twists around a bend and hurries to a red rock, a natural citadel. At its foot is the town. The site arises from the plain of the province of Roman Cilicia in what is now Turkey.[2] Anazarbus was located along two trade routes leading to Syria and Cappadocia. Geography made it important but people did not. The town never equaled the importance and the size of Tarsus, its nearby rival in the spirited urban competitions of the day. Anazarbus' greatest claim to fame was its son Dioscorides, who sometimes noted that flowers and herbs seemed to grow just a bit better in Cilicia than elsewhere.[3] Some later manuscripts referred to him merely as "the Anazarbian" without fear of confusion with any other illustrious citizen, save Oppian, a relatively obscure native son who, a century later, wrote a poem on fishing.

Reconstructing Dioscorides' life is difficult because no one other than Dioscorides himself gives us any helpful information. We say *helpful* information because writers much later than Dioscorides' own time sought to construct a biographical sketch from inferences drawn from Dioscorides' work and from information about others named Dioscorides. Most of these authorities gave these essential details of his life: born with the name Pedanius Dioscorides at Anazarbus, studied at Tarsus and Alexandria, served as physician with the Roman legions, and traveled widely collecting drugs and plants.[4] Some older accounts placed him in Egypt when Cleopatra ruled and Mark Antony dallied there.[5] The latter confuses him with another person by the same name who lived in Cleopatra's Egypt and wrote a commentary on Hippocrates.[6] The word *Pedanius* is found in manuscript rubrics and may have been a name. Greeks normally had only one name, but if one received Roman citizenship, he frequently added a Roman name, perhaps from a benefactor. Three candidates for Dioscorides' first-name benefactor are L. Pedanius Secundus, Roman prefect in A.D. 56; Pedanius Secundus, who was likely governor of the Roman province of Asia in the early 50s; and Gn. Pedanius Salinator, consul in A.D. 60.[7] These possibilities are conjecture, however. All we know from sources other than Dioscorides' own work is his name—Pedanius Dioscorides from Anazarbus.

The preface to the five books comprising *De materia medica* (*The Materials of Medicine*) is a letter written by Dioscorides to Areios of Tarsus, a medical writer on pharmacy whose works are lost but mentioned in later testimonials.[8] Dioscorides graciously dedicated his labor to Areios and explained why he had written the work. In the letter Dioscorides used an expression denoting that he was a student of Areios[9] and that he had been inspired by him to study drugs. Tarsus—no mean city, Saint Paul called it—was an intellectual center that Strabo said surpassed Athens and Alexandria.[10] In particular, Tarsus was a center for pharmacy and pharmacology.[11] "For as it were," Dioscorides wrote to Areios, "since I was a youth,[12] I have shown a continuous interest in the knowledge of [medical] materials and I have traveled in numerous lands—for, as you know, I have lived a soldierlike life." The problem—and it is a big one—is the translation of *οἶσθα γὰρ ἡμῖν στρατιωτικὸν*, which I rendered as "soldierlike life." Others have translated the words differently: "military career," "life of a soldier," and "my soldier's life."[13]

The association of wide travel and militarylike life was enough for many to conclude that Dioscorides was a military physician with the Roman legions.[14] Whereas the ambiguity of the Greek permits translation of a "soldier's life," it is also true that the Greek words are not restricted to this translation. For the following reasons it is by no means conclusive that Dioscorides was a physician with the legions:

1. Little attention is given in his work to wounds, which would be a principal concern for military medical men. In Book I, which covers aromatics and balms used to treat wounds, only 10 drugs are discussed for this therapy, including 6 usages for "drawing together bloody wounds."[15] In the entire *De materia medica* there are 138, liberally counted.[16] These figures are compared with 39 gynecological usages and 24 treatments for regulating dysfunctional menstruation in Book I alone.[17] In all five books, 411 drugs are prescribed for 18 actions for the female urogenital system.[18] Considering the fact that in Dioscorides' day Roman law did not permit soldiers to marry while in service, it would be unlikely that Roman military physicians would

treat mostly women;[19] wound therapy would likely receive emphasis. Dioscorides does not appear to be a specialist in treating the kinds of injuries to which soldiers are vulnerable, whether acquired in battle or in barroom fights.

2. The standing of "physicians" in the Roman legions may have been little higher than that of legionnaires who developed a skill in treating injuries. The existence of "professional" corps of physicians assigned to or employed by the military is uncertain. A lively, informative debate over the standing of Roman military physicians was conducted between John Scarborough and Vivian Nutton. Even if one were to take the best-case argument, accepting Nutton's appreciation rather than Scarborough's depreciation, there is no example that I know of in the records of a Roman medical writer who had a military standing.[20]

3. The places that Dioscorides mentioned in the context of personal observations are mercantile sites and very few are military posts where legionnaires were assigned. Dioscorides often specified plant habitats; he made thirty-eight references to provinces, cities, or mountains in Asia Minor (modern Turkey), twenty-seven to the same on the Greek mainland, twelve to Egypt, nine to Syria, eight to Italy, six to Arabia, three each to Spain and Africa (including Libya, Marmarica, and Ethiopia), three to Persia, two to India, two to Armenia, and one each to Gaul, Somalia (Troglodytia), and the Red Sea. In addition he made numerous references to plants on islands: nine times to Crete, five to Cyprus, two to Sardinia, and one each to the Balearic Islands, Rhodes, Chios, Samothrace, Hyères Islands (off the southeast coast of France), and Cyclades Islands.[21] In the first four books he observed the following places as trade or manufacturing centers for particular products: Petra, a Nabataean caravan city in present Jordan, four references; Egypt, four references, including, specifically, "the merchants of Alexandria"; and one each for Achaia (in Greece), Africa, Barbarian lands, Britain (in reference to mead, the alcoholic drink), eastern Iberia, western Iberia, Palmyra, Pamphylia, and Phoenicia. With the exception of Syria, Iberia, and Gaul, all places in his travels in the Roman Empire were senatorial provinces and not imperial provinces in which the military was stationed. (Egypt had a different status.) Based on the amount of information and its quality, Dioscorides almost certainly visited Petra, the legendary caravan city and capital of the Nabataean Arabs.[22] Petra was outside the Roman Empire and the reach of its legions until A.D. 106. As a soldier, Dioscorides could hardly have visited there.

Dioscorides did not copy these place names from other accounts. He explained that his work differed in part from that of his predecessors because, contrary to some of their methods, he knew plants from examining them in the field and not merely through books. He identified plants and minerals through direct observation and inquiry of the folk in the various regions (Pref. 5). One need not take his word exclusively for this assertion. Where we have fragments of written sources that Dioscorides used, there is little evidence that he copied other people's statements about specific regional habitat or folk practices and nomenclature. Generally, what passes as an observation appears to have been his own.

John Scarborough and Vivian Nutton, who disagreed about Roman military medicine, have turned their considerable talents to the interpretation of the six vexing Greek words, which they have rendered as "you are well acquainted with my soldier's life." Scarborough and Nutton affirm the traditional interpretation that Dioscorides probably did some military service but likely, they think, just for a short term. They base the conclusion on the following evidence: (*a*) it was a common circumlocution to say "soldierlike life" to mean "soldier's life"; (*b*) Dioscorides probably saw too little fighting to stress wound therapy; and (*c*) he could have traveled beyond the Empire's borders to Petra before, after, or during his military service.[23] Their cogently presented evidence leads to a reasonable conclusion that Dioscorides probably was in the military, but likely for only a short term.

Drug Trader?

Accepting for the moment, at least, Scarborough and Nutton's conclusion, let us continue to speculate as to how Dioscorides earned his way in the Roman world while collecting vast information about the materials of medicine. Looking again at the catalogue of plant locations, we see that most are mercantile sites. Could it be that Dioscorides was a merchant who dealt with the drug trade? His interests were in the materials of medicine, and it is true that there was little discussion of medicine as medicine. He remained aloof from the polemical, theoretical controversies among schools of medicine during his time, and in doing so he was perhaps unique among other medical writers of the day who chose sides and defended their ground with vitriol. Dioscorides was more interested in the vitriol itself. His attention was to the identification of plants and minerals; the range of their usages, including nonmedical ones; the methods of preparation and storage; and the techniques for adulteration and testing to detect fraudulent practices. He sometimes related trade information, but there is no concentration on its details. Furthermore, he seldom mentioned packaging and never costs—things one would expect to be among a trader's concerns. Dioscorides was not a drug dealer.

Druggist?

If not a wholesale drug dealer, we ask if he might have been a druggist, that is, in our term, a pharmacist? The Greeks had not one but many words for this occupational group. The most comprehensive term was for the *φαρμακοπῶλαι*, or "makers of remedies," who sold things other than drugs, such as magnifying glasses.[24] Scant though it is, evidence points to these *pharmakopōlai*, or "druggists," as being engaged in health care, even to the extent of preparing bandages in ophthalmological surgery.[25] One *pharmakopōlēs* allegedly performed a sex reversal operation.[26] Nonetheless, the *pharmakopōlai* were not physicians (*ἰάτροι*) and are best described as a member group within the health profession, to use our broad term. The social status of the *pharmakopōlai* was not high, at least it was not in comparison with the high regard for physicians.[27] We do not know the names of outstanding "makers of remedies" who rose above *hoi polloi*.

Occupying an apparently more prestigious position were the "root-cutters," or *rhizotomoi* (*ῥιζοτόμοι*), who may have been distinguished by a greater degree of specialization. Certainly, the ancients from Theophrastus (ca. 371–ca. 287 B.C.) to Galen (September A.D. 129–after 210)[28] referred to *rhizotomoi* as a separate group. For example, Theophrastus said, ". . . we may add statements made by druggists and root-cutters" (*φαρμακοπῶλαι καὶ οἱ ῥιζοτόμοι*).[29] An apparent distinction between root-cutters, or root-druggists, and the *pharmakopōlai* is that root-cutters wrote about their occupation.[30] The term did not seem to be used as disparagingly as was sometimes the case with *pharmakopōlai*.[31] Dioscorides gave a "left-handed" compliment to one of them, Crateuas, when, speaking of the lack of comprehensiveness in earlier books on drugs, Dioscorides said, "Crateuas the Root-cutter and Andreas the Physician—who are apparently more precise in this aspect—omitted many exceptionally useful roots and a few herbs."[32] Crateuas practiced his profession in the court of King Mithridates VI (120–63 B.C.). Dioscorides, Galen, and others generally praised Crateuas and his work, which has survived in fragments.[33]

There was no licensing or regulation regarding any health services in antiquity, nor was there guild control as there was later in the Middle Ages in the West. As a consequence, anyone could sell anything as a drug, and the buyer had to beware. For that very reason necessity required the buyers to be alert for poor products. They needed to measure the quality of a drug and to observe its effectiveness so that, when the medical problem repeated itself, they could know its treatment better. Not having the protection of licensing authority of the state, educational institutions of training and certification, or guild controls, the buyers purchased drugs mostly from those whom they and their friends had come to trust. The community cumulated experiences with the drugs and druggists alike. Probably, in antiquity just as today, most drugs were self-administered but taken in consultation with druggists, friends, and family. It is difficult to exaggerate the sensitivity and alertness to quality drugs and the efficiency of communication about them within the community that must have been present in the towns and countrysides of antiquity in the absence of the institutional protection devices of today.

Sellers specialized with their wares, resulting in a number of other identifiable groups who also could be called druggists. There were the "mixture sellers" (μιγματοπώλαι),[34] the "dealers in scented oils" (μυροπώλαι),[35] and the "ungent makers" (μυρέφοι),[36] to name some.[37] Cosmeticians sold drugs as well as cosmetics. We assume that all of these groups gave medical advice related to drug therapy. Medical assistants (ὑπηρέται) to physicians also were an identifiable group, separate from physicians in training, who may have rendered independent care under supervision.[38]

Since ancient sources do not reveal a complete picture, we might learn from the medical anthropologists who study the selection and training of herbalists in traditional societies.[39] Some learned simple herbal cures and the recipes for compounding them from their parents or friends and then developed the interest to the point of acquiring a reputation within the community. For some, this may have led to a full-time occupation with a place of business. Others assumed a role of part-time druggist—supplier, preparer, dispenser, and adviser. Still others learned the trade skills when they were employed as apprentices.

Dioscorides as Practicing Physician

As noted above, Dioscorides' choice of words indicated that he was a student of Areios of Tarsus. Also, in his dedication to Areios, Dioscorides pointed to Areios' special devotion to those who "practice the same art" (πρὸς τοὺς ὁμοτέχνους).[40] Dioscorides employed the word τέχνη to mean medicine.[41] That term (τέχνη) broadly meant "art" or "skillful trade," but it came to have a more restrictive meaning of "medicine," as in the first Hippocratic aphorism: "The art [of medicine] long, life is short."

Areios wrote a life of Hippocrates that is now lost.[42] In citing Areios a number of times, Galen indicated that Areios wrote on drugs and that once he had been an Asclepiadian,[43] although he later disassociated himself from that group. Asclepiades of Cius in Bithynia (d. ca. 92 B.C.) was a rhetorician-philosopher who turned to medicine allegedly for financial rewards. He became a physician of sufficient importance and controversy that a sect, sometimes spoken of as a school, developed around him in antiquity.[44] In the only specific reference to a sect in his writing, Dioscorides spoke against the Asclepiadians. No doubt he assumed his mentor's attitude.

In summary, Dioscorides was a student of Areios. Areios wrote medical works on drugs and Hippocrates, and once he was an associate member of the medical cult that both he and Dioscorides rejected. These facts indicate that Dioscorides was trained as a physician, having acquired the art from Areios. Not all who wrote on medicine or were learned in the subject were necessarily practicing physicians. As in ancient pharmacy, there was a broad range of specializations and occupations among those engaged in health care and medicine. Dioscorides seemed to have belonged to what we today and the people in his time called the highest type of medical people, the learned physician.

In Dioscorides' time, the Greek physician was closely associated with "learned" or "philosophical" medicine. Although physicians (*ἰατρός, -οι*) referred to their profession as "the art," they did not mean that they thought of themselves only as skilled craftsmen, like carpenters and metallurgists. In the first century, Celsus believed that Hippocrates "in ancient times" had separated medicine from philosophy.[45] Whether this was true or not historically, people believed that the physician's historical ancestor was a philosopher and not a practitioner of anything save pure wisdom. Even though probably only a few of the ancient physicians actually were familiar with the Hippocratic oath,[46] there can be no doubt that physicians (and some lay people as well) considered the medical art to be on a lofty plane. A physician was a *καλοκἀγαθός*, "a practitioner of the noble arts," or "a gentleman in body, mind, and social position."[47] There was a strong professional tradition whereby a medical ethic, known to us as Hippocratic, was transmitted from physician to apprentice, although they did not necessarily share in all of the values that are in the present oath.[48] Greek physicians saw themselves as links in this historical chain whose critical development eighteenth-, nineteenth-, and early twentieth-century historians saw as coming from the "schools" at Cnidus and, to a greater degree, Cos, where Hippocrates himself practiced medicine.[49] Wesley D. Smith believes that there were never competing "schools" at Cnidus and Cos but that scholars misinterpreted evidence while searching to have an ancient founder for medicine, Hippocrates.[50] Classical medicine never had schools in an institutional sense with diplomas or certifying apparata, but there may have been sects in the sense of shared beliefs and practices about how to care for the sick and injured. Students closely identified with their teachers, who were often their fathers, and the association of like-mindedness in medical care. The classical Greek background of Hellenistic medicine is rooted in physicians who learned their skills from those who had gained their knowledge from experience, not from a priest acting as the gods' intermediary.[51] This assertion of history, whether a historical reality or a myth, was a powerful force in directing the self-awareness of medicine's societal role.

Although Greek physicians saw themselves in this chain, they did not have a consensus as to the physiology of the body. By Dioscorides' time, they had separated into various and often bitterly divided schools, but they all regarded one another as physicians (*ἴατροι*). The Greek physician was distinct in at least his own mind, we surmise, from others engaged in health care who had learned medical skills from true craft specialists, such as midwives, surgeons, and eye doctors. Medicine as practiced by the physicians was the art of total health care, though some would stress diet, others drugs, and still others manipulations, all of which were controlled by reasoning (λόγος).[52] Reasoning differentiated medicine from lesser health-related craft skill specialties. In contrast with the Romans, who had a baser opinion of physicians, Greeks, even those in Dioscorides' time, saw the physician and philosopher together in union. One could be a philosopher without being a physician but not a physician without being a philosopher.[53] Dioscorides wrote: "It is, I suppose, obvious to everyone that pharmacology [*ὁ περὶ φαρμάκων λόγος*] is a necessity, closely linked to the whole art of medicine [*ὅλη τῇ τεχνῃ*] and forging with its every part an invincible alliance."[54] Dioscorides connected *medicine and reasoning about drugs* and not medicine and pharmacy, which was an empirical science of preparing and dispensing drugs.

In Book V, Chapter 19, Dioscorides complained that he had to include a section on medicinal wines because its omission would be noted critically by amateur physicians.[55] By reasoning, true physicians, he implied, would know that the drug activity of a medicinal wine was the sum of its constituent parts. Thus, the efficacy of thyme wine (V. 49) as a medicine is predicated on the fact that its activity is the sum of the wine and thyme. Those not in the profession could not be expected to know this; therefore, Dioscorides felt obliged to include the section on composite wines, superfluous though it was to true physicians. By this passage, Dioscorides showed himself to be a physician in the traditional Hellenistic Greek sense and, very importantly, he revealed that his work was intended for all who were engaged in health care, not merely physicians, who were the reasoners about medicine.

Dioscorides revealed himself as being in the chain of Greek doctors, but we must determine whether he practiced medicine in a more indirect way. In the first century A.D., the practicing physician in Greek-speaking areas was recognized as being someone trained in the medical arts. Without a formal certification mechanism, the physician had to be accepted as one who had mastered the skills.[56] These physicians were different from the temple practitioners in the special temples of Asclepios about whom we know little.[57] In the Greek community, as well as in Roman and other ethnic groups, one was a physician if one practiced medicine, and one could practice medicine if he (in rare cases, she) had patients. One way to be accepted by the community to treat patients would be for a person to bring with him an endorsement from an established medical practitioner that his former student or apprentice was trained in the skill.[58]

From the time of Homer, physicians were noted as being travelers. This is evidenced by inscriptions dedicated to peripatetic physicians whose period of residency resulted in an achievement commemorated by local communities.[59] Louis Cohn-Haft said, ". . . travel appears to have been the natural expectation of the physician in every period of antiquity [after Homer]."[60] One Hippocratic treatise, the *Canon*, described a physician as one "who has acquired an exact knowledge of the subject before he set out to travel from city to city." Since Dioscorides was clearly one whose peregrinations led him about the eastern Roman Empire, we surmise that he was a typical, traveling physician who rendered his services widely.

In Greek areas, there was an awareness that the best medical education was acquired in given and well-known cities that were home to famous teachers or that were widely known for political sponsorship of learned activity, Cos and possibly Cnidus, as well as Athens, Corinth, Ephesus, and Assos, were cities and areas to which aspiring poets and scholars could go and expect to find teachers and experts. In the Hellenistic period and early Roman imperial era, Alexandria, Antioch, Tarsus, and Rome were added to this list. Some state-sponsored institutions came into being which officially fostered the gathering of scholars of all sorts, including those in medicine, the most famous ones of these being the Museum (*Mouseion*: "Temple to the Muses"). Ptolemy I (305–283 B.C.) ensured himself a place in cultural history and endeared himself to scholars and bibliophiles, if perhaps not to his subjects, when he founded both the Library and the Museum in Alexandria to promote Hellenistic rule by revitalizing Hellenistic learning.

Once a person had acquired his medical knowledge, he worked to obtain recognition for his learning. Above all, in the period of trial in the community, the residency as it were, the practitioner had to produce some positive results. Communities watched a physician's patients closely, because people in the communities knew one another well.[61] Examinations often were conducted in the open at clinics and not behind closed doors or in the homes of the nonambulatory patients with only family present. If, as a result of the physician's therapy, the patient seemed to benefit, the community members recognized that they had a physician among them. A community could solicit physicians to move to its town, often by offering them recognition as public physicians, in return for which at least part of the physician's practice had to be devoted to the poor for no fee above a possible stipend provided for by the contract.[62] The important point is that the physician was expected to be good at his skill within the limits that people thought possible.

The ability to diagnose and deliver a prognosis was extremely important in establishing a reputation. For this reason, a supreme achievement of classical Greek medicine was the highly refined art of nosography. Merely recognizing and foretelling the course of disease was not the extent of the physician's duty. He was expected to assist nature's curing processes, unless, of course, he recognized fatal signs and was reluctant to risk his prestige with a therapy.[63] Doctors whose patients died were suspect if they had not foretold the outcome.

The ancient physician was not so much a manipulator of natural processes as he was nature's coordinator. Diet regimens, hygiene, and surgery were skilled procedures available, but the emphasis was more on diet than on surgery (which we believe was often performed by specialists, not all of whom were recognized as physicians). Nature provided an effective way to promote curing: drugs. In the philosophy of the Hermetic literature, some of it a product of Dioscorides' time, nature endowed each herb, rock, and animal with a benefit to humans. One needed only to learn the "secret" of each one.[64] We suppose on the available evidence—because there is no way to be certain—that the ancient patient, like the modern counterpart, expected a physician's visit to conclude with a prescription.[65]

Prescribing a drug is no simple task, if it is to be effective—and some degree of efficacy was required to practice, as we noted. A good knowledge of anatomy and physiology would be beneficial, we assert, as did some Greeks, but medicine can be practiced with just an empirical knowlege (ἐπιστήμη) acquired through observation of drug actions. Dioscorides did not write purely about this empirical knowledge. Pharmacology was his subject, but it was disguised because he did not directly discuss the nature of drug actions. Categorizing empirical knowledge and philosophizing on these experiences led to controversy.

"Schools" of Medicine

By Dioscorides' time medical practitioners were neither unified about the nature of disease and illness nor in agreement on a set principle on which to organize experiences and to approach therapy. Perhaps the closest to a general agreement that there ever had been—and this centuries before—was a humoral theory, which postulated that the body's health depended upon a natural balance in the humors, or fluids, of blood, phlegm, yellow bile, and black bile. The humors were based on the four elements of earth, air, fire, and water. Disease and illness were an imbalance in humoral proportions, and the physician's task was to recognize what was out of balance and to assist nature to restoration through his therapy. Despite what Peter Fraser called "some measure of agreement,"[66] there was never complete agreement about the number, designation, or even existence of humors. Among the dissenters was Dioscorides, who did not accept so few as four humors and largely ignored the whole matter.

In respect to drug therapy, Dioscorides wrote: "However, one must admit that the older authors combined the paucity of their information with precision, in contrast to recent writers like Julius Bassus, Niceratus, Petronius, Niger, and Diodotus,[67] all followers of Asclepiades. They have condescended to describe with a mere modicum of accuracy materia medica common and well-known to everyone, but they have noted the properties and testing of drugs only cursorily. They have not measured the activities of drugs experimentally, and in their vain prating about causation they have explained the action of an individual drug by differences among particles, as well as confusing one drug for another."[68] Asclepiades rejected the humoral theory of medicine associated with Hippocrates and projected a medical theory based on atoms. The body's atomic composition could be known only through what the senses told it and through teleology, which is concerned with ultimate causation. A disease then was treated according to its symptoms and what worked. Diet, exercise, and baths were preferable to harsh drugs and surgery—"to cure, safely, swiftly, and pleasantly."[69] Dioscorides rejected Asclepiades and the Asclepiadians, but he did not tell us why. Part of the criticism by others about

Asclepiades is that he was inconsistent in the applications of therapy based on his stated principles.[70]

Roughly in the generation of Dioscorides' father, a new "school" of medicine was developing around Themison of Laodicea and Thessalus of Tralles, who were called the Methodists.[71] Methodists rejected causation and anatomy, and they needed no general or special etiology in their therapies. All illness was a product of one of three conditions: the body's dryness, its wetness, or a mixed condition of various combinations of dryness and wetness. The physician made an excessively dry body wet, and an excessively wet body dry.[72] The object was to cure through a holistic therapy by simple remedies learned through experience. Thessalus allegedly claimed that the Methodists could train full-fledged physicians in six months.[73] A growing demand for physicians in the early Roman Empire could more easily be satisfied through the simplified medical training of the Methodist physicians.[74]

The Roman Empire experienced a growing movement toward various philosophical "schools" that were broad codes of life, such as Epicureans, Stoics, and Neo-Pythagoreans. One notable group was the Skeptics, who formed at least an intellectual link with the Methodists.[75] The Skeptics, as well as the cumulative effect of various other schools of thought, marked a general cultural pattern toward mysticism and away from Hellenistic rationalism.[76]

The Methodists and Asclepiadians developed as a reaction to the rivalry of two earlier "schools," the Empiricists and the Dogmatists.[77] Some of the Empiricists claimed a classical Greek foundation for the "school," but probably it was founded in the third century B.C.[78] The Empiricists did not believe it possible for a physician to penetrate the body's mysteries.[79] Anatomy was rejected (except chance observations of wounds): vivisection was cruel and dissection both disgusting and misleading because they did not believe a dead body could inform one about the functions of a live one.[80] They practiced medicine by what seemed to work with each patient, because each disease or affliction was peculiar to each person. In a curious perversion of the word, Empiricists became authoritarian in defending the precepts of Hippocrates.[81]

In contrast, the Dogmatists appealed to theory and reason; they studied anatomy and etiology of diseases because they asserted that proper therapy rested on a reasonable understanding of what was wrong. Dogmatism and Empiricism were inherently unreconcilable. The Asclepiadians and Methodists tried to find a middle ground.

In Dioscorides' own time still another "school," the Pneumatists, was developing around Athenaeus of Attaleia (fl. under Claudius A.D. 41–54). Athenaeus added a fifth humor, *pneuma*, and based a physiology (whose details are rather obscure to us) on Stoic philosophical principles readily acceptable to the Romans.[82] Medicine in all of its conflicting schools of thought was clearly having to come to an accommodation with religion in the social contexts of the era, after having had a relatively free and independent status earlier.

Dioscorides came from the rational Hellenistic medical tradition, but he is not easily categorized within the swirl of his period's controversies. A century later Galen decried the state of medicine in his day, which, in the word of Philo Judaeus (30 B.C.–A.D. 45), was reduced to *iatrologia*, loosely translated as "lecture medicine."[83] It is enough, Dioscorides said, to observe that former writings on drugs were inadequate partly because the writers allowed disputes to prejudice their observations.

Dating of Dioscorides

An estimate as to when *De materia medica* might have been written is our only means for estimating when Dioscorides lived. In his work he referred to no events, but he named seventeen authors whom he had consulted, and some were contemporaries. In his Preface, as quoted above, he spoke against Petronius and Sextius Niger, both of whom lived in the first century.[84] Around A.D. 10–40, Niger wrote a treatise, now lost, pertaining to drugs. Dioscorides employed it extensively.[85] Petronius *may* have employed Niger's work, but the evidence is not clear. Writing about the herb white hellebore, Dioscorides said that he agreed with Philonides, the Sicilian of the town of Enna, who regarded the drug from the plant as safe if carefully prescribed.[86] This Philonides is possibly the same Philonides of Catana mentioned by Scribonius as having been born at the time of the Emperor Tiberius (A.D. 14–37).[87] If so, he would probably be the most recent author cited by Dioscorides. The great encyclopedist Pliny the Elder, indefatigable in tracing down sources,[88] did not mention or employ Dioscorides' *De materia medica* in his *Natural History*. Since this work was dedicated to Titus in A.D. 77 and published after Pliny's death in A.D. 79,[89] Dioscorides did not write long before A.D. 77, otherwise Pliny would have digested him. Erotian is the first to quote from Dioscorides' work, but the dating for Erotian's work is indefinite, placed variously in the second half of the first century A.D.[90] The final piece of evidence for dating Dioscorides is the mention of Laecanius Bassus in his dedication to Areios. Dioscorides spoke favorably about Laecanius, who he said was prominent and a good friend to both of them. We presume this to be C. Laecanius Bassus, consul in A.D. 64[91] and proconsul to the province of Asia in 79–80.[92]

In summary, Dioscorides probably wrote sometime around A.D. 60–78, a conclusion based on (*a*) the most recent writer(s) quoted or named by Dioscorides (Sextius Niger and, possibly, Petronius and Philonides); (*b*) the first writer, Erotian, to cite Dioscorides' work; (*c*) Pliny's failure to cite Dioscorides; and (*d*) the mention by Dioscorides of Laecanius Bassus.[93]

Sources

Above a photoreproduction machine in the Duke University Library hangs a sign: "To copy from one source is plagiarism, from many scholarship." While modern scholars are cautious about imposing on earlier scholars the values of present research methods, one cannot be disinterested in the question: to what extent did Dioscorides rely on previous authorities without having assimilated their material in some creative way? We want to know how high to erect the pedestal for this author in history.

In seeking to determine Dioscorides' creativity, Max Wellmann studied parallel passages in Dioscorides and Pliny.[94] Pliny often named his sources; Dioscorides usually did not.

One example affords insight. Juba II (before 50 B.C.–d. A.D. 23–25), King of Libya, wrote an entire treatise on a kind of spurge.[95] Pliny credited him with its discovery;[96] Dioscorides, after discussing the physical characteristics of the plant and a method for testing the drug made from it, credited Juba with the discovery of the test.[97] Since Juba's work has not survived, conclusions are impossible especially since practically all the authorities Dioscorides used or could have used are also lost. Only one or two works that Dioscorides used have survived so that we can follow his citations in their original context and not through fragments. Although he did not name him, Dioscorides employed Nicander of Colophon (fl. ca. 135 B.C.), whose works on toxicology were used critically by Dioscorides, as John Scarborough's recent study of Nicander shows.[98] Dioscorides may have used earlier writers on poisons and drugs, such as Diocles of Carystos (4th c. B.C.) and Apollodorus (3d c. B.C.), directly, or he may have known them indirectly through such later authors as Nicander, Andreas, and Sextius Niger.[99] The other surviving work that Dioscorides probably used is Theophrastus' *Enquiry into Plants* (ca. 371–ca. 287 B.C.). Even though Dioscorides cited him directly twice and correctly each time, doubt has been cast on whether Dioscorides actually employed Theophrastus.[100] Theophrastus is the Father of Botany because his writings dealt systematically with plants as plants and because he began a study of plant morphology. But Theophrastus is doubted by some as a possible direct source for Dioscorides. Those doubters suspect that Dioscorides would have relied on Theophrastus' complete work for more of his plant descriptions if it had been available to him.[101] Wellmann believed that Sextius Niger and possibly Crateuas were Dioscorides' sources for Theophrastus' material.[102] In one instance, Dioscorides specifically cited a quotation indirectly and then he named both the original statement and his source. Whereas Meyer and Wellmann may be correct in judging Dioscorides' alleged slippery use of Theophrastus, it is also possible that Dioscorides knew Theophrastus' work directly. As learned as Dioscorides was around libraries, such a celebrated author as Theophrastus would likely have come to his attention.

Dioscorides, as stated above, preferred his own system of organization and, as far as the plant descriptions are concerned, one cannot be certain of the extent, if any, that Dioscorides relied on written sources for botanical descriptions. When he seems to cite other authorities, he is more concerned with usages and nomenclature than botany. Even so, Wellmann's comparisons of parallel passages, notably on the white *chamaileon* (III. 8, possibly *Atractylis gummifera* L. or *Carthamus lanatus* L.), are strong indications that either Dioscorides' knowledge of Theophrastus had been filtered through another source or Dioscorides modified his information to a greater degree than Wellmann was willing to credit him.

Sextius Niger's *De materia medica*, a treatise with the same title as Dioscorides' work, was a principal, mutual source that Pliny and Dioscorides both used.[103] For instance, in the following parallel translated texts, one can see how each handled his source:

Pliny, XXVIII. 34. 131	Dioscorides, II. 71
Sextius gives to cow's-milk cheese the same properties as he gives to that from mare's milk, which is called *hippace*. Beneficial to the stomach are those not salted, that is to say the fresh. Old cheeses bind the bowels and reduce the flesh, being rather bad for the stomach; on the whole salty foods reduce flesh, soft foods make it. Fresh cheese with honey heals bruises, a soft cheese binds the bowels . . . (Jones' trans.)	Eaten without salt fresh cheese is nutritious, easily digestible, good for the stomach; promotes growth of flesh; and has a moderately mollifying effect on the lower digestive tract . . . That which they call *hippace* is horse-cheese, foul smelling, very nourishing analogous to cow's cheese. Some call horse cheese *hippace*.

Other examples are similar. Dioscorides certainly may have employed Sextius Niger as one of his sources for cheese but he integrated much information from other sources as the case with cheese demonstrates—shown above only by the omission of information. Wellmann has some difficulty in sustaining his evaluation of Dioscorides' unfairness in citing his sources, as for instance this section about the yew tree, or holm oak (*smilax* = *Taxus baccata* L.):

Pliny, XVI. 20. 51	Dioscorides, IV. 79
Sextius says that the Greek name for this tree is *milax*, and that in Arcadia its poison is so active that people who go to sleep or picnic beneath a yew-tree die. (Jones' trans.)	The holm oak which grows in Narbonesis [a province of Gaul] has such power that those who rest in its shade or sleep under it are harmed often even to death. One informed of this situation should be mindful of it.

Pliny quoted Sextius Niger as giving Arcadia for the tree's habitat while Dioscorides specified Narbonensis. Max Wellmann said that both locations were in Pliny's and Dioscorides' mutual source and each chose only one to relate.[104] Whereas this is a possibility, it is at least equally possible that this was not the case. Pliny clearly cited Sextius Niger; Dioscorides may have taken his information from another source, written or oral. Elsewhere (*N.H.*, XVI. 7. 19), however, Pliny confused the holly oak (*milax* = *Quercus ilex* L.) and the holm oak. Possibly, Pliny mistook Niger's entry for the wrong tree. The holm oak was a well-known tree and, therefore, it is surprising that Pliny could be that confused. Interestingly, both Julius Caesar, writing earlier, and Galen, writing later than Dioscorides, spoke of the fatal toxicity of the holm oak, or yew tree. Vergil and Theophrastus mention its toxicity, thereby establishing that this was general knowledge.[105] But these examples, and others that Wellmann cites, are tenuous at best in revealing a pattern to Dioscorides' handling of written sources. Pliny's encyclopedic research methods, first copying from this and then copying from that, were well attested to by his nephew, Pliny the Younger.[106] Dioscorides said that his method was to research the usages among those who had written on the subject, to compare the accounts in order to determine what was general knowledge, and to confirm the usages through talking with people about their experiences with them.

Occasionally, when comparing passages, information is evoked that suggests Dioscorides used writings that he did not specifically cite. For instance:

Pliny, XXV. 95. 154	Dioscorides, IV. 79
Anaxilaus is responsible for the statement that if the breasts are rubbed with hemlock from adult maidenhood onwards they will always remain firm. What is certain is that an application of hemlock to the breasts of women in childbed dries up their milk, and to rub it on the testicles at the time of puberty acts as an antiaphrodisiac. (Jones' trans.)	[re hemlock] . . . and quells the milk, prevents the breasts of a virgin growing larger, and produces a reduction [*lit.*: undernourishment] of the testicles of male children.

Probably, though not necessarily, Dioscorides employed Anaxilaus' writings (ca. 28 B.C.); this evidence is all that there is since Dioscorides does not name Anaxilaus elsewhere. Through this type of evidence we postulate that Dioscorides used also the works of Philistion of Locris (4th c. B.C.),[107] Chrysippus of Cnidus (4th c. B.C.),[108] Sostratos of Alexandria (fl. 1st c. B.C.),[109] and, possibly, Diocles of Carystus (4th c. B.C.).[110] Much was written about drugs before Dioscorides.

Rarely, but sometimes, Dioscorides named his source and Pliny did not, as in the following:

Pliny, XXVI. 62. 96	Dioscorides, V. 127
But very high on the list of wonders is the plant Orchis, or Serapias . . . (Jones' trans.)	The other kind of orchis, which some call serapis as Andreas did . . .

As stated above, Dioscorides spoke favorably of Andreas in his Preface. In fact, Dioscorides reserved criticisms of his predecessors entirely to the Preface; in the body of his work, when he cited an author, his purpose was to give particular credit for or authority to his assertion. These instances are usually concerning dangerous drugs. In the chapter on the opium poppy (IV. 64), Dioscorides quotes Diagoras (late 3rd c. B.C.) as citing Erasistratos (ca. 300 B.C.), who cautioned against using opium for ear or eye trouble because it dulls the sight and induces sleep.[111] When Dioscorides quoted Erasistratos through a derived source, he explicitly told us. Andreas, Dioscorides continued, said that opium, if it is not diluted, will actually cause blindness if one is annointed with it. Mnesidemus, an authority unknown in any other source, recommended that use of opium be restricted to its sleep-inducing effect through sniffing it, all other usages being too dangerous. White hellebore (IV. 148) is a drug extensively employed in medical treatments and diet control, but Dioscorides said that he had to agree with Philonides the Sicilian from Enna (1st c. A.D.), who had warned against its abused usages.[112] As we know today, white hellebore is very toxic but has beneficial medical results, as will be discussed below.

The writer who received the most favorable review by Dioscorides was Crateuas. Crateuas was a root-druggist, called in Greek ῥιζοτόμος, or one of the rhizotomi, and attached to the court of Mithridates VI (120–63 B.C.), the king of Pontus who was famous for having successfully immunized himself against all potential poisons. He allegedly took progressively larger amounts of poisons starting with small portions during his youth until he was immune from sly kitchen intrigue at his court.[113] Pliny spoke very favorably of Crateuas' herbal and said that Crateuas himself drew the plant illustrations.[114] As will be discussed in Chapter 5, many of Crateuas' illustrations were substituted for what some scholars presume to be lower-quality drawings in Dioscorides' lost, original work. Dioscorides might not have strongly objected because clearly he appreciated Crateuas' work.[115] He even strove to rescue Crateuas from what he considered questionable statements. Under mercury (III. 125), Dioscorides said Crateuas noted that the seeds of one kind, if drunk, would cause the conception of a female and the seeds of the other kind would produce a male. "It seems to me," Dioscorides apologetically interposed, "that he related these things according to his report of them."

Where we have indications that Pliny and Dioscorides were employing mutual sources, Dioscorides normally omitted what we would call the magical or irrational elements. When he infrequently allowed their intrusion, he did so stating, "It is reported that . . . ," which became Dioscorides' method for placing distance between himself and what his reasoning would not allow him to accept totally.

After following the fragments from writer to writer, Max Wellmann dipped his pen in venom and exclaimed, "Dioscorides is nothing other than a compiler of the first century after Christ!"[116] The entire work must be studied before one can isolate passages here and there for review. Why would innovation in a medical guide to drugs be so highly cherished? Accuracy, not innovation, is the most desirable quality sought. The greatest genius, the most tireless worker, could never in a single lifetime have separated the thousand or so substances that Dioscorides listed with medical benefits from the hundreds of thousands of inert substances nor could he or she determine through personal experiments the almost five thousand medical usages. The best medical authorities, then and now, are searched and researched for critical evaluations of their reports, which are then combined with personal observations and experiment results. The additive is a contribution to knowledge. So it was with Dioscorides. He wrote science, not poetry. All indications point to his work being a critical synthesis of previous scholarship, and this he performed well. He contributed his own experiences with plants, drugs, and their manufacture, which he gathered from his travels and from talking with diverse peoples. Moreover, his effort was on a large scale. The fact that his work survived and was the object of study for the better part of two millennia while other writings on *materia medica* were lost, most of them within a few centuries after composition, was not entirely an accident.

Uniqueness of De materia medica

Max Wellmann's harsh judgment in calling Dioscorides a mere compiler was made in a journal article in 1889. Professor Wilamowitz and the Scientific Society at Göttingen urged Wellmann to produce a critical text of Dioscorides' work, which he undertook undoubtedly with mixed feelings. There were scores of manuscripts, many uncataloged, to be found all over Europe. *De materia medica* was less in size than, say, the works of Aristotle and Pliny but larger than those of Vergil or Homer. Wellmann traveled to Italy, Austria, France, and Spain to seek out the manuscripts in Greek, and letter by letter, word by word, in radically different versions each with innumerable variations, he completed three volumes of a scholarly text by 1914. In many of the libraries one can still see, in the fronts of the manuscripts, Max Wellmann's check-out signature with the date. By 1903, when he wrote an article on Dioscorides for a German encyclopedia,[117] and 1905, when he wrote an essay on the manuscripts for the second volume of *De materia medica*,[118] his sharp criticism had abated, for he had seen the entire work and not just an isolated passage here and there. Even though Dioscorides had understandably not observed the German seminar method for naming his written sources, a method that Pliny had come closer to employing, there were good reasons that medicine had relied so much on Dioscorides' authority for so long.

Dioscorides can best defend Dioscorides both on the matter of his predecessors and on a claim to uniqueness. In his prefatory letter to Areios he said he knew all too well that many others had written on the materials of medicine but that his work would fill a void in comprehensiveness.[119] Some authors fell short of their objectives while others relied exclusively on written accounts. Some—here he specifically names Iollas of Bithynia (mid 3d c. B.C.) and Heracleides of Tarentum (1st c. B.C.)[120]—left out many herbs and omitted metallic (mineral) drugs and aromatic herbs altogether. Even Crateuas, the root expert, and Andreas, the physician, both of whom he acknowledged dealt accurately with their subjects, were incomplete. Crateuas even omitted some useful roots. While the older authorities were few in number, they were fairly accurate; more-recent writers compounded errors, most especially those called the Asclepiadians. The modern writers, he criticized, conveyed detailed information about things already commonly known; moreover, they were too cursory about the properties and testing of drugs, and they argued incessantly about the activities for each drug. Each drug became a controversy. The best of them, Sextius Niger, made errors because he, like the others, relied on written accounts rather than experience to provide the critical test for truth. Niger said that spurge-resin is the juice from olive spurge that grows in Italy, that perfoliated St. John's wort is the same as triangular St. John's wort, and that bitter aloe is mined in Judaea, errors that he would not have made had he looked at them rather than merely read about them.[121]

Dioscorides' predecessors failed to organize their data in a useful way, he said: "Niger and the rest [of the writers on drugs] made mistakes in the organization of their material, some throwing together incompatible properties,[122] others using an alphabetical arrangement which splits off genera and properties from what most resembles them. The result is almost impossible to memorize as a unit."[123]

If we had the earlier works that he criticized, we would know what he meant by collision of incompatible properties. Primitive people first tested drugs by similar and opposite qualities. For example, the plant called *orchis* in Greek, or testicles, because of double root bulbs, was taken as an aphrodisiac,[124] and a plant that was seen growing in rock crevices was thought good for breaking kidney stones.[125] It was thought that qualities which characterized a plant might transfer a similar effect to the body.[126] Opposite qualities served also as a basis for drug testing. Just as one takes something wet when thirsty, so substances that have a strong characteristic, such as a burning taste like hot pepper, would be thought to warm a chilled body. These primitive theories, that is, administration by similarity and by contrarity, were not what Dioscorides was criticising because pharmacy practices had mostly progressed beyond the more simple aspects of these principles. Nonetheless, their vestiges remained in folk practices and learned medicine—even to this day.

We have the titles of Dioscorides' predecessors' works, and they tell us some things: Andreas wrote Νάρθηξ, or *Medicine Chest*; Diodotus, Ἀνθολογούμενα, *Collecting Flowers*; Heracleides, *θηριακά*, *Venomous*

Beasts; Thessalus, *Περὶ φαρμάκων, On Drugs;* Sostratus, *Περὶ ζῴων, On Animal* [drugs]; Crateuas, *Ῥιζοτομικόν, Roots;* Petronius, *Ὑλικά, Materials* [of medicine]; and Philonides, *Περὶ τῆς ἰατρικῆς, On Medicines.*[127] Nicander's *θηριακά, Venomous Beasts,* is organized by types of snakes and remedies for their bites and his *Ἀλεξιφάρμακα, Antidotes,* is organized by types of spiders, scorpions, insects, and myriapods and then remedies for each particular bite or sting. Theophrastus' *Περὶ φυτῶν ἱστορίας,* or *Enquiry into Plants,* is arranged by appearances, such as trees, shrubs, undershrubs, and herbs. Most of Dioscorides' predecessors had obviously not placed together drugs with similar pharmaceutical qualities but instead had organized them by biological characteristics. Some, however, organized by the alphabet. Classification by alphabetical order dated back probably to the library of the Ptolemaic Alexandria. Bolos of Mendes, ca. 200 B.C., wrote a lost work on stones said to be arranged "according to the letter" (*κατὰ στοιχεῖον*), the exact words used by Dioscorides in criticism.[128] Max Wellmann believed that Niger and Crateuas are the prime candidates for the object of Dioscorides' criticism.[129] By listing drugs in alphabetical order, classes and properties of similar classes of plants are torn asunder and our memory has difficulty relating the information. Ironically, Dioscorides' own work was to be alphabetized by others.

How did Dioscorides propose to make a better organization? The answer to this question is complex, very complex indeed. The only explicit answer that Dioscorides gave is as follows:

> I now encourage you, and any who may chance upon my book, not to look at my verbal facility but at my careful practical experience. For I have exercised the greatest precision in getting to know most of the subject through direct observation, and in checking what was universally accepted in the written records and in making inquiries in each botanical region. Furthermore, I shall endeavor to use a different arrangement and describe the classes according to the properties of the individual drugs. It is, I suppose, obvious to everyone that pharmacology is a necessity, closely linked to the whole art of medicine and forging with its every part an invincible alliance. It can also continue to extend its range of preparations and mixtures and its trials on patients, for the knowledge of each individual drug has a great deal to contribute.[130]

Thus, he explained that he grouped things by classes (e.g., aromatics, trees, pot herbs) and then by drug properties. To us, today, pharmaceutical organization by properties seems not only reasonable but also obvious; thus, one would list the laxatives, analgesics, antiseptics, narcotics, and so forth. Heraclides of Tarentum wrote a treatise on laxatives, now lost, and so we know that the method had been devised.[131] This arrangement is not exactly what Dioscorides did. At least, his method was not apparent even to those who devoted most of their lives to his study—and there were many who did.

A paragraph preface to each of the five books explained the broad organizational themes for that book. According to the opening paragraphs of each book, Book I deals with aromatics (or spices), oils, salves, trees, and shrubs (liquids, gums, and fruits); Book II, with animals, animal parts and products, cereals, pot herbs, and sharp herbs; Book III, with roots, juices, herbs, and seeds; Book IV, with herbs and roots not previously discussed; and Book V, with wines and minerals. Broadly and rather crudely, Dioscorides observed what we consider the kingdoms of animal, vegetable, and mineral as well as physical classes, such as aromatic herbs, trees, plants for which the root provides the drugs, pot herbs or foods with medicinal usages, scrubs, whole insects, animal parts (such as urine, blood, liver, and lungs), metals, and precious stones.

His method, in light of his criticism of others and his boastfully superior method, has perplexed many people, including this writer, who once called his method "unfathomable." Since Carl Linnaeus (1707–1778) developed the modern system of botanical classification, scholars have looked back on Dioscorides to see if they could find a key to his system of classification. Some noted, for instance, that Dioscorides grouped together a series in the mint family (Labiates) and another series of the Umbelliferae family.[132] Other sections of the work were puzzling if not mystifying, as when he separated small periwinkle (IV. 7, *κληματίς*, *Vinca minor* L.) from large periwinkle (IV. 147, *χαμαιδάφνη*, *Vinca major* L.) and from *Nerium oleander* L. (IV. 82; *μυκήτων*) as the only three plants he included from the entire Apocynaceae family, or when he separated two irises, *Iris florentina* L. (I. 1;*ἶρις*) from *Iris foetidissma* L. (IV. 22; *ξυρίς*). Four species in three genera of solanaceous plants (*Papaver rhoes* L., *P. somniferum* L., *Glaucium flavum* Crantz, and *Hypecoum procumbens* L.) he arranged in almost consecutive order in Book IV, Chapters 63–65, 67, separated only by *Silene inflata* Sm. in Caryophyllaceae, but then he placed a fourth solanaceous plant in Book II, Chapter 180 (*Chelidonium maius* L.). He placed two closely related genera, the myrtle family and the pomegranate family, together in Chapters 110–112 in Book I, and until comparatively recently, these families were grouped together under one family heading. He placed three members of the birthwort family (Aristolochiaceae: *Aristolochia boetica*, *A. parvifolia*, and *A. pallida*) in consecutive order (III. 4–5), and they are the only plants from that family in his work. In Book IV, Chapters 164–169, eleven plants of the spurge (Euphorbiaceae) family are identified and placed together, but spiny spurge (*Euphorbia spinosa* L.) is Chapter 159 in the same book. How, a botanist would like to know, can one who was able to identify the common features of the other eleven plants fail to recognize those same features in spiny spurge? Instead he separated the chapters devoted to spurges by black hellebore of the Ranunculaceae family, a very different plant in appearance.

John Sibthorp (1758–1796), an Oxford University botanist, devoted much of his life—including the very risk of it, by traveling in rural wild and dangerous areas of Greece, Turkey, and Cyprus—attempting to identify Dioscorides' plants in the habitats known to Dioscorides and then to classify them according to Linnaeus' new system; in short, he wanted to rediscover Dioscorides' system. His journey began just after he was awarded a professorship that would have enabled him to settle down to the secure life of Oxford in that wondrous century that demanded no publication of its professors, much less risk of life in pursuit of knowlege. Sibthorp identified many plants in his travels but he failed to understand the system.[133] He failed to systematize Dioscorides because neither he nor any other botanist since his day could have succeeded if they looked to botany to provide the answer.[134]

Dioscorides' "new and superior" arrangement was not according to botany. What he did, but did not tell us, was to arrange natural products according to the physiological effects that the drugs have on the body. This method would, as Dioscorides suggested, make it easier to remember medical information. His method, he suggested, would provide the framework for new, expanded knowledge in the future. Until the development of chemistry in the eighteenth century, pharmacognosy in the nineteenth century, and recent studies of phytochemistry, one could not have the ready key to decipher Dioscorides, that is, unless his work was approached on the basis that Dioscorides followed in devising it. One has to wonder why Dioscorides thought his method would be apparent when, through the proof of two thousand years' experience with his work, his method was not comprehended, much less the model for arrangement of new contributions to knowledge. It was too intricate, too subtle, and too complex. It required not a knowledge of chemistry but an acute power of observation of physical effects on the body.

Dioscorides provided the clue to his unwillingness to explain his method when he criticized the bitter philosophical debates raging during the first century among competing "schools" of medicine. Their needless prating about the "properties" of drugs had elevated each drug to a level of controversy. Drug properties could be known through clinical observation. His expression was "testing of drugs . . . experimentally." By engaging in argumentation, he would have been sinking to the level of the Asclepiadians, Methodists, Dogmatists, Empiricists, and Pneumatists. The proof for his method would produce the evidence, which, he thought, spoke for itself.

2. ONE PLANT, ONE CHAPTER

DIOSCORIDES ORGANIZED his information in chapters, one per plant, animal, or mineral. Each chapter has a more or less orderly progression for relating information. He did not force his material into Procrustean beds. He followed a general, commonsense formula for organizing information, but, when it was not necessary, he did not force the issue by rigidly adhering to his format. Following the plant's name, synonyms, and picture, he generally would give its habitat and botanical description. If, however, a plant was commonly known, such as garden lettuce (II. 136, *Lactuca sativa* L.), the plant's habitat and description, he must have thought, would be superfluous because it was common knowledge. On the other hand, in the same chapter, he described wild lettuce (*L. scariola* L.), popularly known today as escarole and cultivated, because it was not as well known. If a plant had no harmful side effects, rather than to say, "side effects: none," he said nothing and moved immediately to the next category.

Practically all chapters on plants (except the compound medicines, such as oils) adhere to the following order for relating information:

1. Name of plant, sometimes synonyms, and a picture
2. Habitats
3. Botanical description
4. Drug properties or types of actions
5. Medicinal usages
6. Harmful side effects
7. Quantities and dosages
8. Harvesting, preparation, and storage instructions
9. Adulteration methods and tests for detection
10. Veterinary usages

11. Magical and nonmedical usages
12. Specific geographical locations or habitats

Most chapters would not have all these categories (except for the longest ones) but, generally, information is related in this orderly way. The model chapter on water germander below omits elements 6, 8, 9, 10, and 11 because the plant had no harmful side effects, required no particular instructions for drug manufacture and storage, was not adulterated (probably because of its abundance and relative ineffectiveness as a drug), and had no veterinary, magical, or nonmedical usages. The model chapter on lettuce lacks elements 2, 9, 10, 11, and 12: there is no discussion of habitat because the cultivated lettuce (which even lacks a plant description) was grown virtually everywhere in gardens and wild lettuce's habitat was widespread. In the following chapters translated from Dioscorides, the parenthetical numbers refer to the categories:

III. 111. Water Germander

(1) Water germander [Σκόρδιον, *Teucrium scordium* L.]; (2) grows in hilly and marshy places; (3) its leaves are like those of wall germander [χαμαίδρυς, *T. chamaedrys* L.], larger but not so deeply crenated around their margins; it is like garlic to the sense of smell, but binding [astringent] and rather bitter to the taste; the small stalks are square, from which [grows] a reddish flower.

(4) The herb possesses a warming property [δύναμις]; (5) diuretic when it is green, pounded, and given in a drink; and dried but soaked in wine for snakebites and poisons, for gnawing pains of the stomach [στομάχος], and dysentery and difficult micturition; (7) 2 drachmas [6.82 grams] of weight with hydromel [honey + water]. It cleans out also a thick purulence [πυώδης] from the chest, and it is useful too for cough of long standing, and lesions [ῥήγματα] and convulsions, mixed in a lozenge with garden cress [κάρδαμον, *Lepidium sativum* L.] and honey and dried resin; and having been made into a wax-salve it sooths [παρηγορεῖ] an abdomen long inflamed. And it is also useful for gout smeared on with strong vinegar or being laid on with water; when applied [as a pessary] it causes [κινεῖ] menstruation; it closes up wounds [and] cleans out sores of long standing [and when mixed] with honey, it promotes healing; dried, it retards overgrowths of flesh [ὑπερσαρκώματα]. (11) But also the juice [το χύλισμα] is drunk for "the troubles" as they have been called [τά εἰρημένα πάθη]; (12) the most efficacious is the Pontic and the Cretan.

II. 136. Lettuce(s) (θρίδαξ)

(1) Cultivated lettuce [θρίδαξ ἥμερος]; (4) good for upper tract [εὐστόμαχος], a little cooling [ὑποψύχουσα], sleep causing, softening to lower tract [κοιλίας], increasing lactation. (5) Boiled down it increases nutrition. Unwashed and eaten it is given for upper digestive troubles [στομαχικοῖς]. Its seeds being drunk are good for [those who] continually dream and they avert sexual intercourse; (6) eaten too often they cause dim-sightedness. (8) They are preserved in brine. (5) The stalk growing up has something like the potency of the juicy [χυλοῦ] and sap [ὀποῦ] of wild lettuce.

(1) Wild lettuce [ἄγρια θρίδαξ]; (3) is similar to the cultivated, larger stalk; leaves: whiter, thinner, more rough, and bitter to taste. (4) To some degree its properties are similar to those of opium poppy, thus some people mix its juice with opium. Whence its sap (7) 2 obols [1.14 grams] in weight with sour wine (5) purges away watery humors through the digestive tract; it cleans away albugo [a white opacity of the cornea], misty eyes [ἀχλῦς]. It assists [ποιεῖ] against the burning [of eyes] anointed on with woman's milk. Generally it is sleep inducing and anodyne [ἀνώδυνος]. It expels the menses; [it is] given in a drink for scorpion and venomous spider bites. The seeds, similar to that of the cultivated kind, drunk avert dreams and sexual intercourse. Its juice produces the same things but with a weaker force. (8) The sap extracted in an earth bowl, exposed to sunlight first as it were, and the remaining juice stored.

Note the paucity of words. Even in translation, which expands the verbiage, the economy is plain. Dioscorides feared that his work might be judged by its style (Pref. 5), but he wrote as a man of science—no rapturous descriptions here of flowers—just their location, size, and color. No waste of papyrus.

1. NAME AND PICTURE

The names Dioscorides gave to plants are important. It is not that he "named" the plants for the first time the way a modern taxonomist might receive immortality. Dioscorides' work is important because many plant names were first known to succeeding generations through his authority. Sometimes he introduced plants for the first time, but because most of his predecessors' works are lost, we cannot estimate their number. Theophrastus' earlier, great works in botany did not have continuous use, they being among the "rediscovered" texts of the Renaissance.[1] There will be no generation, East or West, that has not referred to Dioscorides' authority; consequently, his plant nomenclature provides a foundation for modern scientific names. Perhaps, too, it should be mentioned that the Latin translation of Dioscorides' and, to a lesser degree, Pliny's sections on botany are other candidates as contributors to the foundation of plant names in the Latin West.

The problem of identifying plants today by their names is notoriously difficult. If one has only the name, identification is even more of a problem. Dioscorides employed the terms he considered most prevalent in the Greek-speaking world. His nomenclature differed from Theophrastus' terms probably because the names had changed during the more than four hundred years that lapsed between the two men. There was no authority in the period of 350 B.C. to A.D. 60 to act as a corrective. Dioscorides occasionally gave synonyms even in foreign tongues, such as Latin, but his reader is cautioned here: sometime before the fifth century someone added to his text lists of synonyms for many plants—as many as ten or more names for each plant. These synonyms followed Dioscorides' original name at the beginning of each chapter and were thought for at least a thousand years to have been an integral part of his text. They increased his work's usefulness and certainly did not distract from his authority. Just the same, they were not written by Dioscorides. Dioscorides' names often tell us some characteristic of the plant; *σκόρδιον*, for instance, for water germander, means "like garlic," a name first given to it by Lenaeus, who translated Mithridates' work on poisons into Latin.[2] The Greek term for lettuce, *θρίδαξ*, derives its meaning from *τρισ—δάκνω*, meaning "triple sting," alluding to its bitter taste and poisonous nature in the wild state.[3] The Latin term for wild lettuce, *lactuca virosa*, is derived from the name of its milky juice, *virosa*, meaning "poisonous."

The name would not totally identify the plant but a picture of it with its name certainly helped. Although scholars have raised doubts about whether Dioscorides' original text was illustrated, there can be no doubt to me that it was (see arguments below). If it had not been, then Dioscorides' work would have been virtually useless until centuries later when, allegedly, pictures were drawn in his manuscript texts. Dioscorides' plant descriptions are written to supplement a picture, and he wrote to be read and used.

2. HABITATS

Usually, at the beginning of a chapter, special plant habitats are given. Dioscorides often discussed the types of location, such as woods, mountains, plains, and streamsides, and he added specific geographical regions near the end, such as Cilicia, Arcadia, and Mount Parnassus, as will be discussed in (12). The principal reason was to assist in identification. The example of water germander above is rather perplexing because he stated that it grows in marshy places, which is correct, but he also said hilly places, which is not true with today's plant. One modern guide locates water germander on "streamsides, damp meadows, ditches."[4] There is another species of germander, mountain germander (*T. montanum* L.), but its flowers are whitish-yellow,[5] and in the plant description (3) Dioscorides specified a reddish flower, correctly describing water germander. Did Dioscorides combine these two species into one when he said "marshy places and hilly places?" This is an example of some of the problems in dealing with a text so old. One should understand that Dioscorides was not writing a botanical manual but a guide to drugs. In this chapter, as in some others where there is ambiguity, it would matter little to pharmacy whether mountain germander was substituted for water germander. This is not always unimportant, however, because sometimes there are differences between the drug's actions in different species of the same genera—even, for that matter, between plants of the same species, depending on soil conditions, climate moisture, and so forth.

When a plant was commonly known, for example, lettuce, or generally distributed, for example, pennyroyal (III. 31), Dioscorides omitted a description of locations. Rather than say the obvious, he said nothing. No waste of words.

Dioscorides noted that careful consideration should be given to the geographical area where plants were collected because this affects their medicinal properties. As a general rule, he said, plants in mountainous, high, wind-swept, cold, and dry places yield a stronger medicine (Pref. 6). Those growing in flat and wet localities or in shaded and sheltered places are weaker, weaker even than those collected in the wrong season or when wilting (Pref. 6). Dioscorides' observation here is one that modern pharmacognosy and chemistry can partially confirm. As will be discussed below, Dioscorides did not know this through chemical analysis. He observed it in nature. In the individual chapters, however, Dioscorides normally did not give specific directions as to where a plant ought to be gathered here, under the plant habitat section (2), but under geographical locations (12).

3. BOTANICAL DESCRIPTION

Although his objective was not botany as we define the field, Dioscorides' plant descriptions were sometimes very, very good; other times, more seldom, very, very bad. Compare, for instance, his description of water germander:

> Its leaves are like those of wall germander, larger but not so deeply crenated around their margins; it is like garlic to the sense of smell, but binding [astringent] and rather bitter to the taste; the small stalks are square, from which [grows] a reddish flower.

with the following modern descriptions—the first from a popular herbal, the second from a botanical manual:

> The square, hairy stalks are of a dirty color and very weak. The leaves are short, broad, wooly and soft, and indented at the edges. The flowers are small, of purplish-rose colour, in whorls, in the axils of the leaves. It flowers in July and August. The whole plant is bitter and slightly aromatic. The fresh leaves, when rubbed, have a penetrating odour, like garlic.[6]

> A lax, much branched, soft-haired perenn. 20–60 cm with purple or lilac fls. in lax, one-sided, auxillary whorls of 2–6 fls. half hidden among the leafy bracts. Corolla c. 12 mm; calyx lobes equal. Lvs. ½–5 cm lance-shaped, coarsely toothed, softly haired; stalkless lvs. and bracts similar; stolons present.[7]

Dioscorides isolated major distinguishing characteristics of a plant rather than giving complete descriptions. He would use a full range of the entire plant from describing a root system to flowers, fruits, and seeds, provided they were notable. The primary attention went to the leaves, then the stems or branches. He often noted leaf arrangements, how they branched, margins of leaf blades (as with water germander), and the size. Sometimes he gave specific measurements for plant size; more often he related it to the size and appearance of a more commonly known plant and specified the exceptions (as he did with water germander compared to wall germander). In this way we learn the plants that were easily recognized by his contemporaries, ones that could serve as models. For instance, Dioscorides often used white hellebore (IV. 148) as a model, such as "It looks like the white hellebore, except for . . ." He described the leaves of the yellow knapweed (III. 6) as "like those on a walnut, somewhat long, green in color, like those of a cabbage." The pictures of the leaves are often detailed enough to show venation and these pictures trace back to the Dioscoridean original. Types of adjectives used to describe leaves include thick, thin, smooth, hairy, large, small, tough, fleshy, and prickly. For stems, branches, or trunks he often noted their size, color, shoot systems, and, less often, places where they budded (e.g., see the description of flower budding from the leaf axil in water germander). Flowers were noted by their color, size, and abundance, but sometimes he neglected altogether to mention their presence. He apparently recognized the calyx (e.g., II. 185) and stamens (e.g., III. 8, 46). He used the word *pericarp* when describing the crested bunias (II. 110, *Bunias erucago* L.): "It bears the seed in budlike pods [λοβᾶς]. When the seed husks are open there is inside another head-shaped shell [or pericarp, περικαρπιῶν] in which are little black seeds, which, when broken into, are white seeds." Such detail is given because the drug comes from the seed.

Smell and taste figured importantly in Dioscorides' work. Take, as an example, the fine description of the licorice plant (III. 5, γλυκύρριζα):

> The licorice plant is a small shrub with two branches two forearms long [approx. 90 cm], around which stand the leaves thickly, similar to the mastic plant [σχῖνος, *Pistacia lentiscus* L.], fatty and viscous to the touch. The flower is similar to hyacinth [*Scilla* sp.]. The fruit is of the size of a plain-tree apple [*Platanus orientalis* L.], [but] sharper [to the taste]; pods are shaped like lentils, yellowish-red, small. The roots are long, the color of box-wood [*Rhamnus* sp.], like those of gentian [*Gentiana lutca* L.], somewhat astringent, sweet; juice extracted by infusion [or decoction] like [juice of] buckthorn [*Rhamnus infectorius*? Sibth.].

Modern botanists avoid sense comparisons when they can because they are impossible to quantify and have relative values, but Dioscorides could hardly forego such comparisons if he wanted his work to be used by others. His picture of a plant could not tell about taste or smell but his words could and did.

Dioscorides occasionally ascribed sexual gender to plants but, as with all of his fellow Greco-Romans, there was no order to it and usually no rationale. In general, male plants were considered harder, rougher, drier, and more barren, whereas female plants were softer, smoother, moister, and more fruitful.[8] In the cases of fig and date trees, the ancients correctly distinguished between male and female in the same way that modern botany does.[9] Dioscorides employed genders sometimes to distinguish similar species of the same genus, for example, III. 24, 140; IV. 4–5, 74. As Theophrastus had done before him, he gave recognition to popular folk use of gender designations without the imposition of a theory or the study of a method.

As good as some descriptions are, others are poor. For instance, all he said in describing daphne (I. 78, *Laurus-nobilis* L., or laurel) is that "some of it is of a smaller leaf, some of a broader." Today there are two species of the laurel: one has small leaves ("curled, variegated and willow-shaped lvs."); the other, larger ones ("stiff, dull green, lanceolate or oblong-lanceolate, 1–3½ in. long").[10] Dioscorides' picture of laurel (again, I am postulating the picture's presence) gave the details of one species; his words added that there was yet another kind so that the reader could see and know that both were laurel and therefore have the same medicinal effects. To repeat, for many plants, common plants, such as lettuce (II. 136), leek (II. 179), walnut (I. 125), white poplar (I. 81), and garden celery (III. 64), Dioscorides gave no verbal description at all.

Conspicuous in its absence is any reference to growth patterns, such as the time for gestation of seeds, flowering, and the distinction between perennials and annuals. Part of the answer Dioscorides gave in his Preface: "One should not fail to note that plants often ripen either sooner or later according to specific character of the country and according to the climate; some, according to their own particular nature, bear leaves and flowers in winter, while others produce flowers twice a year. It is necessary for someone wishing knowledge in these matters to witness actually when the new shoot emerges from the soil, when the plants are ripe, and when they are fading past their prime, for someone who has chanced upon the sprout alone is not able to know the mature plant, nor having seen the ripened plants to have learned to know the young shoot. Because of the changes in form of the leaves and sizes of the stems, flowers, fruits, and some other specific characteristics, great error is produced by some authorities who have not considered the appearance of plants in their works in this way."[11] Dioscorides' travels had taken him far and he saw too many variations in growth patterns in the different climates and soil conditions to chronicle them all. What of the regions he had not visited, he must have mused? There is no substitute for experience with plants, he said. His books were to supplement experience and not to provide a shortcut to nature's study.

4. DRUG PROPERTIES OR TYPES OF ACTIONS

Following the botanical description and before the specific medicinal usages, Dioscorides normally listed the general property or type of action the drug was expected to have. Water germander had a warming and diuretic action while lettuce was good for the stomach, cooling, sleep inducing, softening, and a lactation stimulant. That the drug properties were intended to have a possibly predictable effect on the body is more implicit than explicit in Dioscorides. Clearly, he must have thought the action of a drug made it a candidate for testing that action in some specific therapy.

Dioscorides was an empiricist, in the modern sense, and not a theoretician. He did not articulate a pharmaceutical theory for drug actions. The drug knowledge of his day had already attempted to organize the millions of drug and chemical experiences into meaningful patterns. This is comparable, or at least it is not dissimilar, to modern drug guides, which classify drugs as analgesics, antipyretics, laxatives, antibiotics, antihistamines, and the like. Some of the Hippocratic writings proposed that drugs had four actions: warming, cooling, drying, and moistening. Aristotle, never one to allow nature to go unclassified, spoke of the four qualities (warm, cold, dry, and wet) that corresponded to the four elements of fire, water, earth, and air. After Dioscorides, Galen elaborated on a pharmaceutical theory that extends qualities to secondary and tertiary ones.[12] Dioscorides did not make these distinctions, nor did he reduce actions to four. We shall examine Galen's theory, but for now the question is whether Galen's theory was a formulation of generally agreed explanations or largely an innovation. Pliny seldom mentioned broad qualities, such as warmness and coldness, and never systematically, but the fact that he did at all indicates that such a move toward theory was developing before Galen and at the time of Dioscorides.[13]

Dioscorides was clearly attempting to produce some order and an inductive medical theory. Book I contains the following properties, with the number for the chapters in which each word was used (when a chapter says it has the same qualities as another drug but fails to specify what they are, those qualities are not numbered here):

Warming (θερμαντικός): 1, 2, 4, 6, 7, 10, 11, 12, 14, 15, 16, 17, 19, 20, 27, 28, 30, 31, 40, 42, 49, 50, 51, 52, 54, 55, 56, 58, 59, 61, 62, 64, 65, 66, 67, 68, 72, 73, 75, 77, 78, 97, 103, 128
Mollifying or softening (μαλατικός): 14, 26, 27, 30, 35, 40, 42, 52, 54, 56, 57, 58, 59, 65, 67, 72, 73, 78, 97, 103, 127
Astringent, bitter, or binding (στυπτικός): 15, 21, 30, 39, 43, 45, 46, 64, 68, 70, 72, 84, 87, 92, 95, 97, 100, 101, 102, 103, 104, 105, 107, 108, 109, 115, 126, 128
Astringent, bitter, or binding (στυφελός): 13, 41, 42, 70, 74, 82, 99, 116, 117, 118, 123
Astringent, bitter, or binding (στῦψις): 20
Diuretical (οὐρητικός): 7, 10, 13, 14, 19, 26, 27, 58, 69, 70, 71, 75, 106, 112, 115, 123
Diuretical (διουρητικός): 4, 8, 12, 16, 17, 114
Drying (ξηραντικός): 7, 13, 14, 15, 64, 68, 97, 106, 107, 110
Cooling (ψύχω): 41, 42, 43, 45, 99, 101
Concocting (πεπτικός): 14, 26, 27, 47, 66
Sharpening (δριμύς): 48, 61, 62, 72

Making thin (λεπτυνικός): 1, 48, 62, 123
Dilating (ἀναστομωτικός): 40, 58, 97
Glueing (viz., joining wounds) (κολλητικός): 64, 73, 121
Sleep inducing (ὑπνοποιός): 15, 54
Relaxing (διαφορητικός): 65, 71
Dispersing or promoting perspiration (διαφορητικός): 73, 78
Stopping of pores (παρεμπλαστικός): 101, 109
Causing thirst (διψητικός): 128
Checking (κατασταλτικός): 110
Cleaning (σμηκτικός): 62
Cleaning thoroughly or emetic (ἀνακαθαρτικός): 71
Decocting (ἀφέψημα): 92
Hardening (σκληρυντικός): 39
Nourishing (τρόφιμος): 128

Discorides lifted pharmacy above the purely empirical, "this for that" level to the important step of determining drug actions. Certainly he intended a relationship between the properties (δύναμες) and the specific medicinal usages. He normally listed the properties, then the usages, but occasionally he explicitly indicated this relationship, as the following excerpts show:

> I. 20. Camel's thorn [*aspalathos*, probably oil from *Alhagi camelorum* Fisch. or related species] has a warming property combined with astringency, *for this reason* it is good for the treatment of thrush when used as a mouthwash; and it is good for the treatment of putrefying wounds on the genitals, and for soaking spreading ulcers, and for the treatment of fetid nasal polyps; and, inserted [into the vagina] in a pessary, it draws down fetuses.

> I. 39. Oil of myrtle. The property is astringency hardening: wherefore mixed with healing [or scar-forming] medicaments, it is effective for burn inflammations [*pyrikauta*], scurfs [*achōres*], branlike skin eruptions [*pitura*], skin eruptions [*exanthēmata*], abrasions caused by friction [= intertrigoes, *paratrimmata*], skin cracks [*ragedas*], lumps [perhaps callosities, *kondulōmata*], joints which have been softened, perspiration, and all [afflictions] that require astringency or the closing of the pores [*puknōsis*].

Would it follow then that all medicines having a warming and an astringency property would have the same force as camel's thorn oil or an astringency-hardening property the same as oil of myrtle? Clearly not.[14] When comparing the same qualities for drugs, there are variations in the specific medicinal actions. A drug that is mollifying or softening, for instance, will often be used as a digestive aid, but not always. The action is sometimes confined to external use as a topical applicant because ingestion would be harmful. Most of the aromatics (I. 1–24) had a warming property and a common use for them was for the upper digestive tract but not the lower. In reviewing the above list of properties, one can see that there was often a grouping in sequence. Cooling drugs, for instance, appear in Chapters 41–45, 99, and 101. This could not be at random but is in consequence of his plan to classify by drug affinities.

For what purposes then were the properties developed? Dioscorides told us at the end of the chapter on oil of myrtle, after he listed the specific dermatologic uses of the oil: the oil is good for "all [afflictions] that require astringency or the closing of the pores." By this we understand that some other illness or affliction needing the therapy of an astringent or condensing drug, such as, say, a ruptured blood vessel, would not automatically be successfully treated by oil of myrtle. But, if a medical person had no other drug known to be effective available, then he could test oil of myrtle. Its property qualified it for testing, making it more likely to be effective than an infinite number of other possible drugs possessing unknown or different properties. A medical person's reasoning ability (λογιστικός) or just common sense would have to inform him that oil of myrtle *might* be good for a small external vessel hemorrhage but not for a large arterial flow.

Dioscorides intended the drug properties to have a broad meaning and some relationship with their medicinal use. Juniper berry (I. 75) "is diuretical; therefore, it is good for convulsion, ruptures, and those who have strangled uteruses." Strangled uteruses are described in great detail by Soranus, a second-century-A.D. author of a treatise, *Gynecology*,[15] and in a shorter manner by Paul of Aegina (6th c. A.D.), which is as follows:

> Uterine suffocation is a rising up of the uterus, affecting sympathetically the most important parts, as the carotid arteries, the heart, and the membranes of the brain. The patients experience, when the attack is at hand, languor of the mind, fear, atony of the limbs, paleness of the countenance and sadness of the eyes; and when the suffocations come on there is deep sleep, mental aberration, loss of the senses and of speech, with contraction of the limbs; the cheeks then begin to redden, and the countenance becomes turgid; but when the attack is going off, some moisture is to be felt about the genital organs; and rumbling of uterus is then gradually relaxed, and thus they recover their understanding and senses. The disease comes on periodically like epilepsy, and is occasioned by the uterus being

> gorged, or from semen or some other matter having become putrid in it . . .[16]

Since both Soranus and Paul associated convulsions and ruptures with a strangled uterus, the question arises whether Dioscorides intended juniper to be for all convulsions and ruptures or just those associated with strangled uteruses. The answer is not clear, nor is it at all clear what a strangled uterus was. A Greek word for uterus is ὑστέρα, or *hystera*. From this name comes our word *hysterical*, a condition to which women supposedly become victims during menstruation. The descriptions of a strangled uterus sometimes resemble chronic cramps, a retroverted uterus, a proplapsed uterus, retention of the placenta, and, perhaps, atopomenorrhea or even vaginitis. Whatever it is, Soranus says of its treatment: "And drinking of water is not only not helpful but sometimes even noxious, since the patient needs strengthening, not metasyncrisis."[17] Thus, a diuretic drug would be harmful. The medical usages for juniper include antiparalysis, diuretic, emmenagogue (i.e., promoting menstruation), and as a uterine stimulant.[18] Its use as a uterine stimulant and diuretic extended to its 1885 listing in the Pharmacopeia of Great Britain.[19] How broadly, then, is the diuretic action of Dioscorides' prescription for juniper to be interpreted? The available evidence indicates that Dioscorides' drug properties were broadly, even loosely, conceived but nonetheless rationally formulated on the basis of close observation of their activity. More research needs to be made in the relationship between properties and specific medicinal action in ancient medicine.

Oak galls (I. 107) are given, Dioscorides explained, "generally where there is a need to bind or to stop or to dry; then one ought to make use of them." He prescribed oak galls specifically for stopping the running of the gums, as an astringent for menstruation, vaginal hernia, and dysentery. The galls contain from 50 to 70 percent of a tannin known as gallotannic acid and around 3 percent gallic acid (3,4,5-trihydroxy-benzoic acid). They have no odor, but their taste is very sharp, sour, and astringent. In veterinary medicine today oak galls are used as a hemostatic, as an astringent in burns, ulcers, and moist eczema, and in diarrhea treatment; for humans, topically as an astringent and styptic. Gallic acid is also sometimes administered in veterinary medicine for diarrhea.[20] The association between the natural substance and its physical effects was made by taste.

Knowledge of drug properties allows one to compare and measure drug experiences. The rhizome of rhubarb (*Rheum officinale* Baill. and other species) has had a long history of use.[21] Dioscorides said of it

(III. 2): ". . . its chief property is its astringency with some heating." The rhizome has anthraquinone derivatives plus tannic acid as do oak galls.[22] Dioscorides included diarrhea among its medicinal usages. The rhizome tastes very acidulous.[23] Today's pharmacognocist will want to know such things as the other chemicals present in rhubarb and oak galls, the amount of each, and the manufacture, quantity, and administration of the drug before definite conclusions are drawn from these examples. These questions will be addressed later but for now it is sufficient to establish a pattern in the relationship between Dioscorides' drug properties and their actual usages. There may be substantial reasons for his observations.

Mace is a drug made from the arillode (the inside covering) of the nutmeg fruit (*Mystica fragrans* Houtt.) and was used until the nineteenth century as an astringent and antidysenteric. Dioscorides said: "Mace is according to the taste very astringent" (I. 82), and he recommended it for hemoptysis (spitting up of blood), dysentery, and lower digestive trouble (such as diarrhea). Galen said secondary qualities—and he included bindingness or astringency as secondary—are known through taste,[24] but, with the exception of the comment on mace, Dioscorides did not say how one would know the quality. In fact, mace is acid to the taste because of the predominance of myristic acid. Mace is an astringent as are oak galls but each has slightly different medicinal usages. The fact that Dioscorides used three different words for astringency may have been intended to indicate distinctive degrees of astringency actions. Galen used two words, one of which was different from Dioscorides' words.[25]

Even though mace comes from a tree of the Ranales order and oak galls from a tree of the Fagales order, they were perceived by Dioscorides as similar though not identical; their medicinal properties produced the similarity. They were grouped in Book I because they were trees. Rhubarb, a small plant, was in Book III because its drug came from its roots and all root plants were in the first part of that book. All three—juniper, oak galls, and rhubarb—were astringent.

Taste did not determine medicinal properties. We understand taste as an indication of the possible presence of many acids (sour, sharp, biting, or astringent), alkaloids and other bases (bitter), salts (bitter salt, sour salt, or, in the case of heavy metals, a metallic taste), and many hydrocarbons (sweet).[26] Toxic substances often are unpalatably bitter but some strong toxins have neither taste nor odor;[27] therefore, Dioscorides could not have relied exclusively on organoleptic tests to produce his organization. Moreover, whole classes of chemicals supplying the active substances of drugs are undetectable through sense perception. Sweet and bitter tastes occur in so many chemical classes that distinction of these classes would seemingly be impossible for the accuracy necessary in medicine.

Wheat meal (II. 85) has "warm and drawing qualities," Dioscorides said, and these properties allow it to "lessen callouses on the sole of the feet." Dioscorides' assertion that it has a drawing quality could not have been based on a sense of smell or taste because wheat meal is neither salty nor astringent. It is warm and drawing by its physiological effects, not by its effect on the organs of sense but on the body as a whole. The medicinal properties were known by "testing," as Dioscorides said in his Preface, by which he meant experience gained from trials on patients. To some degree his properties may have been attempts to detect characteristics that we perceive are there because of the presence of glucosides, tannins, alkaloids, and related substances whose presence can be detected through taste. An organizational scheme by taste and odor would have produced a discernable pattern, but he clearly had no such intention. While Dioscorides gave the senses attention, he did not emphasize organoleptic tests—as seen by the relatively few Greek words to describe them. Taste and odor were factors but not the whole art.

Wild lettuce, or escarole, is bitter to taste but it does not follow that Dioscorides classified it as having an astringent quality and consequently being good for dysentery, watery eyes, and the like. While he noted that it was bitter to taste, he said one of its properties was "a little cooling" rather than astringent. Coolness was the effect, not the physical temperature. Lettuce contains lactucarium, which consists of lactucin, hyoscyamine, and mannite. Hyoscyamine, present in greatest concentration in its seeds, is a tropane alkaloid and a resolution of atropine, which has, as a side effect, blurred vision (Dioscorides said it dulls the sight, as cited above). In 1899, lactucin was said to be discovered as an opium substitute.[28] In truth it was rediscovered, because Dioscorides had already noted it some seventeen hundred years earlier. Opium from the poppy (IV. 64) is described by Dioscorides as having a cooling quality. At first one might find it strange that the opium effect was called cooling when one felt warm with its ingestion. Dioscorides, as Galen did later on, called toxicity from the opium poppy, hemlock, and other toxins as being cooling presumably because their use resulted in a deadening effect or a loss of sensitivity. It was possibly fatal, resulting in a complete loss of innate heat. This is the presumed reason that the extreme toxins were cooling. One would expect, as indeed was later the case, a cooling remedy to be given for a fever, but Dioscorides did not use the cooling property for fever. Wormwood (III. 23, *Artemisia absinthium* L.) is recognized as a febrifuge but Dioscorides said it had a warming property. Thus, when

Dioscorides noted that lettuce, especially the seeds of wild lettuce, was a little cooling, he correctly perceived the physiological effect of hyoscyamine, which is very close to opium. The fact that it was a *little* cooling indicates its quantity. There is a method to Dioscorides' properties.

Even though there is a method, we are hard pressed to explain in terms understandable to our science the basis on which Dioscorides formulated his drug actions. Almond (I. 123) is said to be ἀνωδόνος, that is, "free from pain," or analgesic, but Dioscorides did not list it as a property, as we would recognize it to be, but as a specific medical use. (Note the absence of analgesics from the list above.) Tamarisk (I. 87) was "unequally astringent," a qualification Dioscorides made without explanation, but we may be surprised that he was warning that for some applications it would work and that for others—where one might expect it to be effective—it would not. The damson plum tree (I. 121) affords an example of how Dioscorides made distinctions. Its dried fruit, he said, binds the lower digestive tract (κοιλία). We, of course, know the effect of prunes, but Dioscorides would have us believe that the plant growing in Damascus, good for the upper digestive tract (εὐστόμαχος), staunches the lower tract (κοιλίας σταλτικός). This assertion caused Francis Adams, a nineteenth-century commentator, to explain: "I know not how it is that Dioscorides says that the dried damask-plums bind the bowels, for even those manifestly loosen . . . To us it appears that the only mistake committed by Dioscorides consists in stating his views too succinctly."[29] But then Dioscorides said that the gum of the plum tree has a gluing property and that it breaks the stone (bladder or kidney stone) if it is drunk with wine. Our distance simply does not allow us to interpret how something with a gluing or conglutinating action could be expected to break up or dissolve bladder or kidney stones. We need not have the charity of Francis Adams but merely state that an explanation is not apparent to us. It is enough to note that, as with the plum tree, he observed that drugs coming from different parts of a plant could have different, even opposite, actions.

Dioscorides was neither systematic nor comprehensive in his attempt to classify specific drugs by specific properties. Fruits in general did not have qualities. In fact, with them, he often began the chapter by listing their negative or side effects, dispensing with a description since his readers would already have familiarity with them. The last two books on plants (III and IV), more often than not, have the medicinal property section omitted altogether. There is no explicit reason given. Perhaps he wrote the books in order and by the time he came to Books III and IV he had despaired with the arduous and sometimes impossible task of discerning properties and relating them to specific actions. Perhaps it was the nature of the plants discussed in those chapters.

5. MEDICINAL USAGES

Dioscorides' purpose was to inform people about the medical usages of "the materials of medicine." Understandably, this section accounts for the bulk of information in each chapter. The section also is the most difficult to analyze. Since there are various ways to approach the subject and each method evokes a differing perspective, a number of methods will be used here to discuss this section.

Dioscorides' Plant Drugs and Modern Science

Nowadays, testing a known chemical compound for its precise pharmacological effects is complex. This is true much more so with the crude, natural products that act as drugs. Take, for instance, something common like coffee: a brew made from the extracted juice of the bean of a known plant, its use extensive and yet its detailed chemistry is still being analyzed, its long-range effects debated. How much more difficult is it to form assessments of an ancient peoples' pharmacy? Though difficult, it can be done in a limited but revealing way.

Assessing each of the almost five thousand medicinal usages in Dioscorides is not yet possible. It may never be done. Judgments that are based on current truths are necessary, and our truths today often have short lives. There are numerous levels in which judgments must be made in the evaluations of Dioscorides' medicines. First, there is the reading of the manuscripts in order to determine what he originally wrote. This perilous judgment will be discussed in the next volume. Then there is the translation of technical Greek terms into their equivalents in technical English or other modern languages. Identifications of the plants must be made as to the exact species, and, for Dioscorides, some plants are uncertain. Sometimes we can identify the species, other times a genus or several species, perhaps crossing genera lines, which went under the heading of one Greek word. For a few plant chapters we can only guess among a number of choices as to the probable plant. And there are differences among individual plants of the same species, which depend upon such factors as climate, soil, moistness, parasites, and predators[30]—an observation, incidentally, made in his context by Dioscorides, but one that had to be rediscovered in modern times.[31]

Plants, it is supposed, manufacture some chemicals for reasons, such as to repel certain insects, protect themselves from harsh cold, regulate growth cycles, and combat fungus infections. Other chemicals are waste products of plant metabolism. If habitat conditions change over an extended period, might not the chemistry change? We cannot assume that the chemistry of a given plant today was exactly the same two thousand years ago. Nonetheless, there is rough chemical proximity between plants in different environments and ages. For instance, opium from the poppy is roughly unchanged, judging by Dioscorides' physiological descriptions of its actions then and our knowledge of it as it is today. The therapeutic action of an herb is often different from a medicinal substance that is the active pharmacologic agent. Iodine is released slowly from dried seaweed and can be more effective than in a pure form extracted from the plant when the patient is highly sensitive to the chemical. And the active principle of digitalis isolated from the herb accumulates in the organism with repeated therapy and must be withdrawn after a period of administration, but the drug in its crude herbal form has no such accumulation. The symbiotic relation of chemicals in their natural home can affect test results differently than when they are tested separately.[32] The method of extraction can be decisive in determining efficacy. Some compounds readily dissolve in water, others in alcohol and other liquids. The strength and effectiveness of a drug from natural products are often dependent on the method of manufacture. All these possible variations, however, should cause us to pause any time assertions are made too strongly that a plant has a certain effect.

Plants are not the only factor for potential error. Individual patients produce variable drug reactions according to such things as age, size, sex, and drug tolerance. To evaluate a drug we need to know not only its components but also the quantity, method, and route of administration.[33] Like plants, perhaps our bodies have evolved in their reaction to chemicals. Body size and diet may have affected different responses to drugs between the ancients and moderns. Even when we know the pharmacologically active compound in a natural drug, there are variations between how the body reacts to a pure drug and the same drug in the same amount with similar administration when it is mixed with other chemical components as happens in natural drugs. Then, too, a drug in Dioscorides' day may not be a drug in our sense: it could have been a vitamin that supplied some specific but observable nutritional need in a deficient diet.[34]

Finally, there is a human element in drug administration. In Dioscorides' time as today (but to a lesser degree) drugs were given mostly for symptoms. Symptoms change. Anthropologists note that symptoms and combinations of symptoms vary among cultures or even among classes within the same culture.[35] A Frenchman's liver trouble has no equivalent to a German's. Americans do not have the syndrome the Germans attribute to bad air. An evaluation of a drug's effectiveness necessarily depends upon reasonable judgments formed by accumulating a great weight of evidence and detecting the emerging pattern whereby we may make assertions of probability.

The easiest way to evaluate Dioscorides is to take drugs known today that are derived from plants native to the Old World and seek to find them in Dioscorides. When one does this, the list is impressive; Dioscorides knew amygdalin, belladonna, opium, wild cherry, aloe, tragacanth, castor oil, croton oil, and cassia, to name a few. This exercise is useful in itself for dispelling the 100 percent placebo theory—those drugs work and work in a way that can be verified by modern medicine. In addition, there is the testimony of the seventy or so generations since Dioscorides who took the same drugs, such as opium for a pain and castor oil as a laxative. The method of taking drugs from our present pharmacopoeias and journals and searching their usages in the past is not sound history. It is instead a distortion because the method verifies the present but does not evaluate the past. The numerous other drugs that Dioscorides recommended but that are not found in modern medicine (at least, not easily found therein) must be studied within the context of his whole work.

No discernable theory for disease appears in Dioscorides. He did not subscribe to the Hippocratic theory of humors (χύμοι), although he occasionally used the loose concept of humors in their original sense of "body juices." Oil of mustard (I. 38) draws out old painful humors through the pores; castor oil (I. 32) expels watery humors, which is a way to describe a drastic purgative action; the juice of nard spikenard (I. 7, *Nardostachys jatamansi* D. C.) is good for excessive wetness of the eyelids, which, restated, relieved eyes severely affected by purulent blepharitis.[36] Dioscorides did not subscribe to a balancing (κράσις) of the four humors for good health.[37] The causes, or etiologies, of diseases are seldom mentioned and then largely as harmful side effects. His task was to present relief, not a comprehensive medical text replete with an articulated medical theory.

Beer (II. 87, ζύθος, "barley beer") was diuretic and acted on the kidneys and nerves (νεύρα); but he thought beer greatly irritating (κακωτικός) to the meninges (i.e., membranes investing the spinal cord and brain), producing flatulence and a bad complexion and causing "elephantiasis" (ἐλεφαντίσις). Basing their opinion on Celsus' description, some modern researchers consider the Greek "elephantiasis" to be leprosy.[38] But in the previous chapter (IV. 86), Dioscorides prescribed barley as a cure for leprosy (λέπρα). Probably, "leprosy" in

Greek and Latin meant a disease with a scaly skin with pruritis (severe itching), a condition that could include our leprosy (but not tubercular leprosy) as well as psoriasis and other skin afflictions.[39] "Elephantiasis" possibly meant a chronic swelling of lymphatic tissue, that is, our elephantiasis. Julius Preuss, a historian of ancient Jewish medicine, believes that the Greek *lepra* was the same as the Hebrew *schechin*, which probably meant universal eczema.[40] The Arabic writers identified *lepra* with "elephantiasis" of the Greeks, and subsequently they and Western medieval writers made elephantiasis a type of leprosy.[41] At best we can say that both elephantiasis and leprosy to the ancients were composites of symptoms. If eczema were to have been the affliction, then the scales could be seen as a wort that rises to the top in the brewing process. Vivian Nutton suggests that, if this were the case, barley in the form of beer would not be in the ancients' pharmacy for what we call a medical reason so much as a general allopathic purpose of a sympathetic reaction.[42]

To summarize Dioscorides, barley in its natural form is a cure; barley in another form, beer, is a cause of the same disease. Beer brewing in premodern societies was an involved, technical art. In the hands of the unskilled, a number of problems could have arisen, such as the production of acetic acid. If the temperature was not optimum for enzyme action, the hops could not combat microorganisms.[43] It is not inconceivable that primitive beer could produce dermatological afflictions. Even here we are assuming short-term symptoms and not long-term ones, such as a cirrhotic liver. Therefore, in one of the few instances where Dioscorides gave a cause for a disease, we cannot be sure what it is.

Diseases in antiquity were combinations of symptoms; today they are designated by the microorganisms and other things that cause them, hence they are called pathological. Some historians do not believe, for instance, that, based on descriptions of disease symptoms, influenza existed in Dioscorides' time.[44] Even our common cold seemed less common, again based on medical and literary accounts, but the ancients did acknowledge something like our cold. Dioscorides had individual remedies for coughs, suffering in the chest (*thorax*), headaches, clogged nasal passages, stopped sinuses, and sore throats but nothing for a "cold" as a unit. We are hard pressed to know the actions intended when ancient prescriptions are given for what appear to be cold symptoms or even the precise anatomical region where relief would be expected, such as chest, sinuses, or throat. Beer was mentioned as adversely affecting the "nerves," but the Greek word *neuron* can also mean sinew, tendon, and even penis. Context gives us the *assumed* meaning. Similarly, Dioscorides used the word *thorax* in the following ways: "good for . . ." (I. 73); "cleans away things in . . ." (I. 71, 128); "good for those with thickening stuff in . . ." (II. 112); "pain [or suffering] in . . ." (I. 21, 66; II, 149); "brings out things in . . ." (II. 103); "trouble of . . ." (I. 16); "humors in . . . which are hardly execrable" (I. 71); and "running discharge of . . ." (I. 3, 78). Any of these symptoms might apply to a cold but some can apply as well as to pleurisy, pneumonia, emphysema, and angina pectoris.

Gout

Gout is an example of the different way in which the ancients and moderns regard a disease. The example will also reveal the problems with judging its therapy. Gout (ποδάγρα) to Dioscorides and the ancients referred to a pain and probably a swelling of the feet and other joints.[45] With our pathological conception of disease, we consider gout to be caused by hyperuricemia, an abnormally high production of uric acid, which results in the formation of crystal deposits and tophi (subcutaneous nodules) in joint tissue.[46] Inflammation results along the lines described by the ancients. For acute attacks of gout, the drug of choice today is colchicine, which is obtained principally from autumn crocus (meadow saffron, *Colchicum autumnale* L.), because it breaks the chemical chain reaction that leads to inflammation. Clinical response is within twenty-four hours. Dioscorides' gout would have included gout as we now define it but possibly also other afflictions that have the same symptoms.

Dioscorides had a number of drugs for gout and they tell an interesting and not untypical story. He recommended decoction (i.e., a boiling in water) of white willow leaves and bark (I. 104, *Salix alba* L.) as a warm poultice for gout. White willow bark contains salicin in sufficient amounts to act positively as an analgesic, antiinflammatory, antipyretic, and antirheumatic.[47] Salicin, once swallowed, probably decomposes into salicyclic acid, the base for acetylsalicylic acid, or aspirin, until comparatively recently a primary treatment of gout and probably still today's most widely employed drug for minor gout symptoms. As a topical applicant it would bring quick relief from the pain of gout.[48]

Barley (II. 86), Dioscorides said, was put with quinces or vinegar for gout inflammations. He also said that barley produced "elephantiasis." To us barley is not a drug, but it is a source of a nutrient, pantothenic acid,[49] a B-complex vitamin necessary for life, and it is rich in minerals. Since it is commonly found in the modern balanced diet, its deficiency syndrome is not well established.[50] One must allow that barley may have supplied a vitamin or mineral helpful to gout symptoms because ancient diets were different from today's. Even with this allowance, however, there is no defined reason why barley would be helpful to gout victims.

Under asphalt (I. 73, ἄσφαλτος; three varieties: mineral oil, bitumen, and pitch, according to location), Dioscorides said that a plaster is made of asphalt, barley meal, beeswax, and natron (sodium carbonate) for treatment of gout, arthritis (disease of the joint), and lethargy. Similarly, under figs (I. 128), fig pulp is made into a local applicant for gout with fenugreek flower and vinegar. Although Dioscorides did not say so—he seldom did in these instances—the use of asphalt and figs points to a binding agent; that is, they act as a vehicle for what was considered the active substances. Other uses point to their being thickening and flavoring agents for internal drugs. Returning to the chapter on barley, we find that he said that barley meal, having its juice extracted out by water with pitch (πίσσα) and oil, is good for "runnings of the joints" (τῶν ἄρθρων ῥεύματα). This may be what we call rheumatism, an older term now used for arthritis or tubercular arthritis with draining sinus, or other problems. Since Dioscorides specifically suggested barley meal as an ingredient for local application for "runnings of the joints," did he mean that barley was to be externally applied when he prescribed it (not specifically in a meal) for gout? As a rule, when he did not explicitly state otherwise, the intended route of administration was oral.

What are we to conclude about this apparent confusion regarding barley and asphalt? In different chapters there are slightly different prescriptions and administrations. Is it that Dioscorides was a poor editor who merely copied sources without reconciling differences? An affirmative answer would be too harsh. Dioscorides had no computer or even index cards to sort out these thousands of medical items. Papyrus was much too expensive to use for such checking. His mind had to provide a cross listing and what sorting out there was. Although we do not know for certain, it is likely that ancient authors did not go through many (or any?) drafts of their works. Considering what was involved in such a gigantic undertaking with the distances traveled, the differing languages and cultures, and reconciling folk practices with written authorities, Dioscorides' ability to deal with these problems was wondrous. And, when one compares his work to others, as we shall do, we marvel at this quality all the more.

These usages of willow bark, barley, and asphalt for gout treat the symptoms at best and do not attack the pathological causes of true gout. Indeed Dioscorides has a chapter on the autumn crocus (IV. 83, lily family), the plant supplying our source for colchicine, discussed above as very effective for gout. The only use Dioscorides saw in autumn crocus was as an antidote against mushroom poisoning. In the chapter on the asphodel plant (II. 169, *Asphodelus ramosus* L. and/or *A. albus* L., lily family), some manuscript copies of Dioscorides' text contain this sentence: "And Crateuas the Rhizotomotist said that one drachma [3.4 grams] of the root juice [of the plant] . . . with wine . . . cures [θεραπεύει] the pain of gouts [ποδάγρας ἀλγήματα]." Observe the verb "cures" rather than the milder claims for the analgesics. The asphodel plant contains colchicine in large enough amounts for toxicity,[51] although it is not presently harvested for the drug. For now, we can put aside the question as to whether the sentence was in Dioscorides' original text. There can be no doubt but that the ancients did have the cure for gout, the same one we have as our drug of choice. How could they have used a plant that we do not and not use a plant that we do? It is extremely difficult to answer why some plants' medicinal benefits were discovered, when, and by whom and why others were overlooked for so long. We can speculate that folk practice made the discovery. For all practical purposes, only through this folk discovery could the millions of experiments be undertaken. The next step is the record made when a writer, such as Crateuas or Dioscorides, recognized the discovery and gave his authority to it.

Dioscorides also recommended colocynth (IV. 176, *Cucumis colocynthis* L., Cucurbitaceae family) for gout, and ibn Māsawaih (Mesuë, ca. 954–1015) followed Dioscorides' lead by making it a principal gout remedy.[52] Recent studies show that some plants of the family yield colocynth.[53] It is supposed that Dioscorides and ibn Māsawaih knew the treatment for gout but that the drug was dropped by later practitioners because of its toxicity, only to be rediscovered.[54]

The answer is qualified as to the efficacy of Dioscorides' remedies for gout. One use was as an antiinflammatory agent in a way we can verify, another possibly a dietetic benefit, and another a "true" cure, while some medicines were vehicles for the active drugs. But this is not all. Cabbage (II. 120) is recommended with fenugreek and vinegar because it "helps those with gout in their feet and joints." Fenugreek flower and vinegar were recommended in the chapter on figs, but there is also a chapter devoted to fenugreek (II. 102), in which Dioscorides said that being beaten small, put in melicrate (a honey water), and applied as a topical plaster it is good for internal and external inflammations. What did Dioscorides consider the active substance? Fenugreek, cabbage, or figs? Modern science gives us little information to verify claims about fenugreek or cabbage, even were we to be sure that the Roman cabbage is the same chemically as ours. Cabbage is probably an example of a plant manipulated by humans to breed out or reduce its toxins. One simply cannot make a categorical judgment about Dioscorides and gout therapy. To say that he knew how to cure it needs to be qualified and balanced. To say even that he knew how to treat it effectively needs qualifying because, among other reasons, we are not sure what he was treating.

Neither with gout nor throughout *De materia medica* did he normally make comparative judgments. An exception to demonstrate the rule is when he said that garlic (II. 152) is good for viper bites "as no other thing." He normally did not say that this is the best drug for gout, that the next best, and so forth. His method for dealing with the full range of usages was merely to list under each "simple" medicine all its medicinal usages. His method determined the form for herbals and medicine guides, even today's popular herbals. While he gave willow bark, barley, and asphodel for gout, he also gave eight other medicinal usages for willow, nineteen for barley, and twenty-one for asphodel. We can say that, based on present truths, he got some usages right and some wrong, while many, if not most, remain uncertain or so qualified as effectively to be uncertain.

Ophthalmological Agents

The Romans had considerable trouble with their eyes and paid a lot of attention to them. The words for specialized "eye physicians" (*medici ocularii*) are incised on tombstones. Numerous seals have been found with inverted lettering for stamping eye stick ointments called *collyria*.[55] The term *collyrium* for a special eye medicine (sometimes used for nonocular afflictions as well) derives from a base word meaning "coarse bread." The meaning doubtlessly points to the base substance for early eye ointments. Their extensive use is further indicated by the fact that in one Galenic treatise there are over two hundred collyria prescriptions.[56]

In reading the ancients' descriptions of eye afflictions, modern ophthalmologists recognize such common problems as glaucoma, trachoma, and cataract as well as hyposphagma, nyctalopia, ptilosis and atrophy, strabismus, procidentia, corneal carcinoma, amaurosis, myopia, trichiasis, ectropion, chemosis, emphysema, and psorophthalmia.[57] Again we observe that the ancients described the nervous or functional afflictions by their primary symptoms. Dioscorides often gave only a word or two to describe the problem and then its remedy. A survey inspection of his ophthalmological agents affords insight into the difficulty in evaluating the complexities of *De materia medica*. The Greek term clearly means "eye," so there is not the confusion we have with other organs, such as the uterus, stomach, and various parts of the circulatory system.

Most collyria were given for eye inflammation,[58] but this term would include a variety of things varying from strained eyes to conjunctivitis. Dioscorides had two words that mean "whiteness of the eyes": *λεύκωμα*[59] and *ἄργεμον*, presumably two stages of white ulcers.[60] For one of the two, if not both, leukoma is indicated because it is an infiltration of white pus at the cornea's edge. Being a local infection, it would respond to an astringent or a local antiseptic, especially one having antibacterial action.[61] These "white ulcers" differ from *ἀιγίλωψ* (I. 112, 115), which presumably refers to advanced dacryoadenitis, an inflammation of the lacrimal gland with a fistula.[62] Myrrh (I. 64) is a good example to show the range a single drug was expected to have: "It fills up ulcers in the eye [*ἐν ὀφθαλμοῖς ἕλκη*] that wear away white spots [*λευκώματα*], cleans things that darken the cornea of the eye [*τὰ ἐπισκοτοῦντα ταῖς κόραις*], and cleans roughnesses of the eyes [*τραχώματα*]." The "things that darken the cornea of the eye" may be glaucoma, although other possibilities exist. The "roughnesses of the eyes" indicate trachoma—our word, *trachoma*, is the same as Dioscorides' word. In fact, Dioscorides' use of the word is the first in surviving literature.[63] Myrrh is a gum resin obtained from one of several species of scrub trees of the Rutales family and has local stimulant and antiseptic properties.[64] Although prized in antiquity and frequently mentioned in biblical literature, among other things being one of the three gifts to Jesus from the Magi, its medicinal qualities did not differ from many other resins except that its aromatic qualities were thought especially beneficial to foul-smelling wounds and sores. In modern medicine, myrrh tincture is employed as a topical local anesthetic in the eye where it does not have the harmful side effects of mydriasis or alteration of intraocular tension as do some substitutes, such as procaine.[65] Therefore, even with our inability to understand the precise disorders that Dioscorides meant, if indeed he had definite disorders corresponding to ours, we can be reasonably persuaded that his drug gave some relief to the eyes.

Some other ophthalmological agents are more easily related to modern medicine. The juice of the ammoniac plant (III. 84, *Ferula tingitana* L., Umbelliferae family) is given for "cleaning white spots [*λευκώματα*] in the eyes and dissolving roughness [*τραχύτητας*] on the eyelids." In 1864 the drug galbanum (from *Ferula galbaniflua* Baiss. & Bushe) was melted with potash lye, and an acid called resorcinol or resorcin was identified.[66] Resorcin subsequently became, and remains, an important medicine in eye and skin ointments for its antiseptic, keratolytic, and antifungal properties.[67] Resorcin also comes from ammoniac.[68] One species, *Ferula communis* L., is called Moroccan ammoniac. The example of galbanum is not untypical in that the natural drug in Dioscorides and in subsequent use in medicine should provide the clue for a chemical-analysis search in the nineteenth or twentieth century to synthesize the active compound. As the decades go by, the connection between the pure chemical and its natural home in a plant is forgotten. Soon, too soon, the memory fades. In a real way the drug resorcin was not discovered in 1864; its true discovery is lost in the ancient shadows.

In the first two books alone, Dioscorides named twenty-eight different ophthalmological actions, for example, diseases of the eyes, swollen eyes, pain of the eyes, itchy eyes, crossed eyes (our strabismus), scabs on the eyes, hardening of the eyes, fungus growth on eyelids, wet humors of eyes (emphysema?), misting over of the eyes, sharpening of the sight, black eye, and corrosion of the eyelids. The symptoms are nearly impossible to match precisely with our disorders. Dioscorides recommended onions (II. 151) for *νεφέλιον*, meaning "cloud-like opacity of the eye," which may be a cataract, the first use of the word I have found.[69] Even with examples like galbanum as a drug and cataract as a possible specific affliction, we are unprepared on the basis of the sketchy evidence to evaluate the effectiveness of the bulk of the ophthalmological agents in Dioscorides. Eye ointments were clearly important, widespread, and meaningful to the health of the ancients as judged by the ancients themselves.

Antibiotics

In the previous section I selected the eye as an organ and examined Dioscorides' remedies, but another method is to examine a particular drug action and follow it through Dioscorides' chapters. I shall choose the antibiotics because they received little attention in early medicine and, because their use was probably small, the subject is more manageable.

Twenty-three seals for collyria, or eye medicines, have the word *penicillus* on them, including one labeled "collyrium penicillum."[70] These findings provoked speculation that the ancients knew the effect of penicillin from the blue mold that grew on bread. As observed above, the word *collyrium* is traced to "old bread." Harold Nielsen translates Pliny as specifically stating that "the softest fungus is the brush (*penicillus*) which moistened with mead is useful against an eye tymour . . . ,"[71] but W. H. S. Jones translates the same passage as "the softest kind of sponge is that used for bandage-rolls."[72] Nielsen, however, has argued that there is no persuasive evidence that the ancients knew a crude form of penicillin.[73] Dioscorides recognized *fungi* (IV. 82; chiefly mushrooms but other fungi as well), but his medicinal uses do not suggest antibiotic activity.

The matter does not rest there, however. There are other indications of the ancients' use and knowledge of crude antibiotics. Millet bread (II. 97), heated and put warm into a bag, is good for the pains of colic (στρόφοι). If we presume that a reasonable time period lapsed after the bread was placed in the bag, this would undoubtedly be moldy bread.[74] The problem, of course, comes with the "pains of colic," which seems an unlikely symptom for antibiotic activity. A recent study (1980) of ancient Nubian skeletons reveals the presence of tetracycline (an antibiotic) in the bone. Tetracycline-producing bacteria are commonly found in Nubian soil and certain conditions, such as those found in storage bins, readily produce tetracycline.[75] Egyptian soil and climate are similar to Nubia's and, for that matter, not totally dissimilar to the eastern Mediterranean. Could it be that the grain bases for many of the medicines in Dioscorides (such as barley, above) and for many collyria in particular were there but unrecognized to supply an antibiotic? Penicillin is found in nature as mold in large concentrations in certain plants and this raises the possibility that, when we are searching for the active component in some specified herbal remedy, it was a mold that was active and thus there may have been a primitive use of penicillin. Possibly, too, there needs to be some clinical research to test the historical references. Until then the question of primitive antibiotics from lower plants in Dioscorides remains uncertain.

Antibiotics used in modern therapy come from bacteria or lower plant forms, including fungi, algae, symbiotic lichens, and mosses. There is another, possibly larger, source of antibiotics: higher plants. The number of known antibiotics is large (909 in 1967).[76] A recent (25th) edition of the *Dispensatory of the United States* reports: "New antibiotics are being discovered every week" (p. 1563).

At present no antibiotic from higher plants is used in regular Western therapy.[77] This makes an evaluation of Dioscorides' employment of them difficult. Dioscorides used the plant *lukion* (I. 100) for a variety of things (tonsillitis, infected sores, etc.) for which an antibiotic would be effective. We are unsure whether *lukion* is yellow-berry buckthorn (*Rhammus infectorius* Sibth., Rhamnaceae family) or one of several barberries (*Berberis* spp., Berberidaceae family),[78] but in this case it matters little. Plants of both families contain berberine, a quaternary alkaloid that possesses antimicrobial (antibiotic) activity.[79] Similarly, Dioscorides prescribed birthwort (III. 4, *Aristolochia clematitis* L. and/or *A. boetica* L.) for old sores. We know that the plants contain a broad-spectrum antibiotic agent against bacteria and fungial infections and that it is currently used in folk remedies for colds, chills, fevers, and asthma.[80]

Modern interest in antibiotics from higher plants is currently being awakened (or rewakened?).[81] Until more research is done and clinical experience gained, we shall be unable to evaluate to the degree we would like Dioscorides' remedies where the apparent action was as an antibiotic. Certainly, the circumstantial evidence is there to indicate that he employed them. The proof must be based on a weight-of-evidence basis.

Grime from Gymnasium Walls

An intriguing observation about the medicine called "grime from gymnasium walls" was made by Dioscorides (I. 30). He observed that on the walls of gymnasia or on statues therein there appeared a grime that, when scraped off, was effective "for warming and dissolving inflamed growths [δύσπεπτα φύματα] and suitable [ἁρμόζει] for abrasions caused by friction and for old sores [ἕλκη πρεσβυτικὰ]." What could this be? Why grime found in a gymnasium and not elsewhere, such as a temple or a house? A Greek gymnasium has rubbing rooms, sheltered from the sun, where aromatic oils with olive oil base were massaged into the skin and the excess scraped off. Evaporation and condensation would occur because of the body heat and colder walls. Probably on the walls there grew lower forms of plant life (fungi, algae, lichens) and microorganisms unreached by the sun's ultraviolet radiation. Reduplication of the conditions is nearly impossible because, among other reasons, there were variations in the composition of the rubbing oils and probably even the microorganisms would be different. This particular prescription in Dioscorides was lost to succeeding ages when the peculiar institution of the Greek gymnasium changed.

Dioscorides prescribed "grime from gymnasium walls" for "growths." The word for "growth(s)" is *phuma(-ta)*, which ranges in meaning from our neoplastic lesion or malignant cancer to tuberculous lymph nodes to carbuncle and anthrax. Dioscorides' use of the word points more toward large inflamed growths (he added the adjective "inflamed") capable of "ripening" and disappearing in response to therapy.

Descriptions of *phumata* by Celsus, Paul of Aegina, and Galen indicate that for most occasions carbuncles and anthrax are likely what is meant.[82] Dioscorides treated *anthrax* (ἄνθραξ), which was also probably a carbuncle—a malignant pustule or edema—anthrax, or, possibly, smallpox. Our carbuncle (Latin: *carbunculus*) is commonly caused by the *Staphylococcus pyogenes aureus* bacteria, and our anthrax comes from *Bacillus anthracis* and occurs in the form of woolsorters' disease (pulmonary), mycosis intestinalis (gastroenteric), and a malignant pustule. Whether the ancients, Dioscorides in particular, were distinguishing the same afflictions as our carbuncle and our anthrax is not clear; certainly there were distinctions in words, at least. The author of the Hippocratic work *Epidemics* (III. 7) used *phumata* in the sense of internal and external growths and *anthrax* as a growth occurring mostly in the summer. Humans contact the anthrax bacilli from cattle and sheep, especially through sheep's wool—as one might during the shearing season. The incubation period after shearing would give time for the growths to appear in the summer.

What distinguished *phuma* from other words for growth was the implication of inflammation. The four cardinal signs of inflammation were, according to Celsus, redness, heat, swelling, and pain (*rubor, calor, tumor,* and *dolor*).[83] Galen said that *phumata* suppurate,[84] which fits the description of our carbuncles, and Paul of Aegina (7th c. A.D.) said that carbuncles arise from epidemic causes.[85] Malignant neoplastic lesions appear only as a possibility in some contexts. Whatever the distinction made by the ancients, whether or not they roughly coincide with our equivalents, the evidence points to Dioscorides' "grime from gymnasium walls" for *phumata* as having a bacterial etiology even if the term included tuberculous lymph nodes. We know that the grime from gymnastic walls attacked *phumata* successfully because of the force of the verb Dioscorides used: "dissolves." For the other two therapies, inflammation from abrasions and old sores, Dioscorides gave a lesser claim, "It is suitable for . . ." Why, incidentally, inflammation from an abrasion caused by friction should be different from other superficial inflammations is puzzling. These signs point to some antibacterial action but, whether systemic as through an antibiotic or topical as through an antiseptic, we neither know nor can know.

Drug Actions in the Verb

Critical in reviewing the medicinal action in Dioscorides are his verbs. Some actions are weak, for example, "aids," "is good for," or "cures" (βοηθέω, II. 126) and "is useful" (ὠφελέω, I. 78), while other verbs more precisely relate the drug actions, for example, "joins together"—as in a wound (ἁρμόζω, I. 56), "casts out" or "removes" with force (ἄγω, I. 76), "alters," "sets in motion," "removes" with comparatively less force (κινέω, II. 97), "puts to an end" (κτείνω, I.

78), "destroys completely"—as pain (διαφορέω, II. 99), "brings up" (ἀνάγω, I. 128), "stops" (ἵστημι, I. 7), "makes loose" (λύω, I. 126), "makes soft" (μαλάσσω, I. 64), "holds" (ἐπέχω, I. 117), "swells" or "ripens" (σπαργάω, II. 107), "cleanses" or "purges" (κἀθαίρω, I. 56), "wipes clean" (σμήχω, I. 64), "opens" or "dilates" (ἀναστομόω, I. 56), "hardens" or "prevents" (ἀποστερεόω, II. 136), and "abates" or "calms" (πραΰνω, I. 76). The strongest beneficial drug actions were "treats successfully," is "therapeutic," or "cures" (θεραπεύω, II. 154) and "heals" or "cures" (ἰατρεύω, II. 120), all of which appear relatively infrequently and are verbs that Dioscorides seemed to reserve for well-attested actions. Whereas the lexical range of βοηθέω, θεραπεύω, and ἰατρεύω includes our word *cures*, Dioscorides attached greater force to the last two verbs.

The affliction known to the Greeks as ἀλωπεκία, or fox mange, is probably the same as our alopecia, an affliction that results in baldness or a deficiency of hair but whose etiology is unknown. Hypothetically, it could have a parasitic or neural origin. Onions (II. 151, *Allium cepa* L.) are "for" alopecia because they better stimulate (προκαλέω) hair than does ἀλκυόνειον (a bastard sponge). Garlic (II. 152, *Allium* sp.) "cures" (ἰατρεύω) *alōpekia*, and a type of leek known as *skorodoprason* (II. 153, *Allium descendens* L.) is said to have the same action "for" *alōpekia* as do onions and garlic. White mustard (II. 154, *Brassica alba* Rabenh.) "treats" (θεραπεύω) *alōpekia*. All four were specifically applied as an ointment. The root of the almond tree (I. 123, *Amygdalus communis* L.), when eaten with other things, "puts to an end" (κτείνω) *alōpekia*; the endocarp of the walnut tree (I. 125, *Juglans regia* L.), being burned and mixed with oil, "restores [the hair of]" (δασύνω) *alōpekia*; the hazelnut (I. 125, *Corylus avellana* L.) "restores hair that fell away with *alōpekia*"; various reeds called *kalamos* (I. 85) "treat" (θεραπεύω) *alōpekia*; and radishes (II. 112, *Raphanus sativus* L.) "restore" (δασύνω) *alōpekia*, again in the context of hair restoration.

The intestinal parasitical tapeworm (ἕλμις ἡ πλατεῖα), Dioscorides said, is "shaken out and killed" by a decoction of pomegranate roots (I. 110, *Punica granatum* L.); the root of the mulberry (I. 126, *Morus nigra* L.) "expels" (ἐκτινάσσω) them; and garlic (II. 152) "draws out" (ἐξάγω) the worms.

A user of *De materia medica* would be wise not merely to read about the drug and its use but to pay attention as well to its action as revealed by the verb. Doubtlessly, Dioscorides had not intended a distinction between the anthelmintic actions of "shaken out and killed," "expells," and "draws out." The actions appear the same. In the case of therapy for *alōpekia*, however, there doubtlessly were differences intended. The verbal actions of restores and stimulates clearly in reference to hair growth point to a therapy after a later stage of the affliction has resulted in hair loss, while "treats" and "puts to an end" *may* have meant an earlier time for treatment and stronger results.

Nomas (νομάς) was an internal and external ulcer, boil, or infection that spread. The Greek term probably included such things as our noma, peptic ulcer, and skin infections of bacterial etiology.[86] Again Dioscorides' choice of verbs assists our understanding. Juniper leaves (I. 76, *Juniperus sabina* L.) bring *nomas* to a standstill (ἵστημι);[87] mastic gum (I. 70, *Pistacia lentiscus* L.) is preventative (ἀποτρεπτ [ικός]) of *nomas;* darnel (II. 100, *Lolium temulentum* L.) causes tissue to form around *nomas* (ἔχει περιχαρακτικὴν νομῶν); and plantain (II. 12, *Plantago* sp.) clears out (ἀνακαγχάζω) *nomas* of the stomach. Juniper leaves contain the antibiotic podophyllotoxin[88] and a volatile oil (1%–3%) that is a powerful irritant both internally and externally.[89] Counterirritants are often used for dermatological afflictions because they increase the blood supply to the skin, while a bacterial infection may respond to the antibiotic therapy. Mastic gum contains various acids in a complex chemistry and now is used to form a dental varnish for tooth cavities[90] and as an astringent to arrest bleeding.[91] The sealing actions of mastic could then "prevent" infection, especially one caused by a microorganism. Darnel is highly vulnerable to fungal infections, and it is suspected that the medical actions attributed to it by traditional medicine are mycological in origin.[92] Nonetheless, we cannot explain medically the use of Dioscorides' verb. The verb "clears out," which he used for plantain's action, however, is clearer although not precisely clear. In modern herbals plantain leaves are recognized as having a stimulative action on sores and an arresting action on external hemorrhaging.[93] Plantain has plumbagin, which is antibiotic and antifungal, and its seeds are widely used as cathartics.[94] Dioscorides employed them to remove *nomas* from the stomach. Even if an examination of Dioscorides' verbs does not always lead to a full understanding, it is certainly clear that the verbs presented the medicinal action and were very important to medical knowledge. Dioscorides chose his verbs rationally.

Cancer Treatments

In recent decades, chemotherapy in cancer treatment, using naturally occurring agents, has produced encouragingly successful therapeutic results. Walter H. Lewis and Memory Elvin-Lewis report: "The modern era began in 1938 when it was learned that colchicine was cytotoxic. This alkaloid is obtained from autumn crocus (*Colchicum autumnale*), and it acts by disrupting the spindle mechanism during mitosis, thereby blocking cell division."[95] The modern era may have begun in 1938 but I believe that during the ancient era the plant was employed to treat tumors, both benign and malignant. Dioscorides (IV. 84) recommended that the leaves of autumn crocus (or those of another species having colchicine) be "soaked in wine and administered [topically] to dissolve lumps [οἰδήματα] and growths [φύματα] not yet making pus."[96] Similarly, in 1958 a chemical compound in the squirting cucumber (*Ecballium elaterium* L.) was found to have "strong antitumor activity against sarcoma [cancer]."[97] Dioscorides had recommended it (IV. 150) to "dissolve old lumps [οἰδήματα]." In a later section, suspicions—for that is all that they are—will be outlined to hypothesize that Dioscorides, though crudely and imprecisely, had some recognition of the effects of vincristine from Madagascar periwinkle, a compound recently discovered to be dramatically successful in chemotherapy for Hodgkin's disease and other lymphatic malignancies. But this exercise of cataloging ancient anticipations of modern therapeutic practices is doing what I vowed not to do.

The first question must be: did the ancients have malignant cancers and did Dioscorides recognize them as we now do? The simple answer to the former[98] and the complex answer to the latter are both affirmative. Dioscorides had a number of words whose range of meaning included cancer, that is, hyperplasia of epithelial or glandular cells with infiltration and destruction of tissue. One must observe that today we have numerous technical and lay terms that pass under the name "cancer," a term that should not even be considered a single entity. The common term "lump in the breast" often infers cancer, but, in medical terms, it means only that it may be a malignant neoplasm but more likely is benign, such as a simple cyst.

Already we have encountered two words, *anthrax* and *phuma*, whose meaning may include cancer. Crocus and squirting cucumber were given for *phuma* ("growth") and *oidēma* (οἴδημα). *Oidēma* is defined in one Galenic work as meaning a soft and painless tumor.[99] Estimating whether Dioscorides intended malignancy depends upon the context. *Oidēmata* are "helped" by the root bark of the oak (I. 106, φηγός), which, as stated above, has astringent and styptic pharmaceutical results. Barley (II. 86), cabbage (II. 120), crocus (IV. 84), and squirting cucumber (IV. 150) "dissolve" *oidēmata*; myrrh (I. 87) "stops" them; and the cucumber (*Cucumis pepo* L.) "makes *oidēmata* soft." This last usage goes in the face of the Galenic definition that an *oidēma* is soft. Dioscorides intended a stronger effect for those drugs which "dissolve" or "stop" the lumps than for those which merely "help," implying temporary relief. There were symptomatic signs that differentiated *phuma* and *oidēma* because he used the terms together as two entities, but Dioscorides' distinctions are lost to us. Perhaps he used *oidēma* the way we use the term *edema*, which derives from this Greek word. Edema is a type of neoplastic, benign tumor with water in the tissue and is a characteristic of dropsy (or anascarca). Consequently, Dioscorides' verbs, such as "dissolve," "stop," "help," and "cure," could readily apply. Searching the context of other writers for their word use is of limited value; quite apparently there was little consistency in ancient medicine about such terms.

The word σκληρία, or *sklēria*, meaning "hardness," was another frequent term in Dioscorides where he probably used it to refer to breast carcinoma (I. 108) and uterine cancer (I. 58, 59). He also used it when he recommended liquid pitch (I. 72) for "dissolving *sklēriai* on the fingers," in an apparent reference to callouses. Many benign cysts are quite hard and it is necessary to interpret the context when *sklēria* is carcinoma. Acorns (I. 106) are "good for malignant [κακόηθεις] *sklēriai*." Malignancy would not have exactly the same histiological meaning as today, but on the basis of symptomatic indications of very bad and often fatal growth its meaning is close to ours. Sometimes the adjectives add to the problem: figs (I. 128) "dissolve *sklēriata*" but "with *chalkanthum* they heal [θεραπενεῖ] hard to cure [δυσαλθῆ], discharging [ῥευματικά] malignancies [κακόηθη; actually used as an adjective here without a noun) in the *tibia* [ἐν κνήμαις]." Κνήμα in a Galenic anatomical work meant tibia but, loosely, the word could also refer to the leg in general.[100] Since Dioscorides used figs around a therapeutic theme suggesting cancer, would this be bone cancer, multiple myeloma, or possibly soft tissue sarcoma, which now is occasionally treated by amputation? Any answer would have to be so qualified as to be virtually meaningless.

Certain plants were seen by Dioscorides as providing beneficial results to a variety of dermatological and tumorous afflictions. Bitter vetch and/or horse bean are scrambling, herbaceous plants with small leaves, poisonous seeds, and edible beans when properly prepared.[101] Cows should avoid them, but Dioscorides found them useful. He recommended one or both (II. 108, *Vicia ervilla* L. and/or *V. fava* L.) for "cleaning ulcers with honey, moles [φακόι], skin spots [σπιλόι], freckles [or ?rough spots (ἐφήλοι)], and the rest of the body; it stops boils/ulcers [νομάι], gangrene, or running sores [γάγγραιναι];[102] it softens hardnesses [σκληρίαι] in the breast, malignant ulcers [θηριώδαι], anthrax/carbuncles/malignant pustules [ἄνθρακαι], and *cerium* [yellow and bad skin swelling or ulcer (κηρίον)]."[103] Even though it is probably impossible to define Dioscorides' Greek terms with equivalent modern ones, the range of contexts certainly includes cancers, especially deep-seated, papillary, and superficial epithelioma and nonspecific, metastatic inflammatory lesions associated with cancer in the stage of ulceration. That the vetch plant was employed to treat cancer until the early nineteenth century[104] lends credence to Dioscorides' employment of it for that purpose. Modern science has identified a number of chemicals in the plant, such as vicianin (a cyanogenetic glycoside), choline, guanidine, and xanthine.[105] Eating the bean improperly cooked or even inhaling its pollen produces acute hepatitis and a recent study (1964) has shown that toxic symptoms are pronounced in certain people with genetically determined, biochemical blood deficiency.[106]

In theory, the efficacy of some chemotherapy in cancer is based on the fact that many malignant cell-cycle kinetics for rapid mitotic division are such that they require abnormally high nourishment. Antineoplastic drugs then are "toxins," some of which may enter malignant cells and interfere with their life cycle in one of several ways, resulting in cell death. For a slow-growing tumor, cytotoxic drugs are less effective. Some agents are alkylating compounds that effectively disturb cell function and differentiation. The alleged laetrile therapy for cancer is supposed to work because of the cyanide production made by the apricot plant's extract (*Prunus armeniaca* L. and others) called amygdalin.[107] Amygdalin is, like vicianin found in vetch, a cyanogenetic glycoside.[108] Advocates of laetrile argue that cyanide comes into contact with an enzyme, B-glucuronidase, found in tumor cells and the union kills the cells. While we cannot be certain because of the confusion over the issue, there is evidence to support the hypothesis that Dioscorides' remedy may have had some beneficial results.

Over three thousand plant species have recently (1967) been cataloged for cancer treatments by Jonathan L. Hartwell of the National Cancer Institute in Bethesda, Maryland, in a study embracing the whole history of medicine and folklore.[109] No attempt was made to relate the information to modern studies. At best most of the three thousand plants could have given only temporary relief but a *few were most likely effective*.

While there can be no doubt that Dioscorides included things under these terms that were not our "cancer" and that we have "cancers" he did not recognize, we are certain that he treated cancer. In a medical journal in 1916, William S. Stone, M.D., reviewed the history of chemical therapy for cancer and said that the ancient remedies "have almost invariably been found to consist of arsenic, zinc, or the alkaline caustics."[110] Beginning in 1938 with colchicine, medicine returned to chemotherapy for cancer by coming back to the "alkaline caustics," as Dr. Stone referred to them. Historically, a question is why did Stone and his era reject ancient remedies so quickly without trial? A more pressing question is why, if the ancients had effective treatments for cancer, did they fall into disrespect or, at least, nonuse?[111] Speculative answers will be projected in later chapters where Dioscorides' influence is discussed. For now, we can observe the irony that Dioscorides' chemical cancer therapy is closer to today's than we had previously thought. Rather than to have been so quick to deprecate early medicine, our fathers' generation would have profited from more study and sympathy with ancient medicine. Still our age will not be the last age to judge Dioscorides on his cancer treatments—thank goodness.

Contraceptives

The question as to whether premoderns could control their birthrate by effective contraceptives is broader in its implications than the history of medicine. Restraint, *coitus interruptus*, abortions, and infanticide have always been assumed. Restraint, it is generally agreed, was ineffectual—statistically at least—especially with the ancients whose religion normally did not regulate sexual activity. Evidence in the Roman literature for *coitus interruptus* gives the impression that it was not widely practiced.[112] Abortifacients were available.[113] Their effectiveness is not clearly known, but drug-induced abortions were often dangerous to the mother. Greco-Roman mores did not generally restrain abortions on moral or legal grounds. The prohibition to abortifacients in the famous Hippocratic Oath was probably the production of the Pythagoreans, a small sect, or some other cult and did not apply either to the general population or to the general medical practitioner.[114] Scholars debate whether the Romans practiced infanticide; if they did, it may not have been extensive.[115] The abandonment of a child was considered the equivalent of murder.[116] By the time of Augustus (31 B.C.–A.D. 14) the decline in the birthrate was alarming enough that the government devised policies to encourage marriage and procreation. The Alimentary Laws promulgated in the time of Trajan (A.D. 98–117) were an elaborate device to give government grants for child rearing.[117] The population decline extended well into the Middle Ages and the Christian era. Was it a controlled, deliberate decision by the multitudes to limit births or the result of other factors? The fact that there were government policies to encourage child rearing and that later there were scattered but strong attacks by Christian leaders against contraception, abortion, and infanticide allows us to hypothesize that the decisions not to reproduce abundantly were deliberate. St. Jerome specifically denounced all forms of birth control, and the only praise he could find for the sexual act within the marriage bond was that it was the only method of producing virgins.[118] The degree to which people wanted to control their fecundity and the extent to which it was technically possible and efficient is a historical problem not yet addressed.[119]

Modern science provides less insight than normally is the case for judging early medicine in this area because our culture has restricted the research. There is no compelling reason to test potentially dangerous chemical abortifacients when efficient surgical or mechanical procedures are available and subject to society's control, while the plant remedies are not. In antiquity there was at least some opposition to abortion.[120] Recent centuries of religious objection have undoubtedly had results in eroding western folk practices, the "secrets of women." Even the cataloging of non-Christian practice is difficult because of its sensitivity to the prying anthropologists' eyes.

Dioscorides recommended a number of abortifacients and contraceptives. To manage our analysis, I shall limit the discussion mainly to oral contraceptives. Under various terms for abortions in Greek and Latin the ancients often included contraceptives within the broader meaning of abortifacients. An abortion meant the prevention of live birth, which could be, of course, prevented prior to fertilization.[121] Even so, both Dioscorides and Soranus,[122] the second-century gynecologist, explicitly distinguished between remedies designed to prevent fertilization and those more numerous ones that allegedly aborted a fetus. A few examples taken in order of presentation in *De materia medica* will demonstrate the versatility of Dioscorides' approach to birth control: juniper berries (I. 77) put on the penis or the vulva before insertion cause (temporary) sterility; the bark of white poplar (I. 81) taken with a mule's kidney, "it is reported," takes away conception (ἀτόκιος) and its leaves, drunk after menstruation, have the same effect; hawthorn's root (I. 93, *Crataegus oxycantha* L.), "it is said," causes an abortion (ἐκτρωσμοῖς) when rubbed or anointed three times on the lower abdomen; the chaste tree (I. 103, *Vitex agnus-castus* L.) destroys generation (ἐκλύει δὲ καὶ γονήν); the leaves of white willow (I. 104) cause inconception (ἀσυλληψία); the sap of the Ethiopian olive (I. 105) kills the fetus (ἔμβρυα); the cultivated lupin (II. 109, ?*Lupinus angustifolius* L.) extracts the menstrua and fetus; and the flower of cabbage (II. 120) applied as a pessary *after childbirth* hinders conception.

Some of these preparations may be effective. Juniper berries are a uterine stimulant; that is, when they come into contact with uterine tissue contractions result.[123] While its use has been dropped from our official pharmacopoeias (1885 in Britain) in favor of stronger stimulants to induce labor, mild contractions induced at the time of intercourse might inhibit fertilization or, if the dosage was continued for five to eight days, attachment of a fertilized egg to the uterine wall. Modern studies show that juniper leaves act as an emmenagogue affecting the menstrual cycle;[124] oils from the leaves are uterine stimulants as shown by *in vitro* and *in vivo* tests in animals,[125] and in experiments on the isolated human uterus and Fallopian tubes, the oils cause relaxation and inhibition of movement to an extent that could lead to an abortion.[126] No modern studies have tested juniper for contraception[127] but, based on its physiological effects, it is probable that it would not only interfere with, if not inhibit, conception but also have unpleasant side effects. On the other hand, the alleged sterilization action of the chaste tree has been the subject of related modern investigations as an antifertility agent. In one study, three grams of the seeds of the tree were fed to rats and nine grams to guinea pigs daily for two weeks, but the animals showed no effects.[128] Another study, however, revealed retardation of estrus in female rats.[129] There is at least one modern folk report of its use as a sexual suppressant.[130]

In the literature are unmistakable statements that the bark of white poplar and the leaves of white willow were employed as oral contraceptives. In his study of contraception in the Roman Empire, Keith Hopkins briefly mentioned these two references, as well as five other oral-route drugs and dismissed them, without further comment, as "ineffectual potions."[131] If we look more deeply into the chemistry of these drugs, we find some therapeutic potential but still do not arrive at a full understanding.

Drugs can contain, enhance, or interfere with the hormones and enzymes that regulate much of the body's actions. These drugs are complex molecules and are derived from animal hormones or are synthetically produced. The most widely used oral contraceptive today, the one often referred to as "the pill," is composed of two hormones, estrogen and progestin, which regulate ovarian function as happens with pregnancy.[132] While plants do not produce these hormones, some plants provide the chemical starting materials for hormone synthesis. Progesterone, for instance, is synthesized from diosgenin found in yams (*Dioscorea* spp.).[133] Boleslaw Skarzynski gave a report in 1933 to the Polish Academy of Sciences that "from 65 kgm of the female flowers of the willow, I obtained a semi-crystalline substance" that had "properties which were identical with the properties of trihydroxyoestrin prepared by me from female urine."[134] Skarzynski's report was greeted with scepticism, as was another one in the same year by Butenandt and Jacobi (1933) concerning a study of the date palm and pomegranate, which said that the plants develop female sex hormones.[135] After all, animals manufacture these chemicals in special endocrine glands. During World War II, women in the Netherlands who were forced to eat tulip bulbs because of food shortages developed menstrual upsets and ovulation failures. The cause seems to have been an unidentified estrogenic material in the plant tissue.[136] Of course, malnutrition also will cause anovulation and amenorrhea, but in following up on reports that Burmese and Thai women take orally an extract of the root of *Pueraria mirifica* L. to induce abortion, in 1960 Bounds and Pope isolated a compound called miroestrol, which has medicinally higher activity than estrone. In the 1940s Australian sheep grazing on a type of clover (*Trifolium subterraneum* L.) had sharply reduced fertility. The reason was found to be isoflavonoids in the clover, which induce estrogenic activity in mammals. Other studies hypothesize that certain plants produce the chemical as a means of protecting themselves against predators, especially insects, by interfering with their reproduction.[137]

Dioscorides' use of the white willow as a contraceptive has possible validity, as revealed by recent research. An article in an Indian medical journal reports that in a rough screening test willow bark (no specific species given) interferes with ovulation.[138] One must be cautious because the amounts to be taken were not specified by Dioscorides. A modern scientist would need to know the concentration of active substance in the bark, the amount and route of administration, and the drug's metabolism, but such information is not available. Table 1 shows that the concentration of estriol in willow is low but there are two important cautions here: (*a*) the modern study tested the flower while Dioscorides recommended the leaves and (*b*) regarding the testing procedures for plant estrogens in general, J. B. Harborne (1977) observes, "There is at present the possibility of considerable quantitative variations between plant samples."[139] All these things presume that willow was virtually the same chemically in Dioscorides' day as in our own. Present knowledge of plant estrogenic activity on the human body is not complete, but there is enough evidence to warrant a hypothesis that Dioscorides recorded an effective contraceptive. Still, even Dioscorides was cautious. When he related it, he said, "it is reported," a phrase normally preceding accounts of the supernatural that he received from folklore.

The utility for the bark of the white poplar as an oral contraceptive is less readily seen in modern studies because there has been no testing.[140] Attention, however, is directed to the mule's kidney, which Dioscorides said is to be taken with the bark. A modern source for estrogen, indeed the preferred natural source, is horse's urine. But why was the plant part of the prescription? In the absence of evidence to the contrary and based on the limited modern studies, it is remotely

TABLE 1. *Plants with Human Sex Hormones and Their Contraceptive Use*

Compound	*Plant Source*	*Concentration (mg/kg)*	*Dioscorides*	*Use as Contra-ceptive*
Estrone	Date palm, *Phoenix dactylifera* L. seeds and pollen	0.40	I. 109	no
Estrone	Pomegranate, *Punica granatum* L. seeds	17.0	I. 110–111	no
Estriol	Willow, *Salix* spp. flowers	0.11	I. 104	yes
Estrone	Apple, *Malus pumila* Mill. seeds	0.1	I. 115	no
Testosterone & Androstanedione	Scotch pine, *Pinus sylvestris* L. pollen	0.08 & 0.59	I. 69 (different species)	no

Source: Adapted from J. B. Harbone, *Introduction to Ecological Biochemistry*, p. 85.

possible that the bark contains a chemical starting material for progesterone production. Historically, however, when generations of people relied on a drug for something as readily verified as a contraceptive—full-term pregnancies are not psychosomatic—then we should entertain the possibility that the drug is valid.[141] The burden of scientific proof should not rest only with the negative when historical authorities and tradition assert a fact. In science, all positive assertions are demonstrated by scientific proof, but in history the evidence is more empirical. We can, however, assume that these natural remedies were not completely effective, especially in the absence of controlled preparation, amount, and frequency of administration. Empirically, had the contraceptives been dramatically effective, there would likely have been stronger testimonials in the literature. The basic question is: could premodern people control their reproductive rate through contraception? Evidence in Dioscorides collaborated by modern studies indicates this probability but only to a limited degree.

Dioscorides also knew other means to control births. The examples he gives of hawthorn root, the tears of the Ethiopian olive, and lupin indicate that Dioscorides employed drugs to abort a fetus. In reports published in 1952 and 1953, hawthorn was found to possess therapeutic properties through the action of crataegolic acid and a mixture of sapogenins, sometimes called crataegus lactone. The plant depressed respiration, affected the heart, relaxed the uterus and intestines, and constricted the bronchi and the coronary artery. Drugs from this source currently are used to treat elderly patients with heart disease and patients with mitral stenosis.[142] With such a marked effect on the body, it seems possible that the plant could cause an abortion. Lupanine and possibly other constituents of lupin produce contractions of isolated guinea pig uteri[143] and, in *in vivo* tests, uterine contractions were "very effective" in the second half of the pregnancy of guinea pigs.[144] Since we cannot positively identify the Ethiopian olive, we are unable to evaluate its use as an abortifacient. In all, Dioscorides recommended some forty-six abortifacients.[145] Many of Dioscorides' plants (and other agents) also appear in Norman Farnsworth's list of emmenagogue, abortifacient, and uterine stimulant plants.[146] Based on all that we have seen with other cases, it seems likely that laboratory testing of the abortifacient plants in Dioscorides would confirm at least some as being effective.

Dioscorides distinguished between temporary and permanent sterilizers. The example of the chaste tree points to permanent sterility, and the fern called *thelupteris* (IV. 185, *Agnus castus* or *Pteridium aquilinium* Kuhn?) given to nonpregnant women causes barrenness and given to pregnant women causes abortion. In contrast, the barrenwort's root (IV. 19, ?*Epimedium alpinum* L.) given in large amounts to women causes barrenness but 3 drachmas (12 grams) of its leaves crushed and drunk in wine for three days, beginning three days after the completion of menstruation, keeps women from conceiving. This is an example of an antifertility drug that can lead to permanent sterility or, used in a carefully regulated way, produce temporary contraception. There have been no modern studies to assist our understanding of Dioscorides' sterilizing drugs. A male sterilizer is seen in *periklumenon* (IV. 14, ?*Lonicera etrusca* Santi), which makes men incapable of generation and, interestingly, causes women to hasten birth when its leaves or seeds are drunk for thirty-seven days, but, Dioscorides warned, after the seventh day blood appears in the urine. Pessaries were recommended by Dioscorides to affect fertility but their number is unexpectedly limited. Condoms were not mentioned by him and seemed to have had very limited use.[147]

Modern research points to the necessity of a carefully balanced vaginal chemistry for fertilization to occur and chemical intervention may have noticeable results. Sticky plant gums were given as pessaries, according to Dioscorides (I. 77; III. 34, 130). Hopkins says that these prescriptions would block the os of the uterus or otherwise interfere mechanically with the sperm.[148] I have not identified any clear use of spermatocides in Dioscorides' pessaries. Why this should be true is curious in light of later folk usages of them. There is one mention of an impotency-inducing drug: the water lily's root (III. 132) is drunk to produce impotence for three days and, not unexpectedly, the departure of erotic dreams.[149] Darnel (II. 100) is suffumigated with polenta, myrrh, saffron, or frankincense to help conceptions. Dioscorides thought virtually all aspects of sexuality were responsive to drugs. This is especially apparent in the number of aphrodisiacs he included.[150]

Since Dioscorides did not give comparative values to the various birth control methods, we do not know which were preferred or what drugs were considered most effective. Other ancient sources do not readily yield such private information, but there are sufficient indications that birth control methods were employed, as there are periodic denunciations of them in theological literature. We have some confidence in stating that they were relatively effective, since many of them continue in use down to our own times. But there is no evidence in the works of Dioscorides or any other authority that a medical breakthrough resulted in the reversal of the demographic curve that happened during Dioscorides' lifetime. The will to practice birth control—and here religion is important—is the overriding consideration. After the desire is assessed by the historian, however, we need to know if the people had the means available. Based on Dioscorides, as evaluated by limited modern studies, the probability is that they did have both contraceptives and abortifacients that worked to a degree as yet undetermined.

6. HARMFUL SIDE EFFECTS

Dioscorides was very observant of harmful side effects. By side effects I also mean secondary reactions not intended or desired by the drug administrator. Some drugs were so powerful that the remedy may have been worse than the affliction (e.g., II. 148). Bitter vetch (II. 108), as discussed above, has a cyanogenetic agent and was given for cancer but Dioscorides prefaced his remarks as follows: It "is suitable for therapeutic uses [πρὸς τὴν ἰατρικὴν ἁρμόζει χρῆσιν] but it causes headache [and] disturbance of the bowels; if eaten it draws down blood in the urine." After a discussion of its preparation and beneficial effects to the lower digestive tract, he noted at the end: ". . . but used in excessive quantities in meat or drink, it brings out blood through the bowels and bladder with pains of colic." These are clear, classic symptoms of cyanide poisoning as given in modern toxicological manuals.[151]

The majority of the side effects deal with the digestive system. Balanite oil (I. 34) and the fruit of sycamore (I. 127) are good for the lower digestive tract (κοίλια) but bad for the upper tract (κακοστόμαχος).[152]

Although juniper berries (I. 77) have a general warming effect on the body, a quality usually associated with ingested medicines, they are bad for the upper tract.[153] In contrast, pickled olives (I. 105) are good for the upper tract and bad for the lower. The chapter on walnuts (I. 125) begins with their harmful effects: hard to digest, harmful to the upper tract, engender cholera and headaches, and not to be given to one with a cough. The chapter on hollyhock (II. 118) reveals how refined in descriptions he could be: "bad for the upper tract, good for the lower, and profitable for the intestines [ἔντερον] and bladder [κύστις]." Cabbage (III. 120), if cooked and saturated in salt, is bad for the upper tract and troublesome to the lower—which again suggests that ancient cabbage was more toxic than the modern prototype. But for us it is difficult to understand the anatomical distinctions based on symptoms. Nausea and/or vomiting is a frequent side effect (e.g., I. 40, 52, 78). Radishes (II. 112) breed wind (flatulence) and heat, are welcomed in the mouth, not good for the upper tract, cause belching, and are diuretical. These are comparatively mild side effects.

Some side effects are more ominous. As discussed in Chapter 3, Dioscorides described well and vividly the effects of strong alkaloids, narcotics, depressants, and stimulants in such toxins as atropine, opium, and hyoscyamine. Such information is found throughout his work. The leaf of oleander has the glycoside oleandrin used today as a cardiac stimulant.[154] Dioscorides has a chapter devoted to it (IV. 81; νήριον, *Nerium oleander* L.), including a full plant and habitat description, but his attention was directed to its toxicity in four-footed animals who eat it. For humans he said only that it has a preserving quality and is good drunk in wine against poisonous animal bites. (Incidentally, foxglove, the supplier of the cardiac stimulant digitalis, was not known to Dioscorides, despite at least one modern authority who has attempted to make the claim.)[155]

Some entries in *De materia medica* are there not because the plants possess beneficial qualities but because they have entirely harmful, even fatal, results. A chapter on the strawberry tree (I. 122, κόμαρος, *Arbutus unedo* L.) gives a plant description and then a warning about its kernel: "ingested it is bad for the upper tract and causes headaches."[156] Andromedotoxin is found in plants of the Ericaceae family (to which the strawberry tree belongs) and is a powerful emetic, very toxic, but also useful in diarrhea treatment.[157] Although it is an argument out of silence in the surviving sources, one can speculate that Dioscorides included the plant as a corrective because either some authority or folk use employed its kernel as a drug.

Dioscorides said that wolfsbane (IV. 77, ἀκόνιτον, ?*Aconitum lycoctonum* Auct.), the source of the strong poison aconite,[158] was employed to kill wolves. That much was said in the chapter on the plant. But throughout *De materia medica* there are some seventeen places where antidotes are given for aconite poisoning.[159] The reason for including the plant becomes apparent: one ought to be able to recognize it.[160] Medicines are given not only to combat diseases or to heal afflictions but also to counter the side effects of other medicines. Olive oil (I. 30 [2]), Dioscorides said, is given to dull the effect of "medicines that cause ulcers [*ἑλκούντον φαρμάκων δυνάμεις*]." Although not specifically stated, many drugs that quell upset stomachs doubtlessly were given by Dioscorides because of the nausea generated by another drug.

Neurological side effects were also recognized. Headaches were the most common (e.g., I. 3, 106); others include harm to sight (II. 107, 136) and hearing (I. 79) in specific ways and induction of sleep (I. 66). The latter side effect, perhaps as a narcotic, is mentioned in an intriguing way with an oil called honey oil (*ἐλαιόμελι*), taken from the trunk of an unidentified tree (possibly *Olea* spp.) that Dioscorides said grew in Palmyra.[161] Honey oil (I. 31) can make one inactive but, Dioscorides admonished, do not be afraid to use it as a medicine. Should the patient feel drowsy, keep him or her from falling into a deep sleep. Easier to understand for us are the side effects of mead (II. 88), the fermented drink: headaches, breeder of ill humors, and damaging to the nerves and muscles. We would say "loss of coordination." Dioscorides gave no positive uses for mead.

Some side effects are very specific. Sesame seeds (II. 99) cause the stinking of the breath if lodged between the teeth. Chick-pea (II. 104) is given for jaundice and dropsy but is harmful to an ulcerated bladder and kidney. Quantity is important. Too much basil (II. 140) dulls the sight and in any amount provokes sneezing. Smilax (II. 146) causes troublesome dreams, and onions (II. 151) cause the hair to fall out. Frankincense (I. 68), Dioscorides said, is a good medicine but, if drunk by a healthy person, brings on madness and, if too much is taken, produces fatal results.

While we notice less some of the small claims of side effects, we note that Dioscorides described well the harmful side effects of opium (IV. 64), henbane (IV. 68), and mandrake (IV. 75), all of which have a cooling quality—Dioscorides' way of saying potentially fatal. Somewhat unsettling, however, is the reference in the crocus chapter (I. 26, *Crocus sativus* L.) where the claim is given that 3 drachmas (12 grams) or more cause death, because we are certain that crocus today has no toxic effect.[162] But Dioscorides began the claim with the clause "they say . . . ," not embracing claims derived from folklore but at the same time recording them. One can speculate that, because of the high value placed on the crocus by the ancients, a "rumor" of fatal consequences was perpetuated in order to protect its fragile supply.

7. QUANTITIES AND DOSAGES

Modern pharmacists would have great difficulty with Dioscorides' quantifications. Quantity, frequency, and site of administration are important in evaluating a given drug's metabolism for effective therapy. Regarding those things, Dioscorides was often vague—sometimes he gave us nearly no indication and at other times he related very careful, specific, and insightful instructions. Like most things in his work, there was a reason to be understood within the context of his culture for doing as he did. In the first chapters of *De materia medica* it is not until the fifth chapter, this one on cardamon, that he gave his first quantity: 1 drachma (ca. 4 grams) of the root bark in a drink for "breaking the stone."

Parsley, sage, rosemary, and thyme illustrate his apparent inconsistency in respect to quantity. Parsley (III. 65) seed and root have a diuretic quality and expel the menstrua, but no quantity is given. Nor is a quantity related for sage (III. 33) or rosemary (III. 75) despite the fact that sage has a number of medicinal usages, such as a decoction to stop itching around the genitals. Administration instructions are given in more detail for rosemary: it cures jaundice if it is soaked in water, drunk before exercise and after a bath, with the herb being drenched in wine. Finally, in our four-herb sample, with thyme (III. 38) we have our first quantity: 4 drachmas (16 grams) of its juice drunk with vinegar causes vomiting of blood to cease. A modern guide lists thyme leaves as an antispasmodic in a dose of 2 to 4 grams.[163] The U.S. *Dispensatory* lists thyme for treatment of bronchitis and whooping cough, and this explains why it is an ingredient in some proprietary medicines.[164] Coughing of blood (hemoptysis and hematemesis) is a symptom of a number of things, such as pharyngeal irritation or pulmonary tuberculosis. Whatever its etiology, thyme would probably give some relief in most cases of coughing blood without dealing with the cause. Dioscorides' larger dosage would be attributed to the chronic condition of hemorrhaging or vomiting blood. Among our four-herb sample, thyme is the "strongest" medicine.

Dioscorides had a purpose, albeit unevenly implemented, regarding when he chose to relate quantities. If a medicine was so strong as to be potentially dangerous, he advised his reader about the amount. I shall demonstrate this by taking a number of plants with alkaloids whose specific medicinal actions are discussed in another section. Ten to 15 grains (seeds) of stavesacre (IV. 152, *Delphinium staphisagria*

L.) crushed in honey provokes vomiting "but let him walk who had drunk it." Thapsia (IV. 153, *Thapsia garganica* L.), a strong cathartic, Dioscorides and modern medicine say, is given in the amount of 4 obols (2½ grams) of root bark with 3 drachmas (12 grams) of dill seed or 3 obols (2 grams) of its juice and 1 obol of its sap, "for more is dangerous." Six drachmas (24 grams) of Alexandria laurel or large butcher's-broom (IV. 145, *Ruscus hypoglossum* L.) are given women in child labor, patients with strangury, and during blood extraction; the fruit of the daphne (IV. 146, *Daphne* spp.) is a laxative—"as many as" fifteen berries given in a drink. Presumably, these are for one-time administrations, because for black hellebore (IV. 162, *Helleborus niger* L.), he said 1 drachma (4 grams) or 3 obols (2 grams) to clean fistulas as a three-day applicant. To improve hearing, 1 drachma is put into the ears for two to three days. Three obols (2 grams) of amyris (I. 24) juice reduced to a powder and drunk with water or barley water "for many days in a row causes a person to lose weight." He seldom specified durations, presumably spelling out the long period for weight loss to prevent premature discouragement.

Perhaps the greatest detailed instructions occur in the chapter on the squirting cucumber (IV. 150, *Ecballium elaterium* L.). One-half of a pound (ἡμιλίτριον = 6 Greek ounces) of its root, beaten small with 3 sestes (ca. 1½ liters) of wine, is given in the amount of 3 cyathi (125 cc) every third day until the abdominal swelling has abated. Three semiobols (1 gram) "at least" of the root and also the bark, as much as one-fourth as much, in a small vinegar saucer, purges the bowels, phlegm, and cholera. Elaterin, an extract from the seed of the squirting cucumber, best when two years old, is given most effectively as a laxative in 1 obol (0.66 gram), one-fourth of that amount for children (0.165 gram), with a minimum dosage of half an obol (0.33 gram) for adults. "Anything less is ineffective; more, dangerous," Dioscorides warned. The root of the plant is beaten small in the weight of 1 drachma (4 grams), drunk with honeywater to promote vomiting but, if after supper, one obol (1.32 grams) is sufficient. The distinction between adult and child dosages is not made elsewhere in *De materia medica* but minimum dosages are occasionally found throughout.

Dioscorides clearly took care with the strongest medicines. Experience, as he said in his Preface,[165] was absolutely necessary in determining drug usage. Only experienced medical people would know how much parsley, sage, and rosemary to give because of the innumerable variables having to do with the plants, the patients, and the severity of affliction. Best, he decided, not to recommend a standard dose, especially when there was no imperative established in the culture before his day. Too much or too little and there would be little harm, but not so with the high toxins employed as medicine. For example, with jimsonweed (IV. 73, *Datura stramonium* L.),[166] he stated specifically: "1 drachma [4 grams] in a drink is the quantity that allows one to have fantasies without unpleasantness, 2 drachmas alters one completely for three days, and 4 drachmas being drunk is fatal."[167] Knowing this, he did not leave it unnoted to the inexperienced.

Not all poisons are so clearly instructed as to quantity. While for henbane (IV. 63, *Hyoscyamus niger* L.) he gave a standard dosage, for opium poppy (IV. 64, *Papaver somniferum* L.), the plant that is our best source for morphine, he gave no quantities whatsoever. For corn poppy (IV. 63, *P. rhoeas* L.), another species of poppy, he said that "5 or 6 heads [of corn poppy] soaked in 3 cyathi (126 cc) of wine—boiled down to 2—is given in a drink to whomever would want to sleep." Why this apparent discrepancy in relating information? Modern pharmacologists know that the peak of morphine content in the opium poppy occurs two to three weeks after flowering; harvesting earlier or later yields significantly less morphine while too long of a delay results in a decomposition of the morphine.[168] Dioscorides knew—because he told us in his Preface—that an important variable was when a plant was harvested. How, he might argue, could he specify a quantity when the effective amount varied according to harvesting? Harvesting and preparation are as important as quantity.

8. HARVESTING, PREPARATION, AND STORAGE INSTRUCTIONS

Dioscorides was interested not in plants *qua* plants but plants *qua* medicines, and yet his observations about the plants are so remarkable that today only a few specialized botanists and phytochemists can fully appreciate the depth of his insight. As the example of opium poppy indicated, when and how a plant was harvested had much to do with its medicinal value. In the case of opium poppy, Dioscorides distinguished between the juice of the poppy and an extract of the entire plant.

In his Preface, Dioscorides said: "Before anything else, it is appropriate to consider the storage and collecting of individual drugs in the proper seasons, for these matters in particular determine the weakness or efficacy of drugs." Field southernwood (*Artemisia maritima* L.) contains over 3 percent santonin in the flower heads but only in this amount when the flower heads are unexpanded. Once they mature the santonin rapidly disappears enough so that its anthelmintic principle disappears; that is to say, it will no longer kill intestinal parasites. In the chapter on field southernwood (III. 23), Dioscorides prescribed its use against intestinal worms but he did not give specific harvesting instructions. Instead, in his Preface he told his users that they had to pay careful attention to when a plant was to be harvested.

Dioscorides gave instructions regarding harvesting, preparation, and storage in three different ways: (*a*) general principles applied to all plants and drugs recorded in his Preface; (*b*) specific instructions regarding some plants in the individual chapters devoted to them; and (*c*) separate from the harvesting instructions and ordinarily at the end of the chapter, he sometimes specified in which geographic region the best quality drug was to be found.

General Principles Regarding Plant Environment

Drugs come from various parts of the plant and each has its own rule. Let us compare Dioscorides' rules with those in the introduction to a modern book, *Pharmacognosy* by Varro E. Tyler et al. (1977):[169]

Roots and rhizomes:

> Dioscorides (Pref. 9): Gather roots [and rhizomes] for laying up in storage, as well as roots for juices and root barks when the plants are beginning to shed their leaves.
>
> Tyler et al. (p. 9): Roots and rhizomes should be collected in the fall after the vegetative processes have ceased. Roots, especially if they are fleshy, will shrink and remain spongy after drying if collected during the growing season (belladonna root).

Leaves and stems:

> Dioscorides (Pref. 9): Extract juices from plants by infusion when the stems are recently sprouted, similarly with leaves; but to gain juices and droplike gums by tapping, take the stems and cut them while in their prime.
>
> Tyler et. al. (p. 9): Leaves and flowering tops should be collected when photosynthesis is most active, which is usually about the time of flowering and before the maturing of the fruit and seed (belladonna leaf).

Flowers, fruits, and seeds:

> Dioscorides (Pref. 8): . . . one should gather the medical plants which are like young sprouts [in appearance]—viz. French lavender, wall germander, felty germander, shrubby wormwood, Gallic wormwood, wormwood, marjoram, and plants similar to these—when the plants are swollen with seeds, and their flowers before they fall

off, their fruits while they are ripe, and the seeds when they are beginning to become dry before they drop off.

Tyler et al. (p. 9): Flowers should be collected prior to or just about the time of pollination (rose). Fruits may be collected either before or after the ripening period, i.e., when fully grown but unripe (cubeb, black pepper), or when fully ripe (anise, fennel). Seeds should be collected when fully matured, that is, when most of them have ripened but, if possible, before the fruits have opened (black mustard).

Specialists and nonspecialists alike can readily see that Dioscorides identified the general principles of harvesting medical plants and that there has been no substantial change since his work. As far as we can tell from the surviving documents, Dioscorides' observations were original. No doubt they also reflected the wisdom of those who learned and passed on their experiences about plants to succeeding generations until, eventually, they were recorded by Dioscorides—clearly, concisely, and correctly.

The plants' environments have much to do with medical effectiveness. After stating a general rule that the time of harvesting and the storage of drugs have much to do with the strength and efficacy of drugs, Dioscorides noted in particular (Pref. 6): "For example, herbs should be gathered when the weather is excellent, for it makes a great difference if the collecting is done after recent droughts or heavy rains. Similarly, sites are important, whether they are in the mountains, high up, windswept, cold, and arid, for the properties of such plants are stronger. Those of plants from flat and wet localities, in the shade and not open to the wind, are generally weaker, especially when plants are gathered in the wrong season or when they are decayed through some weakness." Edward Croom has recently brought together the variable factors in the modern evaluation of the efficacy of herbal medicines. Among the factors, plant environment looms important and is often overlooked.[170] The strength and even sometimes the presence of a medicine found in a plant vary according to soil type, available nutrients, moisture, climate, associated flora, and cultivation. Many alkaloid-containing plants have higher concentrations of their pharmaceutically active components in moist regions than in arid ones. High nitrogen content in the soil increases alkaloids. On the other hand, drugs are stronger when found in drier areas, weaker and poorer when found in high vegetation areas, such as moist forests.[171] Dioscorides' observation that generally the strongest medicines derive from plants in high, wind-swept, cold, and arid environments seems more apt for volatile oils than for alkaloids. It is probably not unkind, however, to say that modern science has not researched the effect of environmental factors on plant chemistry with the attention that might be expected. People today say that they can taste where a tomato was grown, that they can identify the region from which cannabis came, and the claim is made that the gaucho can place his approximate location on the pampa by simply tasting the grass.[172]

Conspicuous in its absence in Dioscorides' work, as discussed earlier, is the lack of attention given to the plant's stage of development. In his Preface Dioscorides seemingly left this aspect to the practical experience of the herbalists when he said: "One must not fail to note that plants often ripen either sooner or later according to the specific character of the country and the climate. Some, according to their own particular nature, bear leaves and flowers in winter, others produce flowers twice a year. Anyone wanting experience in these matters must encounter the plants as shoots, newly emerged from the earth, plants in their prime, and plants in their decline." He despaired in accounting for differing climates, probably because in his wide travels he saw the great differences in weather among the regions and because the ancients did not systematically record meteorological information. Occasionally, in an individual chapter, he gave specific information about the harvesting time best for medicines, such as distinctions between ripe and green fruits (e.g., I. 115, 116), but here he gave no generalizations.

When a specific plant had special environmental considerations in addition to or contrary to the general rules, Dioscorides brought them out. *Example*: The best garden myrtle (I. 112, *Myrtus communis* L.) grows on the hills, but the fruit of this kind has the weakest fruit. He observed the best conditions. *Example*: The yellow knapweed (III. 6, *Centaurea salonita* Vis.) loves a rich soil, openness to the sea, weeds, and hillocks. He noted variations in drug efficacy between species. *Examples*: Henbane (IV. 68) grows by the sea and amongst rubbish of buildings; one should use the white (*Hyoscyamus albus* L.), but, if it is not to be found, then the yellow (*H. aureus* L.) but refuse the black (*H. niger* L.), which is worst. The active principles in henbane resemble belladonna and stramonium and the black henbane has the strongest concentrations. It is highly poisonous, more than the white or yellow,[173] and consequently was considered too strong. In the chapter on the inula plant (III. 121), Dioscorides said that there is a third kind (*Inula britannica* L., "softer, thicker in the stalk, more abundant but smaller leaves; grows in moist places") that smells stronger than the other two kinds but it is more unpleasant and less effectual. Sometimes he gave specific warnings about harvesting. *Examples*: Rue (III. 45, *Ruta graveolens* L. and/or *R. montana* L.), Dioscorides said, is gathered about flowering time, but when picked it swells and reddens the skin and imparts an itch and bad inflammation. To gather it, one should anoint oneself (with oil?) on the face and hands. Opium poppy (IV. 64, *Papaver somniferum* L.) must be beaten in a mortar, but, after cutting it, one must prevent the liquid from contacting the skin or clothes. Finally, modern reports even show that there is a diurnal variation in alkaloid content in plants.[174] Dioscorides may have recognized this when, for example, he reported that the yellow knapweed (III. 6) is gathered when the sun is about to rise in the clear season when all things are at the height of growth.

Preparation and Storage Instructions

As with harvesting, Dioscorides gave general preparation and storage instructions in his Preface and specific instructions for special cases in the individual chapters. And, as with the general harvesting directions, Dioscorides' rules are almost identical to today's rules.

Dioscorides said, "The clean roots should be immediately dried out in areas free from moisture, but roots with earth or clay adhering should be washed with water" (Pref. 9). In the 1977 preface of *Pharmacognosy*, Tyler et al. said, "Roots and rhizomes after being thoroughly washed are carefully and completely dried" (p. 11).

Drying is important for flowers and leaves because it more rapidly stops enzymatic action, which breaks down the chemical bonds.[175] Dioscorides (Pref. 9) reported that flowers could be wrapped in papyrus or leaves to preserve their seeds, for those "flowers and parts having a sweet-smelling fragrance should be laid down in a small dry box of limewood [φιλύρινος]."[176] In general, however, Tyler reports (p. 13) that tight, light-resistant containers are best, such as tin cans, covered metal bins, or amber glass jars; wooden boxes should be avoided. Dioscorides (Pref. 9) is rather specific about some kinds of containers: "As for moist drugs, any container made from silver, glass, or horn will be suitable. An earthen vessel is well adapted, provided that it is not too thin, and among wooden containers, those of boxwood. Copper vessels will be suitable for moist eye drugs and for drugs prepared with vinegar, raw pitch, or juniper oil. But stow animal fats and marrows in tin containers."

Careful attention must be paid, Dioscorides said (Pref. 8), to the life expectancy of a drug. Some drugs, such as white and black hellebores, keep for many years, others up to three years; but, implicitly, he said, one must be experienced with each individual drug. Only through careful observation can one know such vital information.

When Dioscorides wrote, he assumed that his readers had experience in drugs and in watching nature. His readers were obviously not expected to be novices who took his scrolls and headed into the field to become druggists and doctors. As was observed above under (7) Quantities, he seldom gave advice on how exactly to collect, store, prepare, compound, and administer a medicine, much less the precise, full diagnostic details. Even so, when he encountered the unusual, he often gave special instructions in the chapters pertaining to each item. The preparation of the drug galbanum from a kind of fennel (III. 86, *Ferula galbaniflua* Boiss. & Buhse) reveals an example of specific instructions. The leaves are put in a cloth bag and suspended in a metal box, not touching the bottom. The box is then put into water and boiled. This causes the leaves to exude a substance, which is strained through the bag and collected at the bottom of the box. There on the bottom is the drug called galbanum.

Normally, when the leaves of a plant are prescribed, no directions are given because he assumed that one would know the "standard" way to handle them as a medicine. The details for the preparation of elaterium (IV. 150), the extract from the seed of squirting cucumber (*Ecballium elaterium* L.), are so elaborate that a large part of a large chapter is devoted to its description. The preparation of daphne (IV. 172) is more simply described: gather the leaves at harvest time, dry them in the shade, beat them (in a mortar, assumed), but take care to remove the strings before administration. The part about being dried in the shade is important, because the sun's rays break down the enzymes. For cinnamon (I. 14), Dioscorides said it was important that it be dried in the shade after being beaten and put in wine, and then stored—in a dark place, it was implied. Tyler, Brady, and Robbers caution modern users of cinnamon about the same thing.[177] Dioscorides was mindful of the plant part in which the most effective drug was to be found. For the drug from the gladiolus plant (IV. 20, *Gladiolus communis* L.), he said that the double roots (rhizome) were not equal in value to one another—the drug from the juice of the upper bulb had more force. The reader, however, should not have the impression that Dioscorides was always so specific about harvesting, preparation, and storage details. Mostly these were matters for the experienced, because environmental conditions varied so much.

9. ADULTERATION METHODS AND TESTS FOR DETECTION

"Nature," Pliny wrote, "has revealed . . . most remarkable properties to mortals, were it not that the fraudulent propensities of man are apt to corrupt and falsify everything."[178] Dioscorides was very mindful that drugs were adulterated, and he sought to warn his readers that they should be alert to this possibility. He even gave specific tests to detect fraudulent practices as well as accidental and natural adulterations. After all, what was at stake was not merely the loss of money, but the very risk to health and even life were an inferior drug to be substituted for a good, effective one. Adulteration means a debasement, and in today's usage refers to a variety of conditions: (*a*) inferiority, a change in a drug regardless of reasons from its "pure" state so that it is in a substandard condition; (*b*) spoilage, a deterioration in the quality or usefulness of a drug; (*c*) deterioration, an impairment in the quality or usefulness; (*d*) admixture, an addition to the drug through accident, ignorance, or carelessness; (*e*) sophistication, addition of another substance(s) with intent to defraud; (*f*) substitution, an entirely different drug sold in place of one requested.[179] Although Dioscorides did not refine his definition, it is clear that adulteration to him included all these conditions. With no government agency as there is in the modern world or trade guilds as there were in the medieval world that could define standards and regulate the purity, the ancient buyer had to beware.

No general rules were given by Dioscorides about adulteration in his Preface, but he gave information for individual drugs in the various chapters. Ernst W. Stieb reports that Dioscorides mentioned forty examples of adulteration.[180] His findings are in Table 2, which shows the relative distribution according to classes and the types of tests for detection. Of the forty adulterations, Dioscorides gave thirty definite methods of detection, and, Stieb reports, "in eight others his qualitative descriptions of the pure substances are probably sufficient for the differentiation of the true from the adulterated sample."[181]

Over 75 percent of the tests were based on sensory-perceptive methods but other testing was also prescribed. Dioscorides cited balsam (I. 19, *Commiphora opobalsamum* Engl. and/or C. *kataf* Engl.) as illustrating the variety of testing:

> [Balsam] . . . is adulterated in numerous ways. There are some who mix with it ointments, such as turpentine [resin], henna oil [*Lawsonia inermis* L.], mastic oil [*Pistacia lentiscus* L.], lily oil [*Lilium candidum* L.], zuchum oil [*Balanites aegyptiaca* Delile], almond[?] oil.[182] However, these things are easily known through testing. One can let pure balsam drop in a woolen cloth. Then wash it and it comes out clean. The counterfeited substances, however, stain the cloth. Or the pure balsam can be dropped in milk and it does what the false substances do not do. If one drops the genuine balsam in milk or water, it disperses smoky and milklike, but the false kind swims on top like oil, forming little balls together, then spreading out like a star. After a period of time genuine balsam becomes thick and it

TABLE 2. *Adulterations and Tests for Them*

Book	*Adulterations Mentioned According to Subdivision*	*Total*		*T*	*V*	*S*	*Ta*	*B*	*C*	*Co*	*Ph*	*O*	*Q*
				Type of Tests Indicated									
I	Aromatics	9											
	Resins	7											
	Pitch	1	19	4	4	14	6	3	4	1	2	2	—
	Shrubs & trees	1											
	Trees	1											
II	Living creatures	1											
	Wool fat	1	3	1	—	1	—	—	1	—	—	—	2
	Dung	1											
III	Juices	2	8	3	3	2	4	—	2	—	—	—	3
	Herbs	6											
IV	Herbs & roots	3	3	2	1	1	—	—	1	—	—	—	1
V	Metallic stones	7	7	3	—	—	2	—	5	—	1	—	2
	Totals		40	13	8	18	12	3	13	1	3	2	8
Subdivision by													
Animal			3	1	—	1	—	—	1	—	—	—	2
Vegetable			30	9	8	17	10	3	7	1	2	2	4
Mineral			7	3	—	—	2	—	5	—	1	—	2

Source: Adapted from Ernst W. Stieb, "Drug Adulteration and Its Detection in the Writings of Theophrastus, Dioscorides, and Pliny," *Journal Mondial de Pharmacie* 2 (1958): 122–123.

T Tactile—includes all references to touch, hardness, density (i.e., "weighty," etc.), friability.

V Visual—includes all references to the use of sight, e.g., color, dustiness.

S Smell.

Ta Taste.

B Botanical—includes all references to parts of plants, such as types of arrangement of leaves, roots, bark.

C Chemicophysical—includes all references to procedures requiring more than ordinary sense perceptions, even if those procedures involve nothing more than the application of heat or solution in a solvent.

Co Comparative—i.e., qualification of purity by reference to other plants or substances.

Ph Pharmacological—references to diminution of "strength" or efficacy of action.

O No tests of any kind mentioned.

Q Cases in which no specific tests for detecting the particular adulteration are mentioned, but in which the qualitative descriptions given seem sufficient to differentiate pure from adulterated samples of the substance in question.

> becomes worse than itself. Those are in error who believe that, if one takes the genuine article and drops it in water, it will sink to the bottom, then rise to the top, and then diffuse. The wood, which is called xylobalsamon, is dearest if it is fresh, has thin stalks, redlike and fragrant and for awhile having a smell like opobalsamon. Regarding the fruit, which also has a necessary use, one should choose the yellow, full, large, heavy, with a biting and burning taste, measured something in smell like opobalsamon. From Petra there grows from a seed, namely ground-pine [*hypericum*], a fruit which is counterfeited [for balsam], which may be recognized because it is larger, emptier, less strong, and tastes like pepper.[183]

The modern reader recognizes that balsam has a latex base and the false balsams an oil base, as the tests were designed to reveal. Still organoleptic tests were important as well in evaluating pure balsam. Under adulteration, Dioscorides also revealed that he included a deteriorated state of balsam. Finally, he corrected a test procedure that he considered wrong (I. 19).

Pliny disclosed that balsam was once a royal monopoly in royal gardens in Jerusalem and Jericho and its value was attested by the balsam trees that were carried in the triumphal procession of Pompey the Great.[184] A pint of balsam purchased in a sale of confiscated property for 300 denarii was resold for 1,000 denarii, a handsome profit. Pliny reported the price of balsam wood at 6 denarii a Roman pound (libra).[185] The reason for adulteration quickly becomes clear.

Dioscorides provided a number of chemophysical tests to detect adulterations. Since these types of tests are likely to be accurate, modern interest centers on them (see Table 3). Although, before Dioscorides, Theophrastus briefly mentioned testing for adulterations, Dioscorides' scale and detail for specific tests surpassed those of his known predecessors.[186]

10. VETERINARY USAGES

The Romans may have surpassed the Greeks in veterinary medicine alone among all of medicine's branches.[187] Such Romans as Varro and Pliny were mindful of the importance of caring medically for animals. They recognized that many of the remedies for humans worked as well for animals.[188] Dioscorides' work gives some confirmation to this but he is not explicit. He failed to apply his drug knowledge systematically to animals. When, however, a medicine uniquely treated animals and not humans, Dioscorides noted the practice near or at the ends of his chapters.

Practically all therapies were for what Dioscorides called scabs of

TABLE 3. *Relative Frequency of Particular Types of Chemicophysical Tests*

Book	*Substance*	*Chemical*			*Physical*					
		Flame Test	*Oxidation*	*Other*	*Solubility*	*Diffusibility*	*Flammability*	*Specific Gravity*	*Fusibility*	*Volatility; viscosity*
I	Balsam			Deterioration; staining		**		**		
	Frankincense									
	bark	*					*			
	gum	*					*			
	manna	*					*			
	Buckthorn	*					*			
II	Wool fat			Formation of lanolin						
III	Aloe								*	
	Opopanax				*				*	
	Galbanum			Purification by solution & diffusion						
IV	Opium	*			*					
	Elaterium						*			
V	Calamine	*	*	Reaction with vinegar	*					
	Pomopholux	*		Reaction with vinegar						
	Verdigris		*		*					
	Soda				*					
Totals:	15	7	2	6	5	2	5	2	2	2
Subdivision by										
Animal	1	—	—	1	—	—	—	—	—	—
Vegetable	10	5	—	3	2	2	5	2	2	2
Mineral	4	2	2	2	3	—	—	—	—	—

Source: Adapted from Stieb, "Drug Adulterations," p. 124.

the skin or itchy condition (ψωρα, *psōra*). This appears to be mange, a broad term that covers a variety of parasitical diseases, all caused by ticks and attacking such animals as cattle, pigs, sheep, and dogs.[189] It is reasonable to suppose that Dioscorides' *psōra* would include our scaroptic mange and psoriatic mange. Dioscorides' remedies were almost all vegetable oils or petroleum: pitch oil (I. 72) cures *psōrai* and ulcers on cattle; juniper oil (I. 77), rubbed on, cures *psōrai* on herd animals, dogs, and oxen and kills lice (φθείροι) on them; mastic oil (I. 4) heals *psōrai* on herd animals and dogs. Modern therapy for mange includes fuel or diesel oil applied to the afflicted skin for acariadic action.[190]

Five chapters show Dioscorides' cross-listing techniques and additional insight into his pharmacology. *Amurca* (I. 102) is the thick sediment of oil formed at the bottom of a vessel—Dioscorides specified a Cyprian brass bowl. It is cooked with lupines and *chamaileōn* and anointed on the skin to heal scabs (*psōrai*) of animals. The use of the oil is consistent with the uses but, here, there is a prescription for *amurca* with two other ingredients. One would expect, then, to find the same information in the chapters on lupin and *chamaileōn*, but Dioscorides did not do it that way—not exactly, that is (see Table 4). Under lupin (II. 109), the only other ingredient mentioned is *chamaileōn melas*. Two plants are called *chamaileōn*, one *melas* ("black") and the other *leukos* ("white"). In the chapter for the black kind (III. 9), the other ingredients mentioned are blue vitriol (or copper sulphate), cedar oil, and pork fat, and, moreover, the therapy is for scabs (*psōrai*) but not explicitly for animals. The plants discussed in the chapters preceding lupin (II. 109), namely vetch (II. 108, *Vicia ervilla* L.), and preceding carthamus, namely white *chamaileōn* (III. 8), are very close chemically to the plant that follows. This is true even though we are uncertain exactly which plant Dioscorides intended by white *chamaileōn*. White *chamaileōn* is identified as either pine thistle (*Atractylis gummifera* L.) or carthamus (*Carthamus lanatus* L.). Both pine thistle and carthamus contain valeric acid and both reportedly kill animals when ingested. Whatever the plant Dioscorides intended, assuming it is correct that it is one of these two, the drug effect would be similar. Sulfur compounds are often added to the antiparasitical medicines for mange control;[191] thus the addition of copper sulfate, a pigment component in the ancient world, is not surprising. Copper sulfate has general antiseptic, astringent, and fungicidal activities[192] and could reasonably be expected to destroy ticks and lice.[193]

Why would there not be more consistency in the cross listing for the various ingredients for mange remedies? As previously observed, the methods Dioscorides employed in gathering his material probably did

TABLE 4. *Mange*

Plant/Product	*Family*	*Location in De materia medica*	*Veterinary Usage*	*Other Ingredients*	*Preparation*	*Administration*	*Comments*
Amurca, plant oil sediment		I. 102	Scabs (*psōrai*) or mange	Lupin, chamaileon	Decoction (cooked)	Topical	Oil used for mange therapy today[a]
Bitter vetch: *Vicia ervilla* L.	Fabaceae	II. 108	1. Fattens cattle (but toxic to humans)	None	Decoction	Ingestion	1. Strongly toxic to animals[b]
			2. Chilblains and itching	None	Decoction	Topical	2. Beans contain dopa,[c] hydrocyanic acid, lycine, xanthine[d]
Cultivated Lupin: *Lupinus hirsutus* L., *L. angustifolius* L.	Fabaceae	II. 109	Scabs (*psōrai*) on sheep	*Chamaileon melas*	Decoction	Topical	1. Toxic when ingested[e] 2. Contains dopa,[f] hydrocyanic acid, lycine xanthine[g]
Chamaileon leukos:[o] (if pine thistle, *Atractylis gummifera* L.;	Asteraceae	III. 8	Kills dogs, pigs, and mice; D. says it is stronger than *Chamaileon melas*	Polenta, water, oil	Mixed with water and oil to dilute	Ingestion	1. Atractyloside 2. Valeric acid[h] 3. Toxic[i]

if *Carthamus lanatus* L.[p]	Compositae						1. Valeric acid[j]
Chamaileon melas: Carthamus	Compositae	III. 9	Removes scabs (*psōrai*) (not specifically for veterinary use)	A little blue vitriol (copper sulphate), cedar oil, pork fat	Mixed	Topical (implied)	1. Contains valeric acid,[k] calendula[l] 2. Promotes erruptions[m] 3. For inflammatory lesions of skin[n]

[a] *Merck Veterinary Manual*, p. 1493.

[b] Kingsbury, *Poisonous Plants*, pp. 362–364.

[c] *Merck Index*, p. 397.

[d] Duke, "Phytotoxin Tables," p. 236.

[e] Blood and Henderson, *Veterinary Medicine*, p. 853.

[f] Duke, "Phytotoxin Tables," p. 227.

[g] Ibid.

[h] Ibid., p. 215.

[i] *Merck Index*, p. 109.

[j] Duke, "Phytotoxin Tables," p. 217.

[k] Ibid.

[l] *Merck Index*, p. 197; cf. uses for "Safflower Oil," p. 928, which comes from *Carthamus tinctorius*.

[m] Ibid., p. 436.

[n] Sayre, *Manual*, p. 435.

[o] Berendes (*Dioskurides*, p. 268) and Gunther (*Herbal*, p. 243) identify *Chamaileon leukos* (= white) as *Atractylis gummifera L.*, but Carnoy (*Dictionnaire*, p. 75) says it may also be a species of *cardopatium* and Schneider (*Lexikon*, 5: pt. 1, 243) allows that it may be *Carthamus lanatus* L. Dioscorides' descriptions do not make it completely clear.

[p] Bailey, *Manual of Cultivated Plants*, p. 1028, designates the family as Compositae, but Duke, "Phytotoxin Tables," p. 217, gives the Asteraceae family.

not permit the type of close editing consistency would have required. From a practical standpoint, by broadening the range of ingredients the number of compounds was increased. The fact that pork fat was prescribed in one instance (III. 90) and plant oil sediment in another (I. 109) would make little difference since the importance lay in the oil (or fat). The inconsistency should be viewed as being supplementary, not contradictory, information. (The plants discussed in the two chapters preceding the antimange remedies, bitter vetch [II. 108] and "white" *chamaileōn* [III. 8], were strong, internal toxins to animals but were chemically related to the *chamaileōn*. This association will be discussed below.)

There are few specific veterinary notices in *De materia medica*. Several observations are related about the nutritious value of certain plants. Sea cabbage (II. 122) helps to fatten sheep while alfalfa (II. 147, *Medicago sativa* L.), Dioscorides noted, is substituted by cattle breeders for ordinary grass. Finally, there are several specific veterinary recommendations for superficial dermatological afflictions. Ulcers resulting from shearing are cured by cedar oil (I. 77); pitch (I. 72) cures boils on cattle; and an unidentified fern called the *lupteris* (IV. 185) heals the necks of yoked animals.

These and other veterinary usages indicate that the level of diagnosis of animal diseases was not highly refined in Dioscorides' work because he seldom distinguished purely veterinary therapies from those for humans. The afflictions mentioned are common. On the other hand, Dioscorides was mindful of veterinary medicine and made it part of his work, because, of course, it was not separated from the general medicinal practice of his day.

11. MAGICAL AND NONMEDICAL USAGES

Magic

"Without health," Sextus Empiricus (late 2d c. A.D.) said, "wisdom cannot develop, skill cannot manifest itself, strength cannot compete in the struggle, wealth is useless, and reason unavailing."[194] For a long period in the history of science, magic was regarded as a contradiction to the rational process associated with science and therefore unworthy of study.[195] Anthropologists assumed the duty and, discharging it well, were the first to cause the historians to retreat from disregarding the irrational.[196] Among the modern historians who have examined the issue, G. E. R. Lloyd advocates viewing magic "less as attempting to be efficacious, than as affective, expressive or symbolic."[197] While heeding his words, one should not lose sight of the phenomenon that magic can be efficacious. Given a compatible set of beliefs, magic can be important in health therapy. Extending Sextus' thoughts, magic can be perceived as instrumental in assisting health, thereby making it possible for humans to avail themselves of reason. Today we know the placebo effect and recognize that a healthy, positive attitude is important when facing the trauma of disease and injury. The assurance of an amulet, relic, incantation, or prayer can be of medical assistance, provided the patient believes in its power—even if only to a limited degree.[198] Part of the reason historians have dropped the challenge to magic is because we have lost confidence in defining magic.[199]

Since primitive times, magic has had a relationship with medicine.[200] Historically, magic often was considered by medical practitioners as a component of medicine. The Greeks made the first explicit attacks on magic, and the learned ones among them sought to separate magic, as part of the supernatural, from medicine, which dealt with the natural world.[201] One Hippocratic writer succintly wrote: "Each [disease] has its own nature [φύσις] and property [δύναμις] and there is nothing in any disease which is unintelligible or which is insusceptible to treat . . . He [i.e., a man with knowledge of the causes] would not need to resort to purifications [καθάρμοι] and magic [μαγεία] and all that kind of charlatanism."[202] Thus, he said, the physician *need not* employ magic provided he can learn the causes of the diseases. Although such rational sentiments fairly characterize the Hellenic and Hellenistic approaches to medicine, the Greeks never succeeded in sweeping knowledge (ἐπιστήμη) clean of phantoms and spirits. People of reason observed (φαίνω) nature (φύσις), but many of the same observed magic (μαγεία) as did charlatans (ἀλαζόνοι).[203] Even during the Hellenistic era, when Greek science was at its zenith, magic was never destroyed. On the contrary, magic adopted the rigorous logical organization and systematization of science and formed systems and disciplines of its own, for example, astrology, alchemy, necromancy, and divination.[204]

In Vergil's *Aeneid* when Aeneas looks upon the plain where Rome will be founded, his father, Anchises, prophesies that Rome, which will come to crush the proud and impose the way of peace, will not be as advanced culturally as some nations that are better at pleading cases of law or engaging in astrological divination.[205] What we call today the pseudosciences were once the hallmarks of achievement, even in Rome's Golden Age during Dioscorides' youth. Prior to Dioscorides' time and continuing through his life, low-level or traditional magic continued seemingly unabated except in aristocratic circles.[206] Also a new, refined, and highly mystical magic developed in the treatises known as Hermetic literature.[207] No less a rationalist than Herophilus of Chalcedon (fl. 320–300 B.C.), the great anatomist and physiologist, said that the drugs were "the hands of the gods" and some herbs were powerful enough to be effective if merely stepped on[208]—perhaps, we suppose, with bare feet. Magic was an integral part of the culture from the beginning of the Hellenistic era, marked by the influence of Aristotle and Herophilus, to the end of Greco-Roman science with Dioscorides and Galen.

Dioscorides came at the end of the period when there was a distinct retreat from rationalism and a marked trend toward magic. Dioscorides stood unobtrusively against the tide. He did not explicitly attack magic, except when he advocated "testing" of the drugs (Pref. 1–2) in "trials on patients" (Pref. 5). Implicitly, he delivered a greater attack against the supernatural than many of his more celebrated predecessors, whose denouncements of magic were strong but who were less consistent than Dioscorides in distinguishing magical elements from rational processes.

Dioscorides distinguished the natural from the supernatural by choice of location in his chapters. After listing the numerous medicinal usages (including quantification, preparation, and localities), he ended the chapter with nonmedical and magical usages. And, whereas for medicinal usages his style was simply a statement that "this was for that," when he related magical folk usage, he placed distance between his own authority and reports that he had heard. He did this some sixteen times with herbs. In this way he could observe folk beliefs without endorsing their authenticity. Since rationality is so important to the history of science, a full listing of the sixteen citations is in order. The listing is by the qualifying subject and verb:

"They say [φάσι] . . ."

of golden drop [*Onosma*; III. 131] that if one with child steps over this herb she makes an abortion.

of gladiolus [IV. 20] that the upper part of the root stimulates sexual drive, the lower part represses it, and the middle part can be given to children.

that aconite [IV. 76] put on a scorpion kills it and hellebore brings it back to life.

"It is said [λέγεται] . . ."

that Christ's thorn [I. 90] placed before doors and windows keeps away *pharmaka* (= "bad drugs"—poisons, spells, or enchantments).

that the chaste tree [I. 103] keeps wolves away if held in the hand.

that alyssum [III. 91] hung on the house is healthy, and some say it is protective for men and animals and, bound in a purple cloth, it drives away illnesses of cattle.

"Some people urge [ἔνιοι κελεύουσιν] . . ."
that chick-pea [II. 104] is touched on each wart in a new moon; it is bound in a linen cloth and commanded to reverse, and this causes them to fall away.

"Some people have recorded [ἔνιοι ἱστορήκασιν] . . ."
that if one beats into small pieces rams' horns and buries them, there will grow asparagus [II. 125].

"Some people carry [ἔνιοι διαφορούσαις] . . ."
plantain [II. 126] as an amulet that dissolves scrofulous swellings in the glands of the neck.

"It is told [ἱστορεῖται] . . ."
that snapdragon [IV. 130] is opposite to "bad drugs/poisons" [φάρμακα] and being anointed with henna oil makes one agreeable.

And, as cited previously, Dioscorides said that drinking one kind of mercury (*Phyllon;* III. 125) conceives male children and the other kind, female. "Crateuas relates this," Dioscorides added, "but he seems to me to relate these things according to his report of them." Dioscorides' high regard for Crateuas caused him to excuse his apparent embrace of an assertion that Dioscorides considered improbable history. But, like Theophrastus in recording medicinal plant uses,[209] Dioscorides considered the record complete when folk usage was included, whether or not he personally could accept the beliefs on rational grounds. Although Dioscorides observed the magical use of the chick-pea to remove warts (II. 104), he had previously listed a prescription for wart removal in a section on various dermatologic afflictions. Dioscorides merely called attention to the folk association of this particular plant to remove warts. When Dioscorides said the ἱερὰ βοτάνη, or "the sacred herb" (IV. 60), was given its name because it was suitable as an amulet, he was not endorsing its use this way but rather explaining its name.

Many more "magical" usages for herbs are described in the writings of Soranus (late 2d c. A.D.), a writer on gynecology who lived after Pliny and Dioscorides. Soranus described an ideal midwife as one "free from superstition so as not to overlook salutary measures on account of a dream or omen or some customary rite or vulgar superstition."[210] Dioscorides did not report all that he heard and read but exercised selective and critical judgment.

Dioscorides deviated from the practice of not endorsing supernatural usage of plants in two or three instances. The exceptions destroy his consistency but should not jeopardize his credibility with the modern reader. He wrote that the bean trefoil (III. 150, *Anagyris foetida* L.) is used as an amulet in childbirth, but discarded afterward,[211] and squill (II. 171, *Urginea maritima* [L.] Baker) "is an *alexipharmakon* [antidote] being hanged up whole before doors." In neither instance is there the normal qualification. Squill was extensively used in ancient medicine and even today is a recognized cardiotonic drug used in both scientific and folk medicine.[212] Its strong physiological effects may help to account for a variety of what we would call magical usages. Its fame can be seen by the reports that squill was the plant used literally to beat a scapegoat out of town.[213] In a Greek pun, Pericles was once called a "Squill-head." Many ancient references to it attest to the fact that magical qualities were associated with it.[214] Pliny reported the same information about squill that Dioscorides did, but Pliny named his source: Pythagoras (ca. 531 B.C.).[215] Allegedly, Pythagoras devoted a whole book to squill.[216] Perhaps it was the eminent authority of Pythagoras that led Dioscorides away from his usual disclaimer. Still there is the matter of the bean trefoil as an amulet. Pliny repeated the assertion, so we are reasonably sure that Dioscorides' source was a written authority; therefore, the "magical" usages for both squill and bean trefoil came to Dioscorides from scrolls, not word of mouth. Even so, one should not lose sight of the fact that Dioscorides did not in these instances qualify his endorsement as he normally did.

A contemporary medical writer, Rufos of Ephesos (fl. to mid 1st c. A.D.), said that amulets were among the "natural remedies."[217] Both Dioscorides and Galen employed stone amulets for what we would call psychosomatic therapy. Even in the rational medicine of the period, powers in amulets were recognized and, by Dioscorides, to an ever so slight degree.

The rule that "magic" comes at or near the end of the chapter has one or two exceptions. A magical use for dock (II. 114, *Rumex* spp.) is within the regular medicinal usage section, but for a reason. Dioscorides said that dock mixed in a concoction with vinegar "is said to dissolve goiter [χοιράς]," but "some use" it as an amulet about the neck. "Goiter" to the ancients implied a scrofulous swelling about the neck;[218] it does not appear to be what is now perceived as goiter. Various species of dock are employed in popular medicine for skin diseases and afflictions today.[219] It also is used in modern Western medical practice for cancer chemotherapy for its antitumoral activity.[220] Dioscorides observed its use both orally and as an amulet, but he did not vouch for either usage. He did, however, specify its use around the neck. Because the active principles in dock are possibly absorbed through the skin when it is administered topically, one cannot be certain that the "amulet" was ineffective. Since plantain (II. 126) was also noted as dissolving swellings when used as an amulet, it is also possible that the affliction was psychosomatic and responsive to suggestive therapy. This was the only specific ailment (except for warts) for which Dioscorides noted a clear medical use for herbs, the other uses being general prophylactics and gender determinants.

One final case demonstrates the fine line of distinctions that Dioscorides drew between the natural and supernatural. The celebrated and powerful black hellebore drug (IV. 162) had been the subject of several reports about its character. Dioscorides said that "they sprinkle the herb about the house in order to clean it." There is no indication who "they" were but Behrendes believed that the sense of the Greek points to a ritualistic or religious cleaning. Dioscorides continued by observing a strange method of gathering the plant: when "they" dig it, "they" stand praying to Apollo and Asclepios and observe the flight of eagles. If an eagle is seen flying in the direction of harvesting, the plant's gatherer will die. Pliny, who related the same story, added that death will come within a year's time.[221] Dioscorides' relation of the black hellebore story affords an opportunity in his work to learn something about ancient herbalists. Other sources indicate the presence of rituals surrounding the collection of certain rare and important herbs.[222] The Jewish historian Josephus, for instance, related the story of how the famed mandrake (*Mandragora* spp.) was pulled from the ground by dogs who died immediately.[223]

From the modern standpoint it seems reasonable to us that those whose livelihood depended on gathering and selling wild herbs would surround their work with ritual, mysteries, and frightening stories in order to protect their business. Like jimsonweed (*Datura stramonium* L.), these plants (mandrake, black hellebore) are not readily cultivated and are found in no abundance in any particular spot. One need not be a Marxist to suppose that these herbalists were keeping the public away from their supplies by propagating these stories. Certainly, the alleged effects of some of these herbs (sleep inducing, narcotic, hallucinatory) were mysterious and their connection with religion understandable. Even with an economic interpretation to explain the stories, one should not necessarily question the sincerity or reality of the folk belief, even by those whose business it was to gather the herbs.

These stories were popular knowledge in the ancient world, as judged by discussion in classical sources. Their relative absence in

De materia medica brings to question why Dioscorides omitted so much while only the black hellebore and dock stories filtered through his pen.

The reference to the gatherers of black hellebore praying to Apollo and Asclepios is the only mention of deity within *De materia medica*. Dioscorides' rationalism was devoid of theology. There was not even a hint that higher beings were directly or indirectly responsible for giving powers to the herbs. Pliny concluded his nineteenth book rapturously by stating that plants reflect the glory of God. Herophilus said, according to Galen: "One is right in saying that the drugs act like the hands of the gods, since it is efficacious for the man who uses them to be trained in logical method and to have by nature a good understanding besides."[224] Galen called himself a "worshipper of Asclepios [θεραπευτὴς 'Ασκληπιοῦ]."[225] In his study of Galen's religious beliefs, Fridolf Kudlien interprets Galen's statement to mean: "For him, Asclepius is clearly not identical with Nature . . . but a real divine person who is very close to him."[226]

We shall see how relatively free Dioscorides' work was of the magical element as the story of his influence unfolds. For now, in summary, we repeat that Dioscorides distinguished between the natural and supernatural, that he included relatively less magic than was found in most other ancient works,[227] and that, when he did include magic, he would not embrace its authenticity (with one or two exceptions). He normally was content to point to the mere existence of folk belief.

Nonmedical Usages

Dioscorides related much more information about nonmedical plant usages than he told us about magic. Some examples include that the bark of poplar (I. 81), broken in small pieces and put in a bed that has been manured, will produce edible mushrooms any time of the year. Wheat flour (II. 128) is suitable for gluing papyrus paper. Nasturtium (II. 128) is good for wreaths, garlands, or crowns. Cedrol from juniper (I. 77) is used to preserve dead bodies but ought not be put on the skin of live ones.

He noted that some plants have special properties as repellants and perhaps as insecticides against specific insects. Modern studies confirm that some plants manufacture chemicals to ward off insect predators.[228] Dioscorides said that the leaves of Italian cypress (I. 74, *Cypressus sempervirnes* L.) keep mosquitoes away by fumigation. Rubbed on the skin, the leaves of tamarisk or aromatic myrrh (I. 87, *Tamarix gallica* L. and/or *Myrrhis odorata* Gaeter) keep away lice and gnats. Citron (I. 115), *malabathron* (I. 12), and wormwood (III. 23, *Artemisia absinthium*, plus other species) will keep moths out of clothes. Wormwood, macerated in oil and anointed, keeps mosquitoes away and—this is fascinating—put in ink, prevents mice from eating the papyrus paper. Mallow and hollyhock (II. 118) are good applied to bee and wasp stings, but a person will not be stung if he or she is anointed with the raw leaves, beaten into small pieces and covered with oil.

Dioscorides saw no medicinal benefits for some of the cereals but nonetheless gave them entries and merely told of their food value (II. 89–91). Rice (II. 89) is more nourishing than barley, but in a bread is less nourishing than wheat. Rye meal (II. 92) eaten as a porridge is good for children. Papyrus root (I. 86) has some food value. Mustard (II. 116) and blite (II. 117) have no benefits attributed to them, medical or nonmedical, which raises the question as to why they should appear at all in *De materia medica*. One can only presume that Dioscorides, knowing they were common plants that perhaps had medicinal virtues ascribed to them, intended his entry to signal his opinion of their negative value.

Dyeing the hair received much attention. Mulberry (I. 126) makes children's hair fair and, on the other end of the age spectrum, wild olive oil (I. 30) delays grey hairs if anointed daily on the hair. Several plants dyed the hair yellow (I. 95, 100, 117); still more plants turned it black (I. 101, 106–109). Dioscorides mentioned a few other plants that dyed the hair but did not specify the color (I. 74, 112, 126).

Of all nonmedical usages, cosmetics account for the majority. The idea that the ancient Greeks and Romans had the clean, unblemished bodies of Apollo and Aphrodite is erroneous. The ancients—including the Egyptians and Mesopotamians—employed considerable makeup and perfumes to assist nature. The Hippocratic notion that nature occasionally needed a helping hand received enormous reinforcement with cosmetics. Painted faces and bodies anointed with strong aromatics were the norm, and the market for the products supported a large number of perfume and unguent makers who, we understand from various literary references, occupied sections of the large ancient cities where they manufactured and sold their wares.[229] Dioscorides, as well as others, mentioned unguent-makers (I. 109, III. 4), and we know that there was a connection between them and the herbalists and medical people. What is uncertain are the details of the nature of the relationship and the degree of separation.[230] Dioscorides recognized cosmetology in his herbal section by making it an integral part of his work.

In Book I, Dioscorides discussed five perfumes and incenses: tree moss (*bruon*, 2, *Usnea* spp.); *agallochon* (22, *Aloexylon agallochon* Bour.

and/or *Thuja* spp.), an aromatic wood from "India and Arabia"; *naskaphthon* (23), the bark of a tree from India; *kankamon* (24, *Amyris* spp.), the tears of an Arabian tree; and *kuphi* (25), an incense preparation. The fact that three came to the Roman Empire as imports partially accounts for the fact that Dioscorides failed to give his usual botanical descriptions. He would have seen only the products and not the whole plant. For each, Dioscorides saw medical benefits, but the medicinal usages seem secondary to their primary use as perfumes. The chapter on *kuphi* (I. 25, κῦφι) points out that it was not a plant but a compound incense preparation.[231] Dioscorides said that in Egypt priests manufactured it, and he implied its ritualistic use. *Kuphi* has the medicinal quality of being suitable for antidotal medicines ("against poison"), and in drinks it is good for asthma. There are various ways to manufacture it and Dioscorides gave one recipe:

> ½ hēmixeston (ca. ½ liter) nut grass (*Cyperus rotundus* L.)
>
> ½ hēmixeston (ca. ½ liter) ripe juniper berries (*Juniper communis* L.)
>
> 12 minas (ca. 14 Greek pounds/4 kilograms) plum raisins, possibly *Delphinium staphisagria* L., or "plump stavesacre"
>
> 5 minas (ca. 6 Greek pounds) purified pine resin
>
> 5 minas (ca. 6 Greek pounds) sweet flag (*Acorus calamus* L.)
>
> 1 mina (15 ounces) camel's thorn [oil?] (*Alhagi camelorum* Fisch.)
>
> 1 mina (15 ounces) camel grass [oil?] (*Cymbopogon schoenanthus* Spreng.)
>
> 12 drachmas (48 grams) myrrh (*Commiphora* spp.)
>
> 9 sextai (504 grams) old wine
>
> 2 minas (30 ounces) honey
>
> Having removed the seeds from the raisins [stavesacre?], pound and triturate them with the wine and the myrrh, and having pounded and sifted the rest of the ingredients, combine them all to soak for one day; then, having boiled the honey until it has a glutinous consistency, mix it carefully with the melted pine resin, and having carefully pounded together the rest of the ingredients, put up for storage in an earthenware vessel.[232]

Virtually the same recipe appears in the Ebers Papyri (ca. 1553–1550 B.C.), showing the remarkable consistency in the recipe for sixteen hundred years.[233]

Perfume prices were high. Pliny told of the security measures used by Egyptian perfume manufacturers, including the stripping and body search of employees at the end of the workday.[234] In a class-conscious age, smell perhaps as much as clothing distinguished the upper classes from *hoi polloi*. Pliny could not help observing the charity of one who paid such a price for others' enjoyment, because he who wore it could not smell it.[235] Even Roman soldiers wore hair oil beneath their helmets, he lamented.[236] Dioscorides gave us the exact formulas for the manufacture of the sixteen classical perfumes as identified by R. J. Forbes.[237] All were ascribed medicinal usages by Dioscorides, and often he did not mention their perfume qualities. Most medicinal usages were for a variety of dermatologic problems and/or as topical muscle relaxants given in the gymnasium as a massage. All sixteen have vegetable oils as a base and would feel pleasant with a dry skin condition: *metopium* (I. 31, almond oil), *balinum* (I. 34, balanite oil), and *omphacinum* (oil of unripened olives or grapes).[238] He gave detailed directions for the manufacture of the first two, but he omitted *omphacinum*,[239] doubtlessly because its method of manufacture was commonly known.

For the manufacture of medicinal perfumed ointments, Dioscorides uses three processes: (*a*) *enfleurage*, the saturation of layers of flowers (or seeds and fruits) in the oil until aromatized, including the removal of the old flowers and replacement with new until thorough saturation occurs; (*b*) *maceration*, the dipping of flowers (etc.) in hot oil followed by the straining of the mixture while still hot; (*c*) *expressing*, the mechanical pressing of flowers (etc.) and mixing them with other ingredients, including oil.[240] The instructions can become rather elaborate. For example, oil of roses (I. 43):

> Take 5 litra [1.8 kilograms] of camel grass [oil], and 20 litra [6.86 kilograms] of [olive] oil. Bruise the camel grass and macerate it in water, soaking it with gentle stirring up and down; strain it into the oil and put 1,000 dry rose leaves in it; stir with up-and-down motion with hands covered in honey and gently squeeze; soak over night and strain; when the sediment has settled to the bottom, change it to a *kraterˉ* [mixing bowl] lined with honey. Put the strained rose leaves in a tub, pour on 8 litra (ca. 2.7 kilograms) of thickened oil, and strain them out again. Keep the oil and repeat each time for seven times, always keeping separate the oil strained out and always put in honey-lined vessels. . . . Optionally, one can thicken the oil by adding sweet flag and camel's thorn or anchusa of good color with salt.

The quantities in this and other recipes indicate that the amounts are rather large, which raises the question of whether Dioscorides' formulas were intended for commercial or domestic use. The amounts seem suitable for use by a medical man in his practice.

The names of the ointments, called oils by Dioscorides, can come from the chief herb, for example, oils of southernwood, sweet marjoram, dill, cinnamon, crocus, iris, balbanum, nard, basil, wild grapes, roses, fenugreek, and marjoram. Or they can come from the place of manufacture, for example, *megalleion*, or oil of Megale, a town in Sicily; *mendesion*, or oil of Mendes, Egypt; and *heduchroon*, which is made in Cos. Dioscorides said that the oil of Megale (I. 58) and *heduchroon* were the same as oil of sweet marjoram, except that resin was added to thicken oil of Megale and that *heduchroon* (I. 58) smelled sweeter. Dioscorides seemed to be giving away the secrets of "brand" names. He said the oil of sweet marjoram was manufactured in Cyzicus; the best oil of iris (I. 56) was from Perga in Pamphylia and Elis of Achaia; and the best oil of galbanum (I. 59) was made in Egypt. *Mendesion* (I. 59) was made of balanite oil, myrrh, cassia, and resin, all of equal weight, and those who put cinnamon in it made a mistake, Dioscorides told us. For oil of nard (I. 62) he gave a cheaper formula for manufacture as well as the more expensive one.

Cosmetics promised about as much in the ancient world as they do in today's. For example, they removed wrinkles (I. 97), gave color (I. 113), beautified eyelids (I. 71, 72, 99, 109), cleaned the face (I. 47, 154), and made the face shine (I. 70). Athenaeus said that there was not a part of the body but did not have its special perfume or cosmetic.[241] Thus, when the charitable person with the expensive smell walked by, Pliny may have been mistaken: the passerby might have been less charitable minded and more health minded.

12. SPECIFIC GEOGRAPHICAL LOCATIONS OR HABITATS

Another means by which Dioscorides specified the environmental factors influencing drug effectiveness—and one frequently employed—was to state the geographical region where plants were found that were the most effective medicinally. This information normally was the last entry in the chapter. In this last section, he conveyed two types of information: the places for the greatest abundance and the places for the preferred medicinal plant. For cumin (III. 60, *Cuminum cyminum* L.), he put the two together: cumin grows most abundantly in Lycia, Galatia, and regions proximate to them, and he added that the most effective drugs from cumin come from these same regions. Acacia (I. 101, *Acacia* spp.) has the power of dulling the strength of sharper medicines, he said. Another kind of acacia, grown in Cappadocia and Pontus, which we cannot identify, has the power to bind but is of less strength than the Egyptian variety; therefore, it is unprofitable to put it into eye medicines. Buttercup (II. 175, *Ranunculus* spp.) growing in Sardinia is especially sharp. Capper (II. 173, *Capparis spinosa* L.) from Africa, especially Marmarica (the desert region between ancient Cyrenica and Egypt), causes inflammations; the kind from Apulia provokes vomiting and that from the Red Sea is extremely sharp, raises pustles in the mouth, and removes skin in the mouth when eaten. These are only a few examples, but to expand on them would just needlessly demonstrate that Dioscorides was very aware that location and the environmental conditions are important to an herbal drug's efficacy.

3. DRUG AFFINITIES

ORGANIZATION OF PLANTS

Iris is a fairly common plant, but the fact that iris (ἶρις = *Iris florentina* L. and/or *I. germanica* L.) was the first chapter in Book I of *De materia medica* made it famous for the long period of Dioscorides' authority. Until now our attention has been on the organization for each chapter. We shall now examine how the chapters were organized in relation one to another. This arrangement, Dioscorides said, distinguished his work from that of his predecessors. Chapter 2 of Book I covers *Acorus*, or *I. pseudacorus* L., a member of the iris family, commonly called yellow flag. Very closely akin botanically to yellow flag is stinking iris (*I. foetidissima* L.), also an iris family member.[1] One would expect then to find stinking iris as Chapter 3 in Book I. But stinking iris is in Book IV, Chapter 22, where it is one chapter away from common gladiolus (IV. 20, *Gladiolus communis* L.) of the iris family. Chapter 3, Book I, is spigne (μέον, *Meum athamanticum* Jacq.), a very aromatic mountain perennial, growing, according to Dioscorides, in Macedonia and Spain. Spigne is a member of the Umbelliferae family. Botanically and even by the layperson's eye, two of these plants are similar, the third dissimilar. Dioscorides, however, saw a similarity that we do not: all cause similar physiological effects.

Dioscorides gave twenty-one medicinal usages for iris and nine each for yellow flag and spigne. Of these, only two usages are shared among all three, but there are many more similarities. All three have a warming quality as a drug action, all are good for torments of the digestive tract (which is a way to say that they are carminatives and cathartics), and all assist, in an unspecified way, in women's disorders (see Table 5).

TABLE 5. *Comparison of Medicinal Usages of Plants in the First Three Chapters*

Iris	*Yellow Flag*	*Spigne*
Warming	Warming	Warming
Purges thick and choleric humors		
	Relieves pain of the liver, side, and thorax	Relieves pain caused by stoppage around the bladder and kidneys
Good for disease of the spleen	Abates the spleen	
Draw out menses		Draws out blood of menses
Women's disorders	Women's disorders	Women's disorders
Torments (of digestive tract)	Torments (of digestive tract)	Torments (of digestive tract)

Over the gulf of two thousand years we have difficulty knowing precisely what Dioscorides saw here. Perhaps the action of iris as purging thick and choleric humors was similar to relieving internal pains, as with yellow flag and spigne? Dioscorides saw each of the three as a purgative (for torments) and as helpful with female disorders, the latter probably a variety of problems mostly related to menstruation. Whereas he saw only the first two as a drug for the spleen, writers after Dioscorides prescribed spigne as a splenetica as well.[2] This tells us that Dioscorides was grouping plant drugs by their physiological effects on the body. A typical natural products drug has, as Dioscorides saw it, not one but a complex variety of effects on the body. He did not group plants according to a principal action; otherwise, he would have placed in order the bulk laxatives, the harsh purgatives, the analgesics, and so on in a way familiar to us. His powers of observation were too acute for such simplicity: each plant has a composite of physical effects. In this case, for instance, iris causes sleep, provokes tears, promotes healing of superficial sores, and relieves a headache, all effects that yellow flag and spigne do not have. Spigne even causes a headache, not cures one. Each is a different drug but they share the chemical ability to affect the body in a discernably similar way.

Why, then, would Dioscorides not have placed stinking iris alongside its botanical kin? We know that generally plants of closely related species of the same genus often have similar physical chemistry. To answer this we have to look back to Dioscorides' gross organization: first, he separated vegetable, animal, and mineral; second, he classified plants by broad appearances. Book I consists of aromatics (Chapters 1–29), oils (30–42), ointments (42–65), resins (64–71), pitch (72–73), and trees (74–129). Stinking iris was simply not an aromatic—its root stinks unpleasantly, while the Florentine iris has a pleasing aromatic quality currently used in toilet powders. Consequently, stinking iris was put in Book IV, Chapter 22, within the category of herbs and roots. Dioscorides faithfully ascribed many of the same medicinal qualities to stinking iris and Florentine iris.

Dioscorides said in his Preface that his organizational method was superior to that of his predecessors for two specific reasons: it was easier to remember and it provided an orderly framework for new knowledge. The human memory associates physical items by broad characteristics, such as animal, vegetable, and mineral, and then by gross physical similarities, such as little herbs, trees, and plants whose roots produce the value. Once he had established these broad categories, he organized the plants by their physiological effects on the body. If one could remember to associate iris and yellow flag then he or she would remember as well their rough affinities as drugs. Dioscorides' organization assisted the memory and, furthermore, allowed substitutions if correctly perceived. In this case one need remember that iris and yellow flag have similar carminative and cathartic qualities and affect menstrual problems similarly—but one should not give yellow flag for a headache. Why, one must ask, did Dioscorides decide to put the Florentine iris with the complex association of plants good for purging, female disorders, menstruation, and torments and not in association with analgesics for headaches? As the evidence unfolds, we shall see that the reason is that Dioscorides identified the principal, most active combinations of effects and associated these together. Even though the Florentine iris is not used in modern medicine, modern manuals of pharmacognosy ascribe only two actions to it: cathartic (purgative) and diuretic.[3] Any analgesic effect must have been minor. Persons simply reading Dioscorides' chapter on this iris, however, would not readily see this pattern and meaning. They would see the thirty-one medicinal usages all stated more or less on equal value and then they would read on to the next chapter, on yellow flag, without realizing a pattern.

There are various alternative methods that Dioscorides could have chosen. In his Preface he explicitly rejected arrangement of plants by both opposite or "incompatible properties" and alphabetical order. Other methods could have been (*a*) morphologic classification, whereby drugs are arranged by the part of the plant or animal from which the active substance derives, such as roots, stems, and fruits; (*b*) taxonomic classification, which seeks to arrange plant drugs by a natural relationship, or phylogeny, which generally breaks down to the genera and family groupings of Carl Linnaeus (although the Linnean classifications were not developed until much later, Dioscorides could have devised a scheme of his own in some fashion); (*c*) pharmacologic, or therapeutic, classification, which groups drugs by function, such as antibiotics and laxatives; and (*d*) chemical classification, which identifies the pharmaceutically active substances and arranges plants by this chemistry. This latter method is what some pharmacognosists recently (1977) stated was the "preferred method of study," but "unfortunately, the present-day status of drug plant investigation is far from complete," thereby making such a method impractical at this time.[4] This chemical method would classify plants by definite types of chemical principles; for example, types of mydriatic alkaloids, oleoresins, tannins, and glycosides tend to have similar metabolic behavior characteristics as drugs.

Dioscorides' method was close to the chemical classification method, but he did not know chemistry. What he knew, he knew from observation of physiological effects. So great was his genius that he actually classified some plants by their active chemical constituents. For example, he grouped together mydriatic alkaloids (atropine, scopolamine), some volatile oils in the Umbelliferae, some alkylating agents with cytotoxic compounds, and acetysalicylic acids. The proof for these assertions gradually will come to light as we explore the organization for vegetable, animal, and mineral drugs. This method cuts across the various methods of modern and ancient classification schemes. Dioscorides employed one element of morphological classification when he grouped the root plants; since chemicals tend to come from the same families or evolutionarlly related families, his method could be seen as taxonomic (such as atropines from the Solanacae family, oleoresins in the Pinaceae, and laxatives in the Liliaceae). For these reasons, modern botanists since Sibthorp have been driven to distraction in attempting to discern a pattern to Dioscorides' method. His method is really more between the therapeutic and chemical classification schemes and it applies to mineral and animal drugs as well.

In order to demonstrate Dioscorides' method, let us take a couple of representative chapters in their associations one with another. The first example will be from the section on aromatics, Chapters 13 and 14, on Cassia and Cinnamon. I select these two because they are examples where, although Dioscorides was wrong, his confusion helps our understanding.

CASSIA AND CINNAMON

When someone today orders cinnamon toast for breakfast, more often than not he or she receives "cassia" toast. Pharmacists, who normally use cinnamon as a flavoring agent, know they can substitute "cassia" but in larger amounts. This is because today there continues a confusion that began long ago, even before Dioscorides. Dioscorides was confused but he, like the modern breakfast eater or pharmacist, had never seen the whole plant but just a powdered bark product from a box or jar. The "cassia" on cinnamon toast and in medicine is a species or two of the genus *Cinnamomum*, most likely *Cinnamomum cassia* Nees/Blume. "Cinnamon" is generally the dried bark of *Cinnamomum loureirii* Nees, commonly called Saigon cinnamon, and/or *Cinnamomum zeylanicum* Nees, called Ceylon cinnamon. The genus *Cinnamomum*, a member of the laurel family, is an evergreen tree found in Sri Lanka, southeastern Asia, Indonesia, and related areas.[5]

Dioscorides described both cassia and cinnamon by the appearance of their barks, the only way he saw them in such market centers as Petra and Alexandria. Dioscorides, Theophrastus, and Pliny all had two names for what they thought were two plants, "cassia" and "cinnamon."[6] Ptolemaic inscriptions specify "cassia" and "cinnamon" as appearing in the perfume *kuphi*.[7] Pliny disclosed that cassia and cinnamon were brought to the Troglodytes (the cave peoples of present Somalia-Ethiopia) by brave men on "rafts" across the seas during the winter months on a journey that lasted five months.[8] An anonymous trade guide to shipping in the Red Sea and western Indian Ocean, written in Greek ca. A.D. 95–130, mentioned only cassia in several places when discussing cargoes at various ports.[9] Modern scholars have supposed this to mean cinnamon, not cassia, but there is more to it: there is a plant genus called *Cassia*, indigenous to Africa although also found in India.[10] From this awareness and Pliny's descriptions comes the modern supposition that cinnamon was delivered from Indonesia in ocean-going double-outrigger canoes (Pliny called them rafts) on seasonal winds to Madagascar and the famed port on the mainland called Rhapta, located somewhere opposite Zanzibar.[11] From there, traders, principally Arabs, trafficked in this and other aromatic drugs to sell them eventually to the Greeks and Romans (see Fig. 1).

We still do not know whether this product was cinnamon, cassia, or

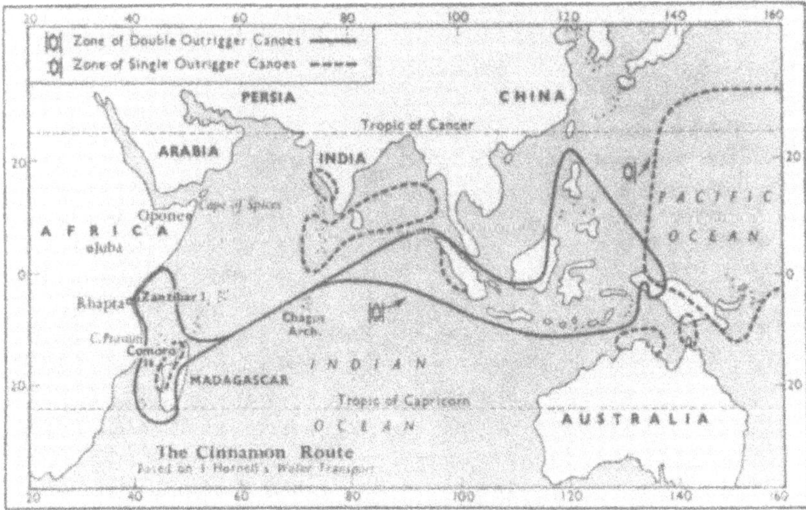

Fig. 1. The Spice Route (The Spice Trade of the Roman Empire, 29 B.C., by J. Innes Miller, p. 172; courtesy Oxford University Press).

both. An inscription of offerings to the Temple of Apollonis Didymei during the period of Seleucus I (350–280 B.C.) confirms that the Western ancients had what they thought were two different products from two different plants.[12] The survival of a list of articles receiving import duty at Roman Alexandria in Egypt shows a listing of cinnamon, Turian cassia, cassia bark, cinnamon bark, and cinnamon leaf.[13] Unfortunately, this list confuses us all the more but at least it makes us cautious about proposing simple solutions, such as cassia = cinnamon, to this identification problem.

The genus of medicinal plants called cassia is a native of southern and eastern Africa. Cassia is a low perennial shrub and does not physically resemble the cinnamon tree. Its leaves and fruit pod produce a famous laxative called senna, which is still employed today.[14] Historians are reasonably persuaded that the medicine senna was a medieval discovery, first described about the ninth century by ibn Māsawaih.[15] Dioscorides described only cassia leaves and bark and cinnamon bark and roots, doubtlessly because that is all one saw of these plants in the ancient marketplace.[16] But since cassia leaves were described, they must have been brought to market for a purpose. However, if we say the ancients knew senna, then why did Dioscorides not describe it as a laxative? Did Dioscorides know plant products of the cassia genus or was his cassia a species of cinnamon or was his cassia both cassia and cinnamon? His full chapter on cassia (I. 13) reflects complexity and a perplexity:

Cassia [κάσσια, κάσια]

> There are many kinds of cassia that are grown in spice-bearing Arabia. It has thick-barked twigs [or shafts], leaves similar to those of pepper. Select that which is pale yellow, fresh, and healthy looking, resembling coral, slender [or thin], long, and hard [or thick massed], like shepherd's pipe,[17] bitter in taste, and astringent with much fiery quality, aromatic, [and] like wine in smell. Such it is called by the inhabitants of the country [or natives] by the name of *achy*,[18] but it is named *daphnitis*[19] by the merchants in Alexandria. Better than this one is the dark, purple, thick kind called *gizir*,[20] having a smell like a rose, most suitable for medicinal usages [πρὸς τὴν ἰατρικὴν] and the kind mentioned not often coming before the first-mentioned kind. The third kind is called *Mosulitis Gatos*.[21] The other kinds are of inferior quality, such as that which is called *asuphe*,[22] black with thin bark, and burst bark, also those kinds called *kitto* and *darka*.
>
> There is also a kind of false cassia, unspeakable in resemblance, which is proven false by taste neither sharp nor aromatic, and it has a bark holding fast to it to the innermost part. One discovers broad tubes [or pipes], soft, light, well sprouting, making a difference from the other kind. But reject that which is whitened beforehand and scabby and having a goatlike smell, and does not have a thick tube but strong and thin.
>
> It has a diuretic, warming, drying, gently astringent quality. It is suitable [as a medicine] for making the eyes sharp [i.e., improving sight] and as an emollient; with honey it removes moles; it brings out the menses and drunk it helps those with spider bites and also being drunk it is good for internal inflammations and inflammations of the kidneys and for women either as a sitz bath or as a fumigant it dilates [the orifice of] the uterus. If cinnamon should be lacking then double the amount of the medicine, it will do the same [as cinnamon]. It is very useful for so many things.

Dioscorides' description of cassia is very poor; the extant, early manuscripts of *De materia medica* do not have pictures of either cassia or cinnamon. All he described were the barks and leaves, the latter, he said, resembling those of the black pepper plant. Indeed pepper leaves do resemble those of cassia in arrangement, venation, shape, and size (although generally slightly smaller), although pepper leaves are relatively dissimilar to cinnamon leaves. The senna drug of the Arabs came from a species of cassia (*Cassia acutifolia* Delile and/or *C.*

angustifolia Vahl.) grown in the Sudan.[23] The Arabs and writers of the Western Middle Ages referred and, in fact, we today refer to Alexandria senna. At times Alexandria senna may have been used to refer to the bark of cassia used as a substitute for senna, which may have had a restricted use for the drug made from the leaves and fruit pod of the same plant. Dioscorides called one kind of cassia *achy*, or *daphnitis* "by the merchants in Alexandria."

Like ancient Greek, the ancient Egyptian language had two words for cassia and cinnamon: *kdy-kdt* and *tiʿsps*, respectively.[24] The famous pharaoh Hatshepsut (ca. 1450 B.C.) brought *kdy-kdt* from the famed land of Punt, generally regarded as in the Sudan-Somalia region. *Kdy-kdt* is translated as cassia,[25] but J. Innes Miller says *kdy-kdt* is cinnamon and related to the Hebrew *qiddah* and *kitto* of Dioscorides.[26] A portion of the cinnamon trade route from Madagascar went up the eastern African coast to Somalia and Red Sea ports to Arabia and Egypt; in other words, cinnamon was a trade product in many of the same ports where cassia was first brought to market. Greek geographers Strabo and Ptolemy pointed to the cassia and cinnamon trade; Strabo said that most of the cassia came from India.[27] In fact, a species of cassia (*C. angustifolia* Vahl. and/or *C. acutifolia* Delile) is found in India and this species is the source of senna.[28]

The kind of cassia called *darka* by Dioscorides and the author of the trade guide provides another insight. The various cinnamon species' barks differ in physical appearance as Figure 2 shows. The bark on the far right is Djakarta or *Cinnamomum burmannii* Blume, which is smooth and closely resembles the bark of *C. cassia* Nees/Blume. Let us assume as a working postulate from this evidence that (*a*) the Greek *darka* is related to the Malay word *Djakarta*[29] and that *darka* cassia is *C. cassia* and, possibly, *C. burmannii* and (*b*) the *daphnitis* of the Alexandrians is *Cassia acutifolia*. Were these postulates true, modern linguistic confusion would be a continuation of ancient confusion. For an example, a list of imported goods detained because of impurities at the Port of New York by the Federal Food and Drug Administration during a one-year period included 19,841 pounds of "cassia" from Indonesia and 22,400 pounds of "cinnamon" from Sri Lanka.[30] Both of these imports, of course, are cinnamon, the "cassia" merely being *Cinnamomum cassia* or, perhaps more broadly, any second-class cinnamon bark.

Thus far our attention has been on Dioscorides' chapter on cassia, but let us now examine in less detail the next chapter, on cinnamon (I. 14, κιναμώμου). As with cassia, he described many "kinds" of cinnamon, with several names proper to the countries where they grow. (The only name he gave, however, is *Mosulum*.) All his descriptive details have to do with bark and root, mentioning only once the size of a

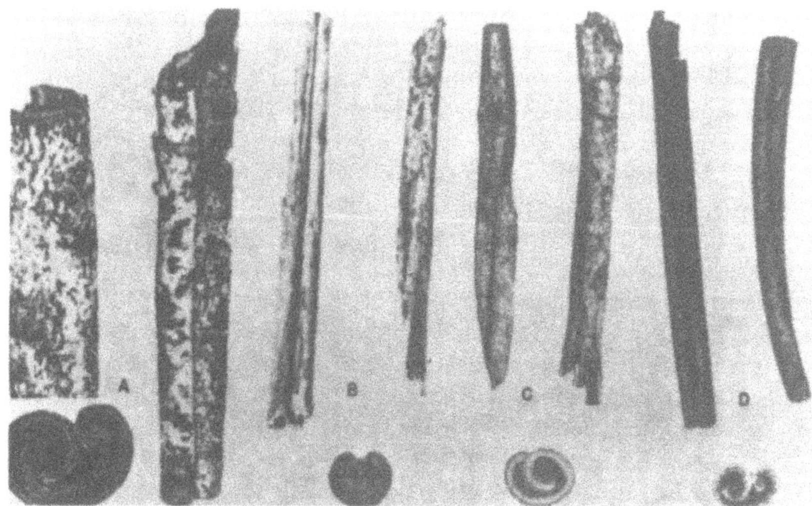

Fig. 2. Cinnamon bark quills in longitudinal and transverse views: *A*, Saigon; *B*, Ceylon; *C*, Cassia; and *D*, Djakarta (*Pharmacognosy*, by V. E. Tyler, L. R. Brady, and J. E. Robbers, p. 123; courtesy Lea & Febiger, Publishers).

kind found in the mountains as being "dwarf." The descriptions are not particularly helpful to us in unraveling the puzzles, but a comparison of the medicinal qualities and usages is helpful (see Table 6).

Plants of the cassia genus have aglycones—specifically, aloe-emodin and/or rhein—which act as an irritant, purging by stimulating the peristaltic movements of the large intestine, and are ultimately excreted in the urine and women's milk. The female genital organ may become hyperemic reflexly (because of the intestinal action) and there may be an increase in menstrual hemorrhage. If pregnancy is present, the result may be an abortion.[31] The plant has cassic acid (rhein), which is antimicrobial for skin afflictions, is an antibiotic, and has a tannin[32]—this much modern medicinal usages testify. In folk or traditional medicine in modern Egypt and India, cassia plants are given for ophthalmia, or eye inflammations.[33] The root is given as a snake bite antidote and for insect stings and bites.[34]

But Dioscorides did not specifically prescribe cassia as a purgative. Galen, who made the same distinctions between "cassia" and "cinnamon," recommended cassia as a purgative.[35] One must marvel that Dioscorides' prescriptions for "cassia" were so similar to modern ones for the cassia genus *except* for the most prevalent usage of all: as a purgative. Having given his pharmacy high marks, we must add a tentative demerit or two here. Even with this failure to recognize the purgative action, we can conclude that Dioscorides' "cassia" seems pharmaceutically to be a drug from the cassia genus of today, but the matter does not rest there.

Plants of the cinnamon genus have an irritant purgative effect by stimulating peristaltic movements.[36] The U.S.A. *Dispensatory* reports: "Cinnamon has a warming, cordial effect on the stomach, is carminative, distinctly astringent and . . . more powerful as a local than as a general stimulant."[37] Its oil (mostly cinnamic aldehyde) is a powerful germicide and it has tannins and terpenes. A modern herbal recommends cinnamon for uterine hemorrhage and menorrhagia.[38]

In summary, plants of cassia and cinnamon genera, one of the laurel family and the other a legume, have remarkably similar effects on the body. We cannot know for sure that Dioscorides' "cassia" was or included species of the cassia genus. Probably it did. The species of cinnamon (*Cinnamomum cassia*) popularly known today as cassia is considered less strong than Saigon cinnamon (*C. loureirii* Nees) and Ceylon cinnamon (*C. zeylanicum* Nees). One pharmacognosy guide even reports that the type of cinnamon known as cassia "contains the most, and Saigon the least, of both tannin and bitter substance." There is reason to suppose that the modern confusion is merely a con-

TABLE 6. *Comparison of Cassia and Cinnamon*

Cassia (I. 13)	*Cinnamon (I. 14)*
Qualities	
diuretical	diuretical
warming	warming
drying	mollifying
astringent (mild)	concocting
Usages*	
improves eyesight	cleans things that darken the cornea of the eye
removes moles	removes moles
provokes menstruation	diuretical
spider bites	difficulty with urination
internal inflammations (esp. in kidneys)	disease of kidneys
dilation of *os* of uterus	dries out menstrua and fetus (orally and as pessary with myrrh)
	nasal discharge of mucus
	dropsy
	coughs

*Twice the amount for all things for which cinnamon is given.

tinuation of Dioscorides' confusion; that is to say, Dioscorides' "cassia" was both various species of the cassia genus and "cassia" of the cinnamon genus.

In view of the pharmaceutical similarity between the two, we can get a glimmer of recognition of Dioscorides' physiological arrangement. He said that, if one does not have cinnamon, then twice as much cassia mixed in medicines will do the same things. Through this muddled confusion about plants Dioscorides did not even know as plants comes the method for the arrangement of chapters. If he could arrange plants with similar physiological effects on the body, the physical appearance of the plants would not matter (except, of course, to those who harvested the plants). One could more easily remember the combinations of effects and this memory would be of great value in the art of medicine.

The example of cassia and cinnamon may partly explain why Dioscorides' successors did not understand his unarticulated method. If one were looking for purgatives, one would not find them as such in the chapters on cassia and cinnamon. Similarly, if one were searching for an arrangement based on any one particular action, the arrangement of chapters is difficult to follow. But if one were looking for a combination of physiological effects resulting from similar chemicals, one has the clue.

PEPPER AND GINGER

Pepper and ginger share several common features with cassia and cinnamon: all are herb products brought by trade from the Far East; all were used as drugs; and pepper and ginger were, like cassia and cinnamon, in two co-joined chapters (II. 159–160) in the sharp herb section of *De materia medica*. Unlike cassia and cinnamon, however, Dioscorides and his contemporaries did not confuse the two products. Pepper and ginger are botanically very different—one dicotyledonous, the other monocotyledonous. The modern classifications of Dioscorides' herbs are as follows:

Pepper

Division: Spermatophyta
  Subdivision: Angiospermae
    Class: Dicotyledoneae
      Order: Piperales
        Family: Piperaceae
          Genus: *Piper*
            Species: *nigrum* L.

Ginger

Division: Spermatophyta
Subdivision: Angiospermae
Class: Monocotyledoneae
Order: Zingiberales
Family: Zingiberaceae
Genus: *Zingiber*
Species: *officinale* Roscoe

Pepper (II. 159), Dioscorides said correctly, comes from the dried, unripe fruits of a "short tree" that grows in India. We would extend his "India" to include the Malay Archipelago and the Indonesian Islands. Ginger comes from the rhizome (root to Dioscorides) of a reedlike plant that grows in China, India, and Africa. Dioscorides said that it grew plentifully in Somalia (Τρωγλοδυτίκη) and Arabia, but likely he mistook Arabia as a producer when it was a transit depot through which ginger traveled.

Dioscorides listed some common medicinal properties for the two drugs: both were warming and concocting; pepper was diuretical, attracting, and dissolving; ginger was mollifying. Both, he said, were antidotal and effective against those things which darken the pupil of the eye. Pepper's usages were more extensive: helped chest problems, coughs, and sore throats (all symptoms of a cold); prevented periodic fever; dissolved strumae; cleaned away white spots on the skin; hindered conceptions; worked as an anodyne; stimulated appetite; and removed torments of the bowels. Ginger, he said, resembles pepper in strength.

In modern usages, the two share qualities as carminatives and diaphoretics, as in tea for colds.[39] In comparison, pepper is uniquely listed as diuretic and as a feeble antiperiodic febricide. It was used into the nineteenth century against malaria.[40] In modern folk usages, pepper is antidotal against snake bites, is a cough remedy, and helps against a toothache.[41] Ginger, in keeping with Dioscorides' special recognition, is of recognized service in serious diarrhea resulting from relaxation of the bowels and was, until recently, given for dyspepsia and flatulent colic.[42] A modern experimental prescription, which includes four drachmas of *Piper longum* L., was taken by four women in twenty-two daily doses each month while abstaining from intercourse; it thereby prevented conception for one year.[43] Folk use for both kinds of pepper (*P. longum* and *P. betle*) was as an oral contraceptive and abortifacient.[44] In summary, then, the combination of modern Western medicine and folk usage for pepper and ginger is nearly the same today as Dioscorides recommended.

The similarity in medicinal usages does not necessarily mean that these two different plants have the same chemistry. Pharmacognosy texts list ginger among the herbs yielding volatile oils and resins and pepper in the alkaloid-bearing plants.[45] Chemically, ginger and pepper share at least twenty volatile (flavor-producing) chemicals. The nonvolatile compounds including alkaloids are not the same but they have similar chemical structures. They both—and here is Dioscorides' key—produce similar physiological effects.[46]

The relationship between ginger and pepper can be pleasantly demonstrated by a medieval recipe for "Ginger Bread" as recorded in two fifteenth-century Tudor cookbooks. The recipe calls for pepper—it has no ginger. I can confidently report that it tastes like Ginger Bread:

Gyngerbrede

Take quart of hony, & sethe it, & skeme it clene; take Safroun, pouder Pepir, & throw ther-on; take gratyd Brede, & make it so chargeaunt that it wol be y-lechyd; then take pouder Canelle, & straw ther-on y-now; then make yt square, lyke as thous wolt leche yt; take when thou lechyst hyt, an caste Box leves a-bouyn, y-stykyd ther-on, on clowys. And if thou wolt haue it Red, coloure it with Saunderys y-now.

1-½ lb. (2 cups) honey

¼ tsp. each saffron and ground pepper

2-½ oz. (5 cups) breadcrumbs

½ tsp. ground cinnamon

18 small bay leaves

6 cloves

Bring the honey to the boil in a pan with saffron and pepper. Remove from the heat and stir in the breadcrumbs so as to make a very thick paste. Simmer on an asbestos mat over low heat for 15–20 minutes until the paste has dried out. Place in 9 × 5-inch loaf tin. Smooth over the top and sprinkle with cinnamon. Make 6 trefoils on the top by sticking groups of three bay leaves together at each group into the surface of the ginger bread. Chill for several days in the refrigerator. Serve in small slices.[47]

TROPANE AND RELATED ALKALOIDS

Until now we have dealt with the arrangement of only two pairs of chapters (cassia-cinnamon and pepper-ginger) and the first three chapters in the work. Dioscorides' method was not solely to pair chapters but also to associate sequences of plants that have like physiological effects on the body. Let us take a specific chemical compound, one having a pronounced effect, and seek to find the plants with that chemical in *De materia medica*. Three such compounds are tropane alkaloids, which include hyoscyamine, atropine, and scopolamine. Chemically, they are nearly the same: hyoscyamine is $C_{17}H_{23}O_3N$, scopolamine is $C_{17}H_{21}O_4N$, and atropine is D-hyoscyamine.[48] Atropine may not even be found in that state in plants but may be formed from hyoscyamine during the extraction process. In either case, all would have equivalent effects. The toxic effects of these compounds are described succinctly as "hot as a hare, blind as a bat, dry as a bone, red as a beet, and mad as a wet hen."[49]

The plants containing these tropanes are found in several chapters in Dioscorides (see Table 7). Botanists will recognize that all these plants are members of the Solanaceae family; an untrained layperson would not see these plants in the field as cousins because their physical appearances are different. Dioscorides did not have other plants from this family elsewhere in *De materia medica*, which emphasizes the rationale of his arrangement. When modern pharmacognosists say that, ideally, plants might be arranged by their chemical effects on the body, as Varro Tyler and others have so stated, this sequence is precisely what Dioscorides used. When one finds tropane alkaloids in modern manuals,[50] one finds the listing of the same plants as in Dioscorides—except, of course, a modern list would be longer, including New World species of Solanaceae.

Before we give Dioscorides a perfect score, there is a vexing problem: Chapter 69, which one can see was omitted from Table 7. The plant is ψύλλιον, which all authorities agree is *Plantago psyllium* L., or fleawort, of the Plantaginaceae family.[51] Fleawort's chemistry is not similar to Solanaceae's chemistry, there being no tropane alkaloids reported.[52] As far as physiological effects are concerned, Dioscorides himself did not list similar effects for fleawort except generally for relief as a topical applicant for various dermatologic problems (including cancerous tumors) and headaches. Dioscorides recommended henbane (IV. 68) and other tropane-type alkaloids for anodynic (pain relieving) actions in topical applications. Modern medical use for fleawort is solely in the management of chronic constipation.[53] There is only a hint of strong action as an applicant in modern folk use where the volatile oil of one species of plantain (*Plantago major* L.) as part of a compounded medicine in an ointment is allegedly helpful for female sterility.[54] How do we treat this interruption of fleawort in our otherwise perfect chemical sequence? As an anomaly, perhaps—one of those frequent imponderables in Dioscorides.

The action that seemed to have linked fleawort with the tropane-

TABLE 7. *Tropane Alkaloids*

Book IV Chapter	*Name*	*Modern ID*	*Common Name*
68	ὑοσκύακος (3 kinds)	*Hyoscyamus niger* L. *H. albus* L. *H. aureus* L.	Black henbane White henbane Yellow henbane
70	στρύχνος	*Solanum nigrum* L.	Black nightshade
71	στρύχνος ἁλικακάβος	*Physalis alkekengi* L. or *P. somnifera* L.	Chinese lantern plant —
72	στρύχνος ὑπνωτικὸς	*Physalis somnifera* L. or *Solanum dulcamara* L.	— European bittersweet
73	στρύχνος μανίκος	?*Datura stramonium* L. *Atropa belladonna* L.	Jimsonweed Belladonna
74	δορυκνίον	*Solanum melongena* L. *Datura stramonium* L.*	Aubergine eggplant Jimsonweed
75	μανδραγόρα	*Mandragora officinarum* L. & other species of *M.*	Mandrake

*There is some disagreement about this identification. J. Berendes (*Dioskurides*, p. 408) quotes older authorities, Rondeletius and Lobelius, as citing *doruknion* as being *Concolvulus monspeliensis* L. and Fraas' identification as *C. dorycinium* L. A. Carnoy (*Etymologique*, p. 112) believes Dioscorides' entry to be *C. oleifolus*. These assertions, however, are unlikely. Pliny (*N.H.*, XXI. 105. 179) used *dorycnion* as an arrow poison in connection with kinds of *struchnoi* plants. All *struchnoi* plants in Dioscorides are positively identified as ones belonging to the Solanaceae family. W. H. J. Jones (Pliny, *N.H.*, *VI.* 287) proposed that the word *dorycnion* derives from δόρυ (spear). The pharmacology as a poison supports Dioscorides' plant as being a Solanaceae plant and not *Convolvulus*. Finally, Nicander (*Alexipharmaca*, 376) used the term δορύκινιον (cf. comments in translations by A. S. F. Gow and A. F. Scholfield, p. 196). Also see Bernhard Langkavel, *Botanik der spaeteren Griechen*, p. 84.

bearing Solanaceae plants is its medicinal property: cooling. As we observed above, few medicines are cooling and, by cooling, Dioscorides did not mean cooling to the senses or perhaps even by symptomatical changes. Jay Arena describes the toxic effects of atropine as follows (with the symptoms for scopolamine being somewhat similar):

> The first manifestation is an almost immediate sensation of dryness and burning of the mouth. Talking and swallowing become difficult or impossible. There is intense thirst. Blurred vision and marked photophobia reflect the pupillary dilation and loss of accommodation. The skin becomes flushed, hot and dry. Tachycardia and fever develop, the temperature sometimes rising to the alarming height of 42.8°C (109°F) in infants. The heart rate may, however, not rise unduly in infants and old people. The desire to void urine is present, but there is difficulty in doing so. These signs and symptoms are often accompanied by marked confusion and muscular incoordination. Mania, delirium and frankly psychotic behavior may develop and continue for hours or days. A rash may appear followed by desquamation especially in the region of the face, neck and upper trunk. Circulatory and respiratory collapse occur with more severe overdosage.[55]

What makes fleawort cooling to Dioscorides is presumably its threat to the vital functions, thereby jeopardizing the very state of organic heat. A cooling action seems to link fleawort with Solanaceae plants in Dioscorides' opinion, but we cannot reconcile this with our knowledge of the plant's chemistry. It seems highly unlikely that fleawort's chemical makeup could have changed so radically in the two thousand years since Dioscorides' time that it did not resemble the chemistry of its own family. Also the prospect is unlikely that Dioscorides' plant is incorrectly identified. Its picture and description resemble fleawort, and there is historical continuity and lack of confusion about its name from Greco-Roman times straight through classical Islamic and Latin Medieval periods down to our own day.[56] The final possibility is that Dioscorides or an unknown manuscript copyist misplaced this chapter but there is no evidence in the various manuscript copies for this having happened. We are thus led back to an anomaly where our science does not assist us in understanding Dioscorides' action. The anomaly of this one chapter should not seriously interfere with our appreciation of Dioscorides' ability to recognize tropane alkaloids and consecutively arrange plants containing them.

In Chapters 68 and 70–75, Dioscorides succeeded in identifying variable physiological actions of a specific class of constituent chemicals (without actually knowing its identity) in connection with other active constituent chemicals in the Solanaceae family. These chapters bear a relationship to contiguous chapters. Chapters 63–67 are devoted to plants of the opium family (Papaveraceae), including the opium poppy (IV. 65, *Papaver somniferum* L.), which contains papaverine.[57] Papaverine is an antimuscarinic agent that acts on the acetylcholine in postganglionic cholinergic nerves and smooth muscles. This class of drugs is employed as mydriatics, cycloplegics, antispasmodics, and antiulcer agents, and it has the following side effects: blurred vision, constipation, dryness of the mouth, and urine retention.[58] Papaverine belongs to a class of drugs that inhibit or block the transmission of nerve impulses at the synapses by occupying receptor sites and act against the actions of acetylcholine. Only a few of these drugs are found in natural products and they include atropine, scopolamine, and hyoscyamine from the Solanaceae family and papaverine from the Papaveraceae. This class of drugs blocks the muscarinic actions, whereas other cholimimetic alkaloids (such as muscarine) compete with the actions by stimulating the neuron.[59] Remarkably, although not coincidentally, Dioscorides grouped together the classes of drugs not only by their action but precisely by the mechanism of their action.[60]

What about the adjoining chapters in the other direction, that is, following the Solanaceae? Chapter 77 is devoted to ἀκόνιτον, *akoniton*, identified in the sixteenth century by Dodanaus as *Doronicum pardalianches* L. (Compositae) but, despite his identification, the actual plant that Dioscorides described and drew is probably wolfsbane (*Aconitum lycoctonum* Auct.).[61] There is more certainty about the next chapter (78), which Dioscorides called "the other *akoniton*," which is monkshood (*Aconitum napellus* L.) and possibly other species of *Aconitum* (Ranunculaceae). This plant (and in lesser amounts other species as well) contains aconitine, a polycyclic diterpenoid alkaloid having chemical similarity with hyoscyamine.[62] The concentration of aconitine is sufficient to make the plant highly toxic. Dioscorides merely pointed to its lethal effect and gave no medicinal uses, but he gave one medicinal use for the first *akoniton*: as an anodyne in eye medicines. Although dropped from modern Western medicine in favor of more effective, less dangerous remedies, aconitine does have an anodyne effect as a local.[63] It seems likely on the basis of pharmacognosy that both Chapters 77 and 78 are devoted to a species of *Aconitum* and that once again Dioscorides succeeded in associating two similar chemicals on the basis of their physiological action.

The next chapter is hemlock (IV. 78, κώνειον, *Conium maculatum* L., Umbelliferae), which has coniine as a strong principle,[64] an alkaloid whose toxic effects are most vividly and accurately recorded by Plato at Socrates' death scene. Dioscorides saw a constructively useful purpose for it; hemlock has an anodynic quality similar to that of aconite, so he put the chapter on hemlock next to *akoniton*.

Thus, in the sequence of Chapters 63 through 78 we have representatives of the Papaveraceae, Solanaceae, Plantaginaceae, Ranunculaceae, and Umbelliferae families, but only those plants whose chemical constitution causes similar physiological reaction. Chemistry, not botany, tied them together. The sophisticated chemistry was detected by Dioscorides entirely on the basis of observation. He observed the actions not of pure chemicals but chemicals in their natural home. Plants of the opium family, for instance, contain many alkaloids whose therapeutic actions are necessarily modified by the presence of other alkaloids and other chemical substances. Dioscorides' ability to associate these related chemicals, much the way modern chemistry does, was truly remarkable and very original.

THE TWO HELLEBORES AND LAXATIVES

The two modern printed editions of Dioscorides by Curtius Sprengel (1829–1830) and by Max Wellmann (1907–1914) disagree about the location in Dioscorides' work of the two hellebores. Following the reading of some of Dioscorides' manuscripts, Sprengel placed white hellebore (*elleboros leukos*) and black hellebore (*elleboros melas*) in sequential order in Book IV, Chapters 148–150,[65] but Wellmann, relying on his reconstruction of the manuscripts, separated the hellebores as Chapters 148 and 162. The Greeks' white hellebore is our *Veratrum album* (Liliaceae family), sometimes called false hellebore, a perennial herb that grows in wet meadows. It has large robust leaves, stands 0.5–1.5 meters tall, with many small perianth white flowers (1.5 cm across) from the stout pedicel. Black hellebore (*Helleborus niger* L., Ranunculaceae family) is a smaller plant with large evergreen leaves and large white or pinkish flowers (3–10 cm across), often solitary, on a stout pedicle. No doubt the Greeks considered the two hellebores as nearly common plants despite their dissimilar appearances. Even Dioscorides made the connection clear when he said that, while some drugs lose their medicinal powers soon after harvesting, others retain their efficacy "for many years, such as white and black hellebore" (Pref. 8). Indeed, modern science verifies at least one similar quality in both plants: they are highly poisonous. Can we determine whether Dioscorides meant for them to be side by side or whether he intended to separate them because of their pharmaceutical qualities? If the manuscripts fail to decide, and if botany is indecisive, then will modern chemistry provide clues? The answer is yes, it will.

In testing Wellmann's reconstruction by separating the discussions of white and black hellebore, the hypothesis is that the chemical qualities of white hellebore more closely resemble those of the plants in the chapters proximate to it, and the same is true of the black hellebore. Chapters 158 through 160 share one common feature: all are laxatives, most varying from strong to drastic cathartics (see Table 8 at the end of this chapter). Laxatives vary according to their action on the body: (*a*) stimulants (stimulate peristalsis); (*b*) bulk-forming agents (absorb water and expand to form a bulk, thereby causing a reflex peristalsis); (*c*) saline cathartics (because of poor absorption, they draw fluid into the intestines through osmotic pressure, thereby increasing peristalsis); (*d*) lubricants (mechanism is unknown; examples: mineral oil, olive oil, and cottonseed oil); and (*e*) wetting agents (lower surface tension of feces and consequently assist penetration of fecal mass by intestinal fluids). We find that all plants in this section of Book IV have a stimulant or hydragogue (wetting) action to produce the purging. Some plants in the section are obscure and their chemistry more obscure still, but most are well known and their chemistry attested. Sometimes their chemistry and the physiological effects are found in modern pharmaceutical guides of current medical practice, others are found in guides to toxic plants, while some are left to science studies.

Let us first deal with an exception that may help prove the rule: one plant is not prescribed as a laxative. Immediately preceding white hellebore (no. 148 on Table 8) is periwinkle (*Vinca major* L., no. 147), which was believed until recently to have supplied an alkaloid employed against cancer. Dioscorides did not employ periwinkle for constipation or cancer (although later in the book he did employ other plants with similar toxic alkaloids for cancer). Observing the use of the juice from the natural product, he recognized effects of the crude drug: headaches, burning of the stomach, torments of the lower digestive tract, and as an emmenagogue and a diuretic. The crude drug would have an effect on the nervous system because of its reserpine component (a rauwolfia alkaloid). Presently, reserpine is given in its purer form for moderate-to-severe hypertension. White hellebore, which Dioscorides associates by placement of chapters with periwinkle, is known to have a hypotensive effect on the body. Its components, veratrum and protoveratrum alkaloids, present in sufficient quantity so as to be effective in the crude drug, act on the afferent receptors of the sympathetic nervous system by sensitizing the nerves and creating by pressure a large amount of afferent nerve traffic. The vasomotor centers of the brain interpret the pressure as real and adjust the sympathetic tone downward and the vagal tone upward, the blood reducing pressure and heart rate (bradycardia). White hellebore, therefore, is given for hypertension. Dioscorides did not recognize hypertension per se, but, if we may interpret, he prescribed the drug for hypertension symptoms. Reserpine from periwinkle and protoveratrines A and B from white hellebore (veratrum) are often used today in combination in more severe cases of hypertension because this rauwolfia alkaloid acts synergistically with hypotensive drugs.[66]

White hellebore, a toxic plant, causes nausea, vomiting, sialorrhea, and substernal pain; consequently, modern drugs containing veratrum alkaloids have agents to counter these side effects.[67] Dioscorides' entry on white hellebore is rather unusual because he became involved in a contemporary controversy about the drug, something he implied in his Preface he would not do. The manner of its use was the center of this controversy. Dioscorides said that he sided with Philonides of Enna in Sicily, who lived about the same time as Dioscorides and wrote a work at least eighteen books long on pharmacy.[68] Dioscorides endorsed Philonides' contention that white hellebore could be taken safely immediately following a drink of pulp or barley water or a small meal by those who have a stifling (πνιγμὸς), or a tensive condition (ἡ ἀσθένεια σώματος).

Immediately following white hellebore (no. 148) are large and small *sesamoides*, plants whose identities are uncertain but were prescribed by Dioscorides as purgatives and, in the case of the larger kind, a dissolver of small tumors.[69] The next plant is more certain; it is the squirting cucumber (no. 150), which is recognized today as a hydragogue cathartic, emetic, and emmanagogue and is employed in the treatment of dropsy and, most recently, sarcoma malignancy (cancer). Saying "recently," however, does not give historical credit to Dioscorides, who employed the squirting cucumber for much the same therapy, including probable malignancies. For instance, when Dioscorides employed it for "headaches of long standing," he was probably referring to headaches resulting from constipation, a condition the plant's juice would relieve. Curiously, however, for a headache, it is administered through the nostrils, making certainty of its use allusive. That the drug was powerful is made clear by the careful instructions Dioscorides delivered for its manufacture and dosage.

The chapters in the block that includes black hellebore, namely Chapters 158 through 170 (narcissus through scammony), have similar and common medicinal qualities. All are purgatives (irritants and hydragogue cathartics), most are skin irritants, many act on the nerves, and most are highly toxic. *Krotōn*, or the castor-oil plant (no. 161), and *Euphorbia*, or spurge (nos. 164–169), are strong skin irritants as recognized by both modern medicine and Dioscorides. He placed black hellebore (no. 162) between the castor-oil plant and spurge.

Clearly, he thought drugs from the black hellebore to have virtually the same action. Spurge (nos. 164–169) and scammony (no. 170) yield resins that are sometimes substituted one for the other, according to a modern pharmaceutical guide.[70] Dioscorides' subtle method was to place the chapters next to one another.

Sometimes it is more useful when assessing ancient medicine to employ early modern medical authorities because they were often still dealing with crude drugs, not pure chemicals or synthetics. In the early 1830s a medical encyclopedia divided purgatives into three categories: *mild* (honey, tamarind, cassia, and manna); *medium* (neutral salt, calomel, ricinoleic acid, rhubarb, and senna); and *drastic* (aloe, jalap, scammony, bryonia, elaterium, various hellebores, gutti gum, euphorbia, and croton oil.)[71] Dioscorides classified aloe under juices in Book III, Chapter 22; jalap and senna are not found in Dioscorides, the former being a Central and South American plant, the latter a drug introduced into Europe later by the Arabs. Otherwise, more than less, the drastic purgatives are grouped by Dioscorides in much the same way as this nineteenth-century guide classified them.

According to Jay M Arena, the toxic effects of delphine in stavesacre (Dioscorides' no. 152) and the veratrin alkaloids found in black hellebore (no. 162) are approximately the same.[72] Both plants have roughly the same effects because the structures of their molecular alkaloids produce similar physiological effects, as, in this instance, aconitine from *Aconitum napellus* (Dioscorides, IV. 77) resembles the veratrin alkaloids in black hellebore. Why then would Dioscorides not place aconite in the same section as stavesacre and black hellebore, the section where he groups plants for drastic cathartics, nerve effects, and skin disorders? A reason appears to be because Dioscorides saw in aconite a plant whose physiological effects were too drastic for human therapy. Consequently, he placed aconite immediately following those plants containing atropine, tropane alkaloids very similar chemically and pharmaceutically to aconitine. Dioscorides ascribed no usage to this aconite plant. Of it, the modern Merck Index says: "Considered dangerous and ineffective," while noting that it had former use in medicine as a febrifuge and gastric anesthetic.[73] Here medicine has returned to where it started with Dioscorides' observations. Significantly, Dioscorides placed in Book IV all those plants which contain strong alkaloids. Thus, Dioscorides observed the chemically similar physiological effects of stavesacre (no. 152), broom (154), narcissus (158), black hellebore (162), castor-oil plant (161), spurge (159, 164–169), and scammony (170). The plants omitted in this sequence, nos. 153, 155, 156, 160, and 163, are missing because either they are not sufficiently identifiable or modern science has yet to test their chemistry and pharmacy.

This juncture brings us back to the question: did Dioscorides associate white and black hellebores? Yes, to some degree, because they have some similar pharmaceutical characteristics, but they are not as closely related one to another as are some other plants. Dioscorides' keen observations discerned similarities and dissimilarities. Max Wellmann's manuscript reconstruction, separating the two hellebores by thirteen chapters, is correct. Now we can add to Wellmann's manuscript study further evidence derived from pharmacy and chemistry, the basis of Dioscorides' organization. Sprengel followed the wrong path through the manuscripts; Wellmann, the correct route. Neither Sprengel nor Wellmann detected Dioscorides' genius.

GENERAL ORGANIZATIONAL PERSPECTIVE

Thus far, we have detailed the organizational relationship of relatively few of the 600–700 plants in *De materia medica*. Without the previous attention to botanical, chemical, and physiological detail, let us now survey some patterns of Dioscorides' scheme to make more sense out of drugs arranged by their affinities.

Abortifacients are in Chapters 156–160, 163, and 165 of Book II, immediately following Chapter 155, devoted to a plant that incites one to love making. In Book III, Chapters 124–126, are plants that influence gender at conception, followed by aphrodisiacs in Chapters 126–130. In Book IV, Chapters 9–11, are plants for joining together the flesh of wounds, which are then followed by plants with an astringent action. Chapters 90–94 in the same book detail plants that dissolve strumae (growths, tumors); two chapters, 93 and 94, are specifically about malignant strumae. Chapters 83–94 deal more broadly with roots and herbs and assert, as a theme among each of the plants' numerous medicinal qualities, that each acts on various types of tumors or swellings—perhaps better characterized as conditions due to mortification and putrefaction of tissues. In Book I, Chapters 105–110, in the section devoted to trees, tumors and growths constitute a theme. But, at the same time, Book I, Chapters 101, 106–109, and 112 have usages for most of the same trees, which dye the hair black; some of these same chapters (100, 104, 106, and 109–112) have the asserted quality of stopping the spitting up of blood. In light of our other findings, one would expect that a phytochemical analysis of these plants would uncover active principles that would respond to these conditions, just as we found that Chapters 84, 85, and 86 in Book III were together because the plants discussed in each chapter had resorcin as a pharmaceutically active compound.

Necessity may be the mother of invention, but near necessity often falls short. Dioscorides needed a computer to organize his material—just as his reader needs one to unravel his organization. Take aloe (III. 22), for example: Dioscorides listed nineteen usages for it with only one being for constipation, one modern use for aloe, but he gave fourteen various usages to promote healing, which is also a recognized modern usage. In comparing usages in related chapters one is stymied when Dioscorides seldom stated the same action in the same words. Chapters 98–105 in Book I seem to have as a consistent theme the plants' use in eye medicines, but this block of chapters also has a large number of prescriptions for wounds, anal fistulas, abrasions, ear trouble, contraception, and abortion. The chapters in this section have "binding" qualities, which, on the basis of other plants examined, would lead us to suspect that a strong alkaloid was present as an active principle.

Occasionally, Dioscorides' organization is simple enough to see readily. In Chapter 85, Book I, he discussed a variety of trees, including one called *suriggias*. This tree is very fibrous, he said, and is suitable for the manufacture of paper (i.e., writing material). The next chapter, 86, is devoted to papyrus. Even with these clues, Dioscorides' method went virtually undetected. Around the turn of this century, the great German historian of pharmacy, Alexander Tschirch, observed in a single sentence without elaboration that Dioscorides' system was a mixture between the chemical and therapeutic, between the morphological and the physiological, but that Dioscorides could not find a correct principle on which to operate.[74] And the physician-historian T. Clifford Allbutt, who wrote on Greek medicine, observed that Dioscorides grouped together the aphrodisiacs.[75] It might be a matter of wonder that Dioscorides' method was not fully seen and was left completely undescribed, but there should be little wonder. It is not easy to see.

Dioscorides even tried to extend his organization across categorical lines, as he said in the Preface, to help people to remember by producing associations. He ended the section on cereals with *amulum*, or milled starch (II. 101). The next section, devoted to pot herbs, begins with the one pot herb that is also milled for its flour (fenugreek). And—following through in this section—Chapters 105 and 107 are devoted to the horse bean (*Vicia faba* L.) and lentil (*Ervum lens* L.), both of which cause bad dreams. The chapter between them is on the Egyptian bean (? *Nelumbo speciosum* Willd.), which does not have this particular quality, but the combination of its qualities was judged by Dioscorides to be closer to the horse bean and lentil than the horse bean and lentil were to each other, hence the order: horse bean, Egyptian bean, lentil. Then, more broadly, comes the section on pot herbs, Chapters 105–109, with emphasis on treatment of dermatologic problems.

Botanists saw some taxonomical patterns in Dioscorides because of his rational use of medicines. Since genera tend to have shared chemical characteristics, Dioscorides often grouped similar species. For example, Chapters 60–89 concentrate on the Umbellifers, which tend to share similar phytochemical features.[76] Possibly, Dioscorides' observations could even supply projects for future scientific research. Earlier we observed that Dioscorides prescribed bitter vetch (II. 108) and lupin (II. 109) for animal mange. Because of this action he associated these two plants of the Fabaceae family. In his study of poisonous plants (1964), John M. Kingsbury observed a similarity in the toxic syndrome produced by animals eating species of these plant varieties. He wrote: "It might be fruitful to search for relationships between vetches and other legumes in which liver lesions or hepatogenic photosensitivity are produced."[77] In other words, Dioscorides recognized a probable chemical relationship between these two plants well ahead of modern notices and a call for future research.

Cabbage and beets provide a tantalizing but unclear revelation into Dioscorides' method for making observations. Cabbages (II. 121–122, *Brassica oleracea* L. and *B. cretica* Lam., Cruciferae family) and beets were said to share some similar physiological effects, including that, when the two are mixed with *nitrum* (soda carbonate) and put in the nostrils, they clean them. This may be relief of sinus congestion and is the only mention in Dioscorides' work of this action through nasal administration. Cabbage and beets share a few chemicals: guanidine, hydrocyanic acid, acetaldehyde, and oxalic acid.[78] In an isolated state the last two will irritate the mucous membranes.[79] I am uncertain of the exact action Dioscorides forecast, but, in any case, he saw a similar effect when the plant juices of these two natural products are mixed with sodium carbonate.[80] We may always be uncertain, because, as we speculated previously, the ancients' cabbages appear more toxic than our garden variety.

Another example of association is with heatstroke (σειρίασις), a term found in Books I–III only in two contiguous chapters. Scrapings of the gourd (II. 134, κολόκυνθα) and melon (II. 135, πέπων) were placed on the foreheads of children for heatstroke. Dioscorides grouped pot herbs with a cooling quality in Chapters 131–132 and 135–136. Presumably—and we must presume because Dioscorides did not state it explicitly—the plants in the chapters that omitted

TABLE 8. *Hellebores and Drug Affinities (All in Book IV; numbered according to Wellmann's reconstruction)*

Dioscorides' Plant	*Modern Popular Name*	*Modern Scientific Name*	*Family*	*Dioscorides' Therapeutic Usages*	*Some Active Components*	*Modern Therapeutic Pharmacy Usages*	*Popular Modern Herbal Usages*
144. μυρσίνη ἀγρία	Butcher's-broom	*Ruscus aculeatus* L.	Liliaceae	Removes obstructions (stones in urinary tract) Diuretic Emmenagogue (stimulates menstruation) Strangury (painful and interrupted urination) Jaundice Headache	Steroid Saponins (incl. ruscogenin)[a] Azetidine-carboxlic acid[b] B-sitosterol	Antiinflammatory and vasculotropic activity[b] Stimulates central nervous system[c] Investigated as competitive cholesterol inhibitor[d]	Laxative Diuretic Deobstruent (removes blockages) Diaphoretic (stimulates sudoriferos glands) Scrofulous tumors Clears chest of phlegm[e]
145. δάφνη Ἀλεξάνδρεια	Alexandrian laurel	*Ruscus hypophyllium* L.	Liliaceae	Assists in childbirth labor[f] Strangury Vesicant (draws out blood)			
146. δαφνοειδές	Daphne	*Daphne mezereum* L. *D. gnidium* L. *D. laureola* L.	Thymelaeaceae	Purgative (through bowels) Emetic (promotes	Mezereum Daphnin	Digestive aid Skin irritant Vesicant[g] Epispastic (producer of	Abortifacient[j]

				Emmenagogue Headache Provokes sneezing		riform discharges by exciting inflammation)[h] Stimulant Toxic symptoms: purging, nausea, vomiting[i]	
147. χαμαιδάφνη	Periwinkle[k]	*Vinca major* L. or *V. herbaceae*[k] Waldst. & Kit. or	Apocynaceae	Headaches Burnings of stomach Torments (of abdomen) Emmenagogue Diuretic	Reserpine Vincamine Vincine[l]	Hypertension Sedative Hypoglycemia Local anesthetic[n] Purgative[o] Dysentery & hemorrhoids Improves intellectual capacity in patients with cerebrovascular disorders[p] Diuretic[q]	Astringent Hemorrhoids Menorrhagia Laxative[r]
		Catharanthus roseus G. Don—formerly *Vinca rosea* L.	Apocynaceae		Vincristine (leurocristine) Vinblastine[m]	Acute lymphocytosis Leukemia Hodgkin's disease Carcinoma Lymphosarcoma[m]	

TABLE 8 (*cont.*)

Dioscorides' Plant	*Modern Popular Name*	*Modern Scientific Name*	*Family*	*Dioscorides' Therapeutic Usages*	*Some Active Components*	*Modern Therapeutic Pharmacy Usages*	*Popular Modern Herbal Usages*
148. ἐλλέβορος λευκὸς	White or false hellebore	*Veratrum album* L.	Liliaceae	Emetic Glaucoma[s] Emmenagogue Abortifacient For those with a stifling or a hypertensive condition[t] (Kills lice)	Protoveratrine A and B Veratrine Veratridine Jeruine[u]	Emetic Hypertension[u] (decrease in both systolic and diastolic blood pressure) Abortifacient[v]	Skin diseases, e.g., scabies, Kills lice Errhine Sternutatory Amaurosis and chronic affections of the brain[w]
149. σησαμοειδὲς τὸ μέγα	Possibly upright mignonette Aubretia Black or false helleborine Sesamoides	Possibly *Reseda alba* L. *Aubrietia deltoide* *Veratrum nigrum* *Sesamoides pygamer* Sheele[x]		Purgative—mixed with *Veratrum album*			
150. σίκυς ἄγριος	Squirting cucumber	*Ecballium elaterium* L.	Cucurbitaceae (gourd)	Hypertension (difficulty in breathing)[y] Cathartic Emetic Emmenagogue Abortative Dropsy Dissolves old	Elaterium Elaterin	Powerful purgative (hydragogue cathartic) Emetic Emmenagogue Dropsy[aa] Cancer—sarcoma[bb]	Hydragogue cathartic Emetic Diuretic Dropsy *Oidēmata*, esp. due to kidney disease[cc]

				Breaks small swellings Gout Cleans various skin afflictions[z] Sciatica (pain in hips) Mouthwash for toothache Headache			
151. [considered interpolation]							
152. σταφὶς ἀγρία	Stavesacre	*Delphinium staphisagris* L.	Ranunculaceae	Cathartic[dd] Emetic Itching *Psōra* (skin affliction) Expectorant Toothache Pneumatic gums *Aphthas* (?) in stomach Kills lice	Delphinine Delphisine Delphinoidine Staphisagrine Staphisine[ee]	Cathartic[ff] Emetic Toxic symptoms: parathesia, nausea, vomiting, hypotension, weak pulse, and convulsions[gg] Insecticide Parasiticide	Insecticide Emetic (drastic) Cathartic Applicant for skin erruptions[hh]
153. θαψία		*Thapsia garganica* L.[ii]		Cathartic Emetic Antiasthmatic Expectorant Various skin afflictions			

TABLE 8 (*cont.*)

Dioscorides' Plant	Modern Popular Name	Modern Scientific Name	Family	Dioscorides' Therapeutic Usages	Some Active Components	Modern Therapeutic Pharmacy Usages	Popular Modern Herbal Usages
154. *σπαρτίον*	Broom	*Spartium junceum* L. *Cytisus scoparius* Link[jj]	Leguminosae	Purgative Emetic[kk] Sciatica	Sparteine Scoparin Cytissine[ll]	Emetic Cathartic Diuretic Antiarrhythmic[mm] (cardiotonic)	Cathartic Cardiotonic Diuretic Dropsy[nn]
155. *σίλλυβον*	Saint-Mary's-thistle	*Silybum marianum* Gaertn. (*Carduus marinus* L.)	Compositae	Emetic			Promotes lactation Demulcent Cancer treatment[oo] Widely used in homeopathic medicine[pp] Nitrate poisoning of animals[qq]
156. *βολβὸς*	? Horseradish tree	Possibly *Moringa oleifera* Lam.	Moringaceae	Gout Skin afflictions[rr] Emetic Laxative (but harmful to stomach) Astringent	Ptrigosperim[ss] Ephedrine[tt]	Irritant dermatitis Toothache Antibiotic activity[uu] Hypotension Sympathomimetic vasocon-	

157. *βάλανος μυρεψική*		?[ww]	?Moringaceae	Emetic Purgative (oil "binds" intestines) Various skin afflictions[xx] Gout Splenetica			
158. *νάρκισσος*	Narcissus/ daffodil	*Narcissus poeticus* L. *N. tazettz* L. *N. pseudonarcissus* L.	Amaryllidaceae	Emetic Burns Sprains and dislocations Pain around joints Various skin afflictions[yy]	Calcium[yy] oxilate Colchicine[zz]	Toxic symptoms:[aaa] gastric lavage, vomiting, and wide-quick pulse Chemotherapy for cancer Irritant dermatitis	Emetics Febrifuge Swelling Infected ears Boils Sprains Stiff or painful joints[bbb]
159. *ἱπποφαές*	Spiny spurge	*Euphorbia spinosa* L.[ccc]	Euphorbiaceae	Cathartic	See below, nos. 164–169, for spurge plants		
160. *ἱππόφαιστον*		Uncertain[ddd]		Cathartic Because of purging good for orthopnoea, epilepsy, and sprains/pains at joints			

TABLE 8 (*cont.*)

Dioscorides' Plant	*Modern Popular Name*	*Modern Scientific Name*	*Family*	*Dioscorides' Therapeutic Usages*	*Some Active Components*	*Modern Therapeutic Pharmacy Usages*	*Popular Modern Herbal Usages*
161. κίκι/ κρότων	Castor-oil plant	*Ricinus communis* L.	Euphorbiaceae	Cathartic Emetic Cleans acne and freckles[eee] and stops *erysipelas* Helps as application on tumors, eye inflammations, and mammary glands swollen with milk	Castor oil Ricinoleic acid[fff] Ricin[ggg] D-galactosyl[ggg]	Cathartic[fff] Chemotherapy for cancer Spermicide[hhh] (vaginal jelly)	Laxative Ingredient for soap (in India) Increases flow of milk for mothers as external (in Canary Is.) Ophthalomic surgery as solvent[iii]
162. ἐλλέβορος μέλας	Black hellebore	*Helleborus niger* L.	Ranunculaceae	Cathartic Epilepsy Hypertension ("atrabilious state")[jjj] Arthritis Paralysis Emmenagogue Abortifacient Variety of skin afflictions Hard of hearing	Helleborin Hellebrin (or Helleborein) Veratrin	Cardiotonic Drastic hydragogue cathartic Emmenagogue[kkk] Toxic symptoms: parathesia, nausea, vomiting, hypotension, weak pulse, and convulsions[lll]	Drastic purgative Emmenagogue Anthelmintic (expels worms) Nervous disorders Hysteria[mmm] Abortifacient[nnn]

163. *σησαμοειδὲς τὸ μικρόν*	Bear's foot	*Helleborus lividus* Aiton *Reseda sesamoides* L. *Passerina hirsuta* L.		Purgative Dissolves tumors (*phumata*) and old sores (*oidēmata*)			
164. *τιθύμαλλος* (seven kinds) 165. *πιτύοσα* 166. *λαθυρίς* 167. *πέπλος* 168. *πεπλίς* 169. *χαμαισύκη*		*Euphorbia* (various species)	Euphorbiaceae (spurge)	Cathartic[ooo] Emetic Depillatory Toothache (put in cavities) Variety of skin afflictions and good against sores and tumors[ppp] (Side effect: strong on bronchial tubes)	Euphorbium Caoutchouc Diterpine esters[qqq]	Emetic[rrr] Cathartic Vesicant Antiasthmatic (expectorant; diaphoretic) Bronchodilator[sss]	Cathartic Emetic Vesicant Dropsy Errhine[ttt] Toothache (put in cavities)[uuu]
170. *σκαμμωνία*	Scammony	*Convulvulus scammonia* L.	Convolvulaceae	Cathartic Sciatica Abortifacient Dissolves tumors (*phuma*) Removes scaliness on skin (*lepra*) Headaches long in duration	Scammonin	Hydragogue cathartic[vvv]	Drastic cathartic[www]

TABLE 8 (*cont.*)

[a]D. Panova and S. Nilolov, "Steroidal sapogenins and sterois of Ruscus aculeatus var ponticus (woronov)," *Farmtsiya* 29 (1979): 25–29 (*Chemical Abstracts* 92 [1980]: 312; 92: 211816h; also see *Chemical Abstracts* 80 [1974]: 3764u).

[b]Hubert Sesse, Jean Ray, and Jean Pierre Tarye, "Pharmaceutical Composition with Antiinflammatory and Vasculotropic Activity," *France Demande* 2, 377, 20 (Cl. A61k37/48), August 11, 1978, Appl. 77/1,290, January 18, 1977, 13 pp., through *Chemical Abstracts* 91 (1979): 9494A.

[c]Lewis and Elvin-Lewis, *Medical Botany*, pp. 19, 373.

[d]*Merck Index*, p. 951.

[e]Grieve, *Modern Herbal*, 1:129; cf. Schneider, *Lexikon* 5: pt. 3, 198–200.

[f]Although there is no confirmation of this action in modern literature, Pliny (*N.H.*, 24. 81. 132) says that *chamaedaphne*, or periwinkle, assists childbirth, thus showing that Dioscorides possibly saw this as a similarity between *daphne* and *chamaedaphne*.

[g]Lewis and Elvin-Lewis, *Medical Botany*, p. 80; cf. Edmund N. Gathercoal and Elmer H. Wirth, *Pharmacognosy*, pp. 496–497.

[h]*Merck Index*, pp. 695–696; Sayre, *Manual*, pp. 311–312.

[i]*Dispensatory*, p. 1757.

[j]Lewis and Elvin-Lewis, *Medical Botany*, p. 323; another species, *Daphne genkwa*, has reported abortifacient qualities as a uterine stimulant (Farnsworth et al., "Sources of Antifertility Agents," p. 575).

[k]Sprengel identified Dioscorides' *Chamaidaphne* as *Ruscus racemosus* L. and this was accepted by Berendes (*Diokurides*, p. 444). Gunther (*Greek Herbal*, p. 539) slightly modifies the proposal by suggesting *R. Hyppjyllum*. However, Carnoy (*Dictionaire Etymologique*, pp. 74–75) identifies the plant as *Vinca herbacea* Waldst. & Kit or *Vinca major* L., both periwinkles, and Sir Arthur Hort (Theophrastus, *Enquiry*, 111. 18. 13, 2:281) translates *chamaedaphne* as periwinkle. Pliny's term *chamaedaphne* is translated by W. H. S. Jones (*N.H.*, 7:498) as either periwinkle or *Ruscus*. However, Dioscorides' description is appropriate to periwinkle: "Chamaidaphne . . . develops stems, single branched, a cubit long [1', 5½" / 44 mm], straight, thick-skinned, and smooth, and its leaves are like these of *daphne*, but more delicate and greener; its fruit [i.e., buds], which grow out into leaves, rounded, reddish." The stems of the greater periwinkle are long, slender, and about 4–5 cm, which is roughly a cubit; its leaves are 2–4 cm, ovalar with a rounded base, smoother, smaller, and more green than daphne's. The vinca alkaloids are shown to have no antitumor activity; however, confusion arises when vincristine and vinblastine are synthesized from a plant of a related but different genus, *Cartharanthus roseus*, native of the Old World tropics, especially Madagascar and India. In 1948, M. Pichon observed that what was called *Vinca rosea* L. should be *Cartharanthus*. We have no way of knowing whether people in Dioscorides' time confused the similar plants. Almost certainly, *Cartharanthus roseus* would have reached the Roman world as a trade item while the vincae were more readily available. In at least one instance, natives of Natal were reported to be taking *Vinca major* for diabetes, while we now believe they were taking *Cartharanthus roseus*, which is an antidiabetic remedy. See Norman R. Farnsworth, "The Phytochemistry of Vinca Species," in *The Vinca Alkaloids*, ed. William I. Taylor and N. Farnsworth, p. 114. See also William T. Stearn, "A Synopsis of the Genus *Vinca*," in *Vinca Alkaloids*, pp. 19–94, esp. pp. 19–20.

[l]N. Farnsworth, "Phytochemistry of Vinca," pp. 95–179.

[m]B. Oliver-Bever, "Vegetable Drugs for Cancer Therapy," *Quarterly Journal of Crude Drug Research* 11 (1971): 1668–1671, 1677; Paul Calabresi and Robert E. Parks, Jr., "Chemotherapy of Neoplastic Diseases," in *The Pharmacological Basis of Therapeutics*, ed. Louis S. Goodman and Alfred Gilman, pp. 1284–1287; Lewis and Elvin-Lewis, *Medical Botany*, pp. 130–134; Goth, *Medical Pharmacology*, p. 660.

[n]Milos Hava, "The Pharmacology of Vinca Species and Their Alkaloids," in *Vinca Alkaloids*, pp. 305–338.

[o]Toxic effect of vinblastine observed by Arena (*Poisoning*, p. 368) and Calabresi and Parks ("Chemotherapy," pp. 1286–1287).

[p]*Merck Index*, pp. 1107–1108.

[q]Schneider, *Lexikon*, 5: pt. 3, 400.

[r]Grieve, *Modern Herbal*, 2:629–631.

[s]Kaufman (professor of ophthalmology, University of Wisconsin) wrote to me (May 27, 1981) that he could not see "any way in which any of the veratrum alkaloids would be helpful in the treatment of any of the different kinds of glaucoma."

[t]Dioscorides' words are *πνιγμός* and *ἡ ἀσθένεια σώματος*, which can mean "a stifling condition" associated with shallowness of breath and "a tensive condition."

[u]Gordon K. Moe and J. A. Abildskou, "Antiarrhythmic Drugs," in *Pharmacological Basis*, pp. 716–720; *Dispensatory*, pp. 1486–1492; Lewis and Elvin-Lewis, *Medical Botany*, pp. 188–189; *Merck Index*, p. 1104; Arena, *Poisoning*, pp. 436–437. In addition to the veratrum alkaloids, the jervavine components also act for hypertension (*Merck Index*, pp. 555–556).

[v]Farnsworth et al., "Sources of New Antifertility Agents," p. 568 (with refs.).

[w]Grieve, *Modern Herbal*, 1:391.

[x]Identifications vary widely: *Reseda alba* (André, *Lexique*, p. 291); *Reseda mediterranea* L. (Sprengel and Berendes, *Dioskurides*, p. 448); *Aubrietia deltoides* and *Veratrum nigrum* (Carnoy, *Dictionaire Etymologique*, p. 242). Schneider (*Lexikon*, 5: pt. 3, 180) is uncertain. There is a plant called today *sesamoides* (of the same mignonette family as reseda), whose description could also fit Dioscorides' description, especially since he mentions white flowers (Polunin, *Flowers of Europe*, no. 375). Dioscorides only prescribed its use with *Veratrum album*; it is very difficult to determine the intended plant from the description or the pharmaceutical usage.

[y]*Duspnoos* is a symptom of hypertension, but there is no modern recognition that the plant acts as a hypertensive agent. John Crellin suggests that Dioscorides may have been referring to a condition attributable to pulmonary edema.

[z]Specifically, in Latin terms *vitilgo* (a psoriasis), *leprosy* (a scaly condition), *impetigo* (a kind of eczema), *melas* (black spots—a psoriasis), and *skilos* (spots) on the face. Notably, Dioscorides said "cleans" and not a stronger verb like "cures."

[aa]Frederick B. Power and Charles W. Moore, "Chemical Examination of Elaterium and Elaterin," *Pharmaceutical Journal and Pharmacist*, October 23, 1909, pp. 501–504; Trease, *Pharmacognosy*, pp. 358–359; Sayre, *Manual*, p. 417; H. Kraemer, *Botany and Pharmacognosy*, p. 387; Gathercoal and Wirth, *Pharmacognosy*, p. 704; Schneider, *Lexikon*, 5: pt. 2, 45–46.

[bb]David Lavie and Shlomo Szinai, "The Constituents of *Ecballium Elaterium* L. II: a-Elaterin[1,2]," *Journal of the American Chemical Society* 80 (1958): 707–710; D. Lavie and Shlomo Szinai, "The Constituents of *Ecballium Elaterium* L. III: Elatericin A and B[1,2]," ibid. 80 (1958): 710–714, reporting "strong anti-tumor activity against sarcoma."

[cc]Grieve, *Modern Herbal*, 1:241.

TABLE 8 (*cont.*)

[dd]Dioscorides noted its extreme toxicity by describing its dosage carefully (10 to 15 grains of seeds) and by stating that light exercise should immediately follow ingestion.

[ee]*Dispensatory*, p. 1869; Kraemer, *Botany and Pharmacognosy*, p. 428; Driver and Trease, *Chemistry of Crude Drugs*, p. 92.

[ff]No longer in use in U.S.A. because of extreme toxicity.

[gg]Arena, *Poisoning*, pp. 505–506.

[hh]Grieve, *Modern Herbal*, 2:771.

[ii]Sprengel and Berendes (*Dioskurides*, p. 453) identified this plant as *Thapsia garganica*, but that identification is a candidate for II. 156 of *De materia medica*.

[jj]The entry may be either the Spanish broom (*Spartium junceum*) or Scotch broom (*Cytisus scoparius*), both members of the Leguminoseae family. Both have sparteine and similar physiological properties. See Kraemer, *Botany and Pharmacognosy*, p. 637; Gathercoal and Wirth, *Pharmacognosy*, p. 370; Schneider, *Lexikon*, 5: pt. 3, 282–283. Duke ("Phytotoxin Tables," pp. 220, 234) says both species contain cytissine; cf. *Dispensatory* pp. 1660–1661.

[kk]Dioscorides says it purges like hellebore but without its danger and its seeds purge downward, which implies that the juice from the root provokes vomiting.

[ll]*Dispensatory*, pp. 1887–1888; see also n. dd, above.

[mm]Gathercoal and Wirth (*Pharmacognosy*, p. 370) and Kraemer (*Botany and Pharmacognosy*, p. 637) say that sparteine has physiological properties that are the same as digitalis (*Merck Index*, p. 363). Sparteine and scoparin are not, however, mentioned in McIlroy's chapter on cardiac glycosides (*Plant Glycosides*; cf. Schneider, *Lexikon*, 5: pt. 3, 282–283). The *Dispensatory* (p. 166) says cystisine "produces a primary rise and secondary fall of the blood pressure through its effects upon the sympathetic ganglia, and causes vomiting, primary stimulation and secondary depression of respiration."

[nn]Grieve (*Modern Herbal*, 1:124–130), who says under *Cytisus scoparius*: "*Substitutes*. It is essential that true Broom be distinguished from Spanish Broom (*Spartium junceum*), since a number of cases of poisoning have occurred from the substitution of the dried flowers of spartium for those of true Broom." The ambiguity in interpreting Dioscorides continues.

[oo]Grieve, *Modern Herbal*, 2:797.

[pp]Schneider, *Lexikon*, 5: pt. 2, 262–263.

[qq]Kingsbury (*Poisonous Plants*, pp. 435–436) reports that animals eating it have symptoms of nitrate poisoning.

[rr]*Psora* (itching), *lepra* (scaly condition), *alphos* (white psoriasis), *vitiligo* (psoriasis), *phakos* (moles), *melas* (dark psoriasis), *ionthos* (acne), *ephelia* (freckles), *exanthemata* (eruptions in hair on face?).

[ss]Lewis and Elvin-Lewis, *Medical Botany*, p. 361.

[tt]Duke, "Phytotoxin Tables," p. 228.

[uu]Lewis and Elvin-Lewis, *Medical Botany*, pp. 80, 252, 361.

[vv]*Merck Index*, p. 410; *Dispensatory*, pp. 500–506.

[illegible] Dioskurides, p. 455; Gunther, Herbal, p. 555; Theophrastus, *Enquiry*, IV. 2. 1), but the plant seems to be of the moringa family.

[xx] *Psora* (itching), *lepra* (scaly condition), *alphos* (white psoriasis), *melas* (dark psoriasis), *phakos* (moles), *ionthos* (acne), *ephelia* (freckles), *exanthemata* (eruptions in hair on face?): cf. nn. rr and yy.

[yy] *Ephelia*, *alphos*, cleans dirt from ulcers and breaks boils. Lewis and Elvin-Lewis (*Medical Botany*, pp. 78, 80) identify the action with calcium oxilate found in crystals in the outer layers.

[zz] Ibid., p. 135, naming pseudolycorine in *N. tazetta* for cancer therapy, but Duke ("Phytotoxin Tables") says that colchicine is found in the narcissus group.

[aaa] Arena, *Poisoning*, p. 506; Lewis and Elvin-Lewis, *Medical Botany*, p. 60; Schneider, *Lexikon*, 5: pt. 2, 350–351.

[bbb] Grieve, *Modern Herbal*, 1:246

[ccc] Sprengel, Berendes (*Dioskurides*, p. 456), and Carnoy (*Dictionaire Etymologique*, p. 145) make this identification, but Gunther (*Herbal*, p. 556) believes it to be *Hippohae rhamnoides*, or sea buckthorn.

[ddd] Identifications vary: *Cirsium stellatum* (Sprengel); *Centaures spinosa* L. (Berendes, *Dioskurides*, p. 457); and *Euphorbia spinosa*, *E. Acanthothamnos*, or *Poterium spinosum* (Carnoy, *Dictionaire Etymologique*, p. 145).

[eee] Croton oil is a powerful skin irritant (Gathercoal and Wirth, *Pharmacognosy*, p. 436), but is not therapeutically used today.

[fff] Edward Fingl, "Laxatives and Cathartics," in *Pharmacological Basis*, pp. 981–982. Castor oil mixed with beer was a standard laxative for the ancient Egyptians (Lewis and Elvin-Lewis, *Medical Botany*, p. 271; Schneider, *Lexikon*, 5: pt. 3, 171).

[ggg] Lewis and Elvin-Lewis (*Medical Botany*, p. 135) list ricin from the castor plants as current therapy for cancer. D-Galactosyl- is a lectin that Lewis says "contact[s] functional cell membrane glycoproteins bearing polysaccharide side chains . . . [and] can combine to form bridges between cells, causing agglutination in vivo . . . [which induces a] preferential killing of tumor . . . cells" (p. 96).

[hhh] *Physicians' Desk Reference*, pp. 519, 813, but Farnsworth et al. ("Sources of New Antifertilty Agents," p. 549) report no inhibition of implantation in tests with rats.

[iii] Grieve, *Modern Herbal*, 1:172–173.

[jjj] A free translation for μελαγχολικός.

[kkk] *Merck Index*, p. 519; Kraemer, *Botany and Pharmacognosy*, pp. 495–496; Gathercoal and Wirth, *Pharmacognosy*, pp. 265–266; *Dispensatory*, pp. 1711–1712.

[lll] Arena, *Poisoning*, p. 506; Lewis and Elvin-Lewis, *Medical Botany*, p. 31.

[mmm] Grieve, *Modern Herbal*, 1:389.

[nnn] Farnsworth et al., "Sources of New Antifertility Agents," p. 572.

[ooo] The usages here are for the first "kind" of spurge that Dioscorides discussed.

[ppp] Dioscorides: "It takes away itching, *akrochordos* [a wart with a thin neck], large warts, *leichenas* [several sorts of eruptions, including ringworm], as an applicant." The vesicant action of euphorbium could be expected to account for these therapies. Today the use is limited to veterinary practice. For sores and tumors, he says: "It is appropriate for *pterugia* [inflamed nails], *anthraka* [hardness], *phagedena* [cancer or gangrene], *gaggraina* [cancer or gangrene], and *surigga* [fistula]." Diterpene esters common to many euphobiaceae are carcinogenes.

TABLE 8 (*cont.*)

[qqq]Lewis and Elvin-Lewis, *Medical Botany*, pp. 37, 121; *Dispensatory*, p. 1688.

[rrr]Lewis and Elvin-Lewis, *Medical Botany*, p. 278.

[sss]Sayre, *Manual*, pp. 284–285; Gathercoal and Wirth, *Pharmacognosy*, pp. 438–439; *Merck Index*, p. 446; Kraemer, *Botany and Pharmacognosy*, p. 317; and Flückiger and Hanbury, *Pharmacographia*, p. 560, who are more detailed in their chemistry but their experiments, personally peformed, are more than a century old.

[ttt]Grieve, *Modern Herbal*, 2:764.

[uuu]Current folk practices in South Africa, Central America, and India call for its sap being put in tooth cavities as Dioscorides prescribes it (Lewis and Elvin-Lewis, *Medical Botany*, p. 253); for other folk usages, see Watt and Breyer-Brandwijk, *Plants of Southern and Eastern Africa*, pp. 401–433.

[vvv]Gathercoal and Wirth, *Pharmacognosy*, pp. 592–594; *Merck Index*, p. 935; Driver and Trease, *Chemistry of Crude Drugs*, p. 130.

[www]Grieve, *Modern Herbal*, 1:102–103.

a specific of quality, including 134 on the gourd, had a cooling action as well.

Dioscorides cannot be nominated for a posthumous Nobel Prize in chemistry. Even with his organization by drug affinities, he did not perform perfectly. Viper's bugloss, or blueweed (*Echium vulgare* L.), and heliotrope (*Heliotropium europaeum* L.), both belonging to the Boraginaceae family, contain pyrrolidizine alkaloid. Dioscorides placed viper's bugloss in Book IV, presently numbered Chapter 27, near other species of *Echium*; he placed heliotrope in the same book but widely separated, in Chapter 190. Even so, when both plants are drunk with wine they assist those bitten by poisonous snakes. While he thought the physiological effects of the two plants not sufficiently similar to associate them in close proximity in his work, he nonetheless recognized their similar effects. Whether we are able to confirm or even to reject the specific effect, in this case as an antidote, we must recognize him for what he was: a rational user of drugs. Otherwise he could not by coincidence time and time again observe similar actions of similar drugs. He was neither a trickster with placebos nor an encyclopedist who collected a census of usages. Astutely and acutely, he observed nature by synthesizing how plants operated on the body.

4. ANIMALS, WINES, AND MINERALS

ACCORDING TO a 1976 report, the sources of modern Western drugs are as follows: (*a*) chemical synthesis, 50 percent; (*b*) microorganisms, 12 percent; (*c*) minerals, 7 percent; (*d*) higher flowering plants, 25 percent; and (*e*) animals, 6 percent.[1] Approximately 10 percent of Dioscorides' drugs came from animals and 10 percent from minerals (102 chapters).[2] Because many synthesized drugs are or were once based in natural plant products, the percentages of Dioscorides' animal and mineral drugs are roughly similar to the modern distribution. Dioscorides was not the first to discover animal and mineral drugs; the recipe literature of older Egyptian and Sumerian works shows that they were an integral part of medicine then, possibly with a greater weight being given to animal-product drugs. Closer to Dioscorides' time, Sostratos (1st c. B.C.) had written an entire tract devoted to animal drugs.[3] As claimed in his Preface, Dioscorides believed his work to be the most comprehensive; he included drugs from all three of what we call kingdoms—animal, vegetable, and mineral. He implicitly recognized the kingdoms by separating the three through his organization.

ANIMAL DRUGS

Many of us have the unpleasant image of puppy dog tails, elephant dung, and chameleon blood when we picture animal products used in old medicine. Dioscorides did not completely spare our modern squeamishness, as when he recommended chameleon blood (II. 79) as an eyelash depilatory. There is no dog's tail in Dioscorides, but, while he also had no mention of elephant's dung, he specified forty-six usages for the dung of various animals (II. 80).[4] Some of these usages for dung sound about as antiseptic as the processed cow manure in plastic bags sold in garden shops. Fresh cow manure, Dioscorides stated, was wrapped in leaves, warmed in hot ashes, and then applied to inflammations arising from wounds. Again, we must look beyond our wriggled noses in evaluating and appreciating Dioscorides on animal drugs. As an example already mentioned, we get a substance from horse urine and label it estrogen; Dioscorides would only have listed usages for horse urine.

Comparing ancient and modern animal-derived drugs is even more difficult than when dealing with plants, but insight can still be afforded. It is easier to take earlier, modern pharmacy guides, which were written before the substantial impact of modern chemistry. Lucius E. Sayre's *A Manual of Organic Materia Medica and Pharmacognosy* has a section on animal drugs.[5] Sayre discussed some twenty-nine animal drugs, beginning with cantharis, or Spanish fly, and ending with civet. Of these twenty-nine, Dioscorides had twenty but did not have fauna indigenous to the New World. In other words, the principal animal-derived drugs have a historical continuity of over two thousand years. Though some animal drugs have steadily and helpfully served humans, beginning with Egyptian medicine and ending with the twentieth century, there has been a very long, gradual reduction in the use of animal products.

In the section on animals (Book II, Chapters 1–84, by Wellmann's count), Dioscorides included 506 medicinal usages. He divided this section into two parts. He devoted the first part (Chapters 1–69) to specific animals and discussed either whole or small animals or specific parts—such as goats' hooves. There are 156 different medicinal actions out of the total of 244 medicinal usages, revealing the section's diversity. The second part (Chapters 70–84) concerns animal products, such as milk, fats, suet, and honey, and outlines some 262 medicinal usages. This part has some of the longest chapters in the entire *De materia medica* because here Dioscorides gave more attention to preparation instructions.

Identifying specific animal species in this section of *De materia medica* is accomplished principally by the pictures in the manuscripts.[6] The problem with this method is that many of the animal pictures almost certainly were not Dioscorides' pictures (as we shall see in Chapt. 5); therefore, all we know is the species of fish, caterpillar, or rat that the manuscript illustrator had in mind when he drew it many hundreds of years after Dioscorides. Based on the limited—very limited—knowledge of the pharmacognosy of unrefined animal drugs, the exact zoological species is normally of little consequence pharmaceutically when we can be reasonably certain of the family of animal and usually know the range of possible species.

Dioscorides attempted the same organization with animal drugs as he did with plants, but his results were mixed. With far fewer animal-derived drugs, there were fewer pharmaceutical analogues to match. Even so, he made some astute observations.

Chapter 1 is devoted to ἐχῖνος θαλάσσιος, or sea urchin (*Echinus* sp.), and Chapter 2 is about ἐχῖνος χερσαίας, or the hedgehog (*Erinaceus europaeus* Archil.). Thus the Greek word ἐχῖνος meant both animals, with the distinction coming from the adjectives for "sea" and "land," making it "sea urchin" and "land urchin," or hedgehog. The nomenclature satisfied Dioscorides' wish to make associations easy to remember—but what about drug affinities? Like Chapter 1, Chapters 3–11 are all on shelled water animals, such as snails, mollusks, and crabs. The hedgehog seems to be an intrusion, especially when, as we shall see, Chapters 1 and 3–11 have the same chemical theme. The answer is fascinating—again a mixture of the familiar and the bizarre, as by now we have come to expect.

Dioscorides specified that the shells of each of the animals in this block (I, 3–11) were to be burned. When this happens, they are reduced to a white powder, calcium oxide (CaO), popularly known as quicklime, burnt lime, or calx. When mixed with water, as Dioscorides sometimes prescribed, calcium hydroxide, $Ca(OH)_2$, results. Both forms are employed in medicines, especially for caustic, dermatological actions and digestive disturbances, but they are used less often today than formerly.[7] Quicklime made from sea urchin, Dioscorides believed, has the following medicinal qualities: good for the upper and lower digestive tracts (εὐστόμαχος, εὐκοίλιος) and as a diuretic. Dioscorides specified its medicinal usages as follows: sea urchin's raw shell is "burned and mixed with other useful things for *psōra* (itchiness), acting as a cleanser, and it cleans running ulcers and halts excrescencies of the flesh." Because Dioscorides did not specify what the "other useful things" to be combined were, we presume this is probably not true soap, although soap was developed about Dioscorides' time.[8] In its pure form, quicklime has a caustic action.[9]

The use of quicklime continues in the sequence of Chapters 3–11. The sea horse (II. 3) is burned whole (which would make the residue include other materials beside quicklime) and then put in various salves for alopecia, or fox mange.[10] Chapter 4 is devoted to two kinds of sea animals and two parts of each: the shell of the purple murex (*Purpura* sp.), "being burnt, has the property of drying and cleaning [καυστικώτεροι] the teeth, checking the excrescenies of the flesh, and cleaning and healing ulcers [ἀνακαθαρτικὴν ἑλκῶν καὶ ἀπουλωτικήν]." Next he wrote a rather important observation: "And the whelk [sea snail], being burned the same way, is even more caustic when filled with salt and burned in a plain earthern pot. It is good for cleaning teeth and as an applicant for burns. But one should allow the medicine to harden as a scab shell and then the burn would fall off. It is made into quicklime [ἄσβεστος] and I shall discuss it in the section on quicklime." As he promised, Dioscorides has a chapter on quicklime in Book V (115, ἄσβεστος) in the section devoted to minerals.[11] Here he gives detailed instructions on how to manufacture quicklime out of common marble, certain types of stones (λίθοι καλάκοι), and the shells of sea animals. Remarkably, even though Dioscorides saw the differences between the animate and inanimate materials, he observed, correctly, a common chemical base. He concluded: "All quicklime [regardless of source] has the same properties of being fiery [or inflammatory], biting, caustic, and escharotic. But mixed with certain other things, such as grease or oil, it becomes digestive [πεπτική], mollifying, dispersing, and cicatrizing. The most powerful is that which is fresh and unwetted."

Dioscorides described the characteristics of quicklime on the body in much the same way as do modern reference works. And, indeed, quicklime mixed with oil, such as linseed oil, is more digestible, and it is employed in today's medicine in such a form.[12] Pure quicklime is also stronger, therefore less employed in medicine than that which has been wetted, producing calcium hydroxide.[13] Dioscorides' observations cannot be said to be chemical theory but certainly they were a science of chemistry and a direction that, if pursued by others, would have served as a foundation for chemical theory. When one adds other observations, such as that the red earth of furnaces (V. 158) has the same property (δύναμις) as shells and that butter has the quality of oil (II. 72), one can conclude that Dioscorides provided a foundation for chemistry on which a structure was long in coming. He was attempting to reduce the multiplicity of phenomena to a working knowledge (τέχνη). In so doing he cut across the animal, vegetable, and mineral barriers to find common behavioral themes for matter. These themes—physiological reactions—were ultimately structurally imbedded in the chemical elements and compounds. He saw, organized, and recorded, but he did not explain more than he thought necessary in using the information.

One reason his successors failed to build on his method was his lack of consistency in fully realizing the implication of his observations. If he saw quicklime as the active substance common to the drugs coming from these animals and minerals, then he ought to have had the same physiological reactions listed in each chapter. While there is similarity, there is not precise congruence. If, for instance, he saw quicklime as a cleanser of teeth as he specified in Chapters 4, 8, and 9, why did he not mention this usage in the other chapters where quicklime is the drug product? One reason is that he usually factored into his prescriptions the whole animal, which would produce differing impurities. *Examples*: Chapter 4 on the purple murex and whelks has, in addition to the burned shells (quicklime), a drug good for the upper tract made from the columella, or fleshy part.[14] In Chapter 8 on the *onux* (*Stombus lentiginosus*, plus *S.* spp.), shellfishes, Dioscorides said that the whole animals burned with their shells were good for suffocation of the uterus, epilepsy, and the same usages as for purple murex and whelks. In his brevity he neglected to exclude specifically the columella in the drug's manufacture. The burned shell of river crabs (10, *Cancer pagurus*, plus *C.* spp.) was good for the bite of a mad dog, fistulas on the feet and anus, and two types of tumors, but the shell, ground and raw with milk, was good against the bites of snakes, scorpions, and spiders. The river crab shell in ass's milk was good for consumption and those who swallow the poisonous sea-hair coralline; with basil in a topical applicant the drug kills scorpions. As these examples show, Dioscorides had more than one substance that he attempted to place in sequence by its effects. He had a general theme for the quicklime portion of the chapters: all usages were for dermatologic, hair, antidotal, and digestive agents.

Even with varying substances taken into account, he would give some different usages, especially dermatologic ones, such as sea urchin shell (1) for *psōra*, ulcers, and excrescencies; snail shells (9) for white spots and freckles; and river crab shells (10) for fistulas and tumors. A contributing factor doubtlessly would be found in his sources (both written and oral), were they available. As we found the case to be with similar herbs, the experience gained with one particular action did not necessarily extend the same action in another herb that was an analogue. This is not uncommon today where, in theory, two drugs have the same pharmceutical action but, lacking clinical testing of one drug for a particular affliction for which the other is known to be good, there is no recommendation for the untested remedy in the guides. While quicklime made from the snail was known through experience and authority to be good for white spots, at best Dioscorides implicitly pointed the way for testing it for this affliction when he observed that it was the same substance that came from burning shells and when he placed the chapters in sequence, meaning the drugs were affinitive. Even so, Dioscorides placed out of this sequence the cuttlefish (II. 21, *Sepia officinalis*), whose shell is burned as a remedy for white spots, freckles, and itchy scales and as a cleaner of teeth.[15]

Our erstwhile hedgehog (II. 2) intruded in the sequence because its skin was burned and the ashes anointed to assist with fox mange, the same usage as for the sea horse (II. 3), and its flesh is a good digestive aid, the same as for those animals yielding quicklime (II. 1, 3–11). This placement met Dioscorides' criterion for drug affinity. The reason the hedgehog, or "land urchin," came second was because it was easy to remember the association with "sea urchin" (II. 1).

With fewer combinations to manipulate, Dioscorides attempted to arrange animal drugs by the same method he used with plants, as the chapters on quicklime show. Egg whites (II. 50), grasshoppers (II. 51), locusts (II. 52), and the ossifrage bird (II. 53) were all good for urinary and kidney problems. Millipedes (II. 35) and cockroaches (II. 36) were good for the earache.[16] Ass's hooves (II. 42) and spavins of horses (II. 43) were good for epilepsy.

Dioscorides also continued to handle his material about animal drugs with the same critical perspective he had used with plants. He corrected a number of misconceptions on the viper (II. 16, *Columber* sp.).[17] Pliny reported: "From the viper are made the lozenges called by the Greeks *theriaci*.[18] Lengths of three fingers are cut off from the head and tail, the intestines drawn with the livid part that adheres to the spine, the rest of the body, with the vertebrae extracted and fine flour added, is thoroughly boiled in a pan of water with dill, and the mixture dried in the shade and made into lozenges, which are used in making many medicaments."[19] More briefly, Dioscorides clarified: ". . . one must, when it is skinned, cut off the head and tail because they are without flesh. The cutting off the extreme parts is but a fable." Apparently, then, there was some legend about three-finger lengths that Pliny specified in the size of the portion and Dioscorides rejected totally. Where Pliny said that eating viper flesh will keep away lice,[20] Dioscorides asserted the story was wrong. Dioscorides appeared uncertain about the lore that those who eat its flesh live a long time. In relating the story, the skeptical Dioscorides employed his usual method of disassociation by using, "They say . . ." Just in case it might be true, he gave the recipe for cooking viper meat. Since we today are the grandchildren of the Enlightenment, there is no need to repeat the recipe.

The appreciation of Dioscorides' critical talents is afforded with the comparison of his prescriptions with Pliny's. Pliny denounced magic but he related considerable supernatural information.[21] As previously seen, Dioscorides was not invulnerable to some lapses—as we today would characterize magical intrusions—but in general he was the model of a rational Greek.

Poisons were especially combatted by animal-dung antidotes. The ancients and medieval peoples must have been especially vulnerable to snake, spider, scorpion, mad-dog, and viper bites judging by the attention given them and the number of ways to prevent or to counter them.[22] In the first section on specific animals, the following chapters contain drugs that were considered antidotal for both specific and general poisons: 5, 10, 19, 22–26, 28, 30–32, 41, 46, 49–50, 66, and 68–69. The following antidotes for snake bites: river crabs (10), hippopotamus' testicles (23), castoreum from the beaver (24), dried weasel meat (25, possibly *Putorius putorius*),[23] frogs (26), a fish called *kobios* (30, ?*Gobius fluviatilis*),[24] boar's liver (46), and chicken-hen meat (49). Eating bedbugs was good specifically for asp bites;[25] the white of a chicken egg (50) was for a bite of the snake called *haimorroidos* (?*Echis carinatat* Wagler).[26] Two spoonfuls of burned ashes of river crabs (10) with one spoonful of the root of gentian (?*Gentiana lutea*) drunk in wine for three days had a measurable effect on those bitten by a mad dog. The roasted liver of a mad dog (47) eaten by those bitten by one decreased the afflicted one's fear of water. (Modern medicine notes that hydrophobia occurs in 43 percent of the patients with rabies.)[27]

Dioscorides used a drug coming from the poisonous animal as an antidote to its own toxin: "earth scorpions" (11) were "a remedy for those hurt by it." Similarly with sea dragons (13, *Trachinus draco*) and Spanish fly (61). A lizard called *skigkos* (66) was eaten to combat a bite by it while the shrew mouse (68, *Sorex araneus*) was chopped up and applied to a bite made by the mouse. Occasionally Dioscorides used the word *ἀντιφάρμακον*, *antipharmakon*, to mean a general antidote (II. 25–62), while at other times he used the words *θανάσιμον φάρμακον*, *thanasimon pharmakon* (II. 24, 70).[28] The Greek word *pharmaka* meant both "drugs" and "poisons," the subtlety of which should not be lost in the modern world.

Some of the *pharmaka* are interesting. The testicles of a hippopotamus are more interesting for what Dioscorides did not say about them than for what he said. In earlier medicine such bizarre medicines were prescribed on the principle of similar quality, whereby a virile organ like testicles would be expected to produce a similar, masculine reaction in those who take it as it had in the animal. Dioscorides did not accept this principle as a working postulate—only things that worked, worked. Exceptions to the rational use of medicines occasionally filtered into his work. We would suspect, for instance, the basis on which the judgment was formed that old shoe leather (II. 48), burned and reduced to a powder and applied to the feet, helped blisters arising from wearing shoes. The development of pharmacy was advanced in the direction that we know it when, step by step, minor things, such as hippopotamus' testicles, were given for snake bite rather than for virility. These small incidents do not have the drama that, say, Copernicus had in overturning Ptolemy's universe, but, nonetheless, the accumulations of these little observations are the unnoted changes in history. Humans were accumulating experience by observing nature. The change was more steady than sudden, evolutionary rather than revolutionary, a change made more by anonymous people than celebrities.

Of all the antidotes the one with the most specificity was junket from milk (II. 70) in the animal-products section. Junket, milk curds and cream, was good for bites, stings, and burnings from "deadly poisons," especially Spanish fly, *pituokampe* (a stinging caterpillar), salamander, *bouprestis* (a blister beetle), henbane (*Hyoscyamus* sp.), *doryknion* (*Solanum melongena* L. and/or *Datura stramonium* L.), *akoniton* (*Aconitum* sp.), and meadow saffron (*Colchicum parnassicum* L.). Similarly, he prescribed chicken egg whites (II. 50) as an antidote. Modern toxicology recognizes both junket (or even whole milk) and egg whites as "generally useful household antidotal substances."[29] They interfere with the poison's absorption and act as demulcents.

Junket's use as an antidote for Spanish fly reveals the Greeks' double-nature conception of *pharmakon*, a medicine-poison. Dioscorides had a full entry on the Spanish fly, a popular name for the drug cantharidin, which comes from several species of beetles. Identifying exactly what species is largely fruitless because the active substance cantharidin is found in so many beetles that pharmaceutically it makes little difference even though some species have higher concentrations.[30] Dioscorides gave detailed instructions about the preparation through drying of the blistering beetle and then he added a paragraph about the *bouprestis*, which he said had the same properties: septic, warming, and causing ulcers. Recently, John Scarborough identified *bouprestis* as *Meloe variegatus* Donou, a species of blistering beetle that has cantharidin in it but in less concentration.[31] What Dioscorides thought to be two drugs with roughly the same properties, we see as one, Spanish fly. It cures, he said, cancer (*carcinoma*) and *lepra* and *leichenes* (skin afflictions), it provokes menstruation, and it helps dropsy by acting as a diuretic; the wings and feet of the beetles are an antidote for those who drink Spanish fly. Thus, the blistering beetle produces a *pharmakon*, a "drug," which at once is a medicine and a poison and provides its own antidote. The drug cantharidin today has a similar standing; in a regulated way, it is a helpful medicine but it is also a poison.[32] For Dioscorides' use of Spanish fly for *carcinoma*, presumably malignant tumor, it is possibly significant that Spanish fly was also taken for malignant diseases in Chinese folk medicine.[33]

The drug castoreum from the beaver (II. 24) is an example of where Dioscorides as well as other ancient writers knew a drug but were confused about its origins.[34] Castoreum comes from the preputial follicles of both sexes of the beaver. The small follicles lie between the cloaca and pubic arch of the animal and can be seen only by removing the skin and cutting into the animal. The watery decoction had a strong, peculiar, and nauseous odor. Dioscorides said castoreum came from the beaver's testicles, an assertion repeated by other writers. They were all mistaken about the beaver's anatomy but they were not mistaken about the pharmaceutical effects of castoreum. Dioscorides said that it provoked sneezing, was an emmenagogue, stimulant, and antispasmodic, expelled the fetus and afterbirth, and was an antidote against deadly poisons and the chamaeleon thistle (*ixia*). Although castoreum has been dropped from recent pharmacopeias, this compares similarly with twentieth-century usages of castoreum, thereby making it unlikely that the ancients' castoreum was from the beaver's testicles.[35] The smell is unmistakable. The conclusion must be that Dioscorides and the other ancient writers simply had not skinned a beaver and their knowledge was from second-hand sources, who might have acted to protect their market by keeping secrets.

Animals can be a source for hormones, vitamins, and nutritional aids. Modern chemists have great difficulty determining hormonal structure. Most of our hormone drugs come from chemical synthesis and not natural products.[36] While there is no clearly identifiable use of a hormone as a drug in Dioscorides' animal section, the possibility cannot be ruled out that some of the recipes have hormonal actions. Some uses we recognize as nutritional merely because Dioscorides said they were. He said *silouros* (II. 27), a river fish, was nourishing[37] and that goose grease (II. 76) took away weariness. He prescribed fish soup (II. 33) to mollify the digestive system.[38] Even our familiar chicken soup for colds may have had an equivalent use when he recommended chicken broth (II. 49) for "tempering humors in a bad state."

Many of the animal products were emollients, sweeteners, and vehicles for other drugs in compounded medicines; fats and honey are clear examples. The chapter on animal fats (II. 76) is eight pages long in Wellmann's printed edition. Here, as in the other chapters on animal products, Dioscorides discussed the product in general and then individual sources for the same product coming from various animals, for example, gall (II. 78) in general and then the gall of a sea scorpion, eagle, and bear. The products discussed are milk (70), cheese (71), butter (72), wool (73), lanolin (74), rennet (75), fats and suet, including various perfumed fats (76), marrows (77), galls (78), blood (79), dung (80), urine (81), honey and sugar (82), beeswax (83), and beesglue (84).

Information on amber was strange but medically accurate. Amber is petrified rosin found abundantly in Europe along the Baltic shores.[39] In Greek there were three words that meant amber. Amber is vegetable in origin, a fact of which Dioscorides had some awareness—in Book I, Chapter 83, he said that the tears (i.e., rosin) of black poplar (*αἴγειρος*) drop into the Po River and subsequently harden into amber (*ἤλεκτρον*), called by some *χρυσοφόρον*. Here Dioscorides alluded to the Greek legend that amber was formed by trees transformed from the sisters of Phaeton, the son of the Sun, whose body fell into the Po River and over whom his sisters wept tears until they turned into poplar trees.

Amber was also once thought to be lynx's urine. In the chapter on urine (II. 81), Dioscorides wrote: "The urine of the lynx, which is called amber [*λυγγούριον* = *lyncurium*], is thought, as soon as it is pissed, to grow into a stone. That is but a foolish story. It is called by some amber [*ἤλεκτρον*] because it draws feathers to it." The Greek *ἤλεκτρον*, or *ēlektron*, the word from which we derive the word for electricity, alludes to the static electricity produced by rubbing amber. This would "draw feathers to it." The name "lynx's urine" also has an explanation. Amber was traded to the Phoenicians by the Ligurians and conveyed to the Greeks, who called it by the name the Phoenicians, from whom they purchased it, told them. Later when some "rational" Greeks came to explain the name *luggourion*, it sounded like *λύγξ* for "lynx" and *οὖρον* for "urine." Dioscorides rejected the myth that amber was actually lynx's urine.

Amber is principally succinic acid and has some medicinal use. In the plant section Dioscorides said that amber, ground and drunk, stopped the flux of the upper and lower digestive tracts. In the animal section he said virtually the same things, except he added that one drank it with water. Dioscorides wrote to a wide audience and he doubtlessly knew that some people would know amber by one word and others by another. The story connected with one word made it a vegetable and the other, a mineral. Dioscorides communicated to all and was fairly consistent in his critical information. Pliny said: ". . . .heaven knows, the medical profession is the only one in which anybody professing to be a physician is at once trusted, although nowhere else is an untruth more dangerous."[40] Dioscorides saw his way through myth and fantasy, and he related his medical information accurately enough that, here at least, it was helpful and not dangerous.

WINES, WATERS, AND MEDICINAL DRINKS

Before Dioscorides, St. Paul said it: "Stop drinking nothing but water; take a little wine for your digestion, for your frequent ailments" (1 Tim. 5:23). Wine was not just for pleasure; it was a drug supplying the base for a number of herbal and mineral additives, which were taken, as St. Paul asserted and Dioscorides detailed, for digestion and a large number of afflictions. A long tradition exists in the West for "a little drink for medicinal purposes," even when others suspect some imbibers' sincerity.

Dioscorides began Book V with a review of the first four books and then announced his intention to complete his discourse on *materia medica* by treating "wines and metals [minerals]." Strictly speaking, the first section deals with vines, wines, waters, and vinegars.

The vines of the cultivated grape (V. 1, *Vitis vinifera* L.) and wild grape (V. 2, *Vitis sylvestris* Hegi) are treated with the normal organization of herbs. The leaves, tendrils, juice of stems, and fruits (including skin, pulp, and seeds of ripe and unripe grapes) supplied the drugs, with the grapes of the wild grapevine having some different usages. The vine tendrils and juice (V. 1) are drunk for dysentery, hemoptysis, depressing sexual drive, and as a general aid to the stomach. Raisins (V. 3) are for a cough, among other things, and the juice of unripe grapes (V. 5) has extensive medicinal effects.

The Greeks and Romans were true lovers of wine. Dionysius, the Greek god of the vine, steadily rose in the pantheon. Pliny discussed some 150 wines and varieties of grapes.[41] Vintners were highly respected and their vineyards known by their seals. Dioscorides saw so many medicinal uses for various wines that we today have difficulty in making the fine pharmaceutical distinctions. Dioscorides' discussion of wines is divided into two sections: wines (Chapters 6–19) and wines with various additives (20–73). In the first section he included not only pure wines but also some additives to wine, as well as waters and vinegars by themselves. Chapters 6–19 are organized in the following way:

Wines in general: age, color, flavors (e.g., sweet, sharp, seawater)
Wines by location
Types: wines from wild grapes, old wine and honey, honey mead, water mead
Other medicinal drinks: water, seawater, seawater with honey, vinegar, vinegar and honey, vinegar with salts, vinegar and thyme, vinegar and squill, wine and squill, and wine and seawater.

If there is a general theme to wine as a medicine, it is as an aid to digestion, a diuretic, and an antidote by inducing vomiting. Occasional dermatologic usages are given, undoubtedly in part because of the antiseptic action of its alcohol. But Dioscorides began by particularizing how wines differ one from another. Old wines (V. 6) are more harmful to the nerves (and muscles?) and other senses but are pleasant to taste. Unless one is strong, a person should avoid old wines. New wine, on the other hand, is inflative, is harder to digest, causes bad dreams, and is more diuretical. The most healthy wine is that of middle age. White wines are best for the stomach in contrast to dark wines, which are worst, and the claret, which ranks in the middle of this spectrum; consequently, white wines are best for healthy persons as a drink as well as a medicine for the ill and sick. One should not fail to take into account the quality of these wines for, by inference, Dioscorides seemed to say that a poor-quality white wine might be less preferred as a medicine than a good-quality dark red.

The differences in wine flavors are related to differing medicinal properties. Sweet wine, for instance, is relatively inflative and hard on the digestive system but it is less inebriating and less harsh on the kidneys and bladder. Sharp wine is more diuretical and inebriating and it causes headaches. New wine is good for digesting meats but it is binding in the bowels.

The location where the grapes were produced and the wine manufactured is an important factor. Italian wines he thought best, especially the Falernian. In the second century B.C., the Greek mainland and island wine industry became depressed and Italian wines rose in prestige.[42] For various wine-producing locations Dioscorides elaborated on numerous medicinal distinctions to a point where only a medieval scholastic or a connoisseur could appreciate his subtleties.

Good drinking habits are important to health, Dioscorides cautioned (V. 6). The quantity that one should drink varies by the drinker's age, the time of the year, and the quality of the wine. Peculiar tolerance for wine and experience with it were variables in determining how much wine was healthy and how much too much. One should not drink to the point of inebriation because all drunkenness was harmful, most especially that which was continuous. Dioscorides described alcoholism. There is an exception to the rule about drunkenness: to be moderately drunk for several days can, in some circumstances, actually be helpful because it improves the inner state of the person, purges vapors that annoy the senses, and opens up the pores. If one resorts to this therapy, Dioscorides cautioned, one should drink much water while drinking alcohol and continue to take in water while detoxifying.

In antiquity the poor drank a third grade of wine called *deuterias*, which was prepared by mixing or cooking wine lees with some water.[43] Dioscorides (V. 6) said that *deuterias* was a good substitute for those sick persons who should not be drinking regular wine. In instructing its preparation, Dioscorides did not recommend cooking.

The Romans and Greeks did not have sugar to sweeten their wines but they had an additive that sweetened the wine but brought with it a deleterious consequence recognized by Dioscorides. They boiled down grape juice or, in some cases, wine to varying degrees of concentration and added the product to wine. Dioscorides called the additive σίραιος (V. 6) and strickly boiled wine, ἕψημα (V. 6). In Latin the concentrations were called *sapa, defructum*, or *defritum*.[44] All classical writers who describe these additives agree that lead vessels were preferred for boiling.[45] The most recent scholar to study this practice, Jerome O. Nriagu, reports that such a process would result in lead toxicity. Heavy drinking of the "flavored wines" would result in chronic lead poisoning. Dioscorides reported (V. 5, 6) that ἕψημα wine caused a pounding and fiery head, drunkenness, flatulency, slowness to dissipate, and ill effects to the upper tract. In general, he said that such wines were pernicious. Nriagu finds that, for this description and others where lead is a suspected by-product of the adulteration manufacture, Dioscorides was describing the symptoms of lead poisoning.[46]

The remainder of the first section (V. 7–19) on wines is devoted to various medicinal drinks, predominantly those made with a wine or vinegar base. Honey and wine were often used through *De materia medica* as a vehicle for other drugs, but the two mixed together also stood as a drug. Old wine and honey, called *melitites* (V. 7), was given to those who had a long and continuous fever with an accompanying weak stomach. A kind of mead (V. 8, *oinosmeli*) was made from hard wine and honey, by which we presume a second fermentation. Dioscorides said that it ought not be drunk after eating meat. Pliny quoted Pollio Romilius' answer to Augustus Caesar's question about the secret to his longevity: "By honey wine within and by oil without."[47] Very popular as a drink and as a medicine in antiquity was *melicraton*, or water mead (V. 9).[48] This was a mixture of honey and water allowed to ferment. Among its usages was one for coughs.

Having discussed water mead, the subject of water was introduced and Dioscorides used the association to discuss the medicinal qualities of water (V. 10–11). A general discussion of water was difficult, Dioscorides lamented, because its nature varied so according to its location. The best is pure and sweet and has no medicinal effect on the body except to pass through it without trouble. Seawater (V. 11) is hot, sharp, and bad for the stomach but, just the same, it has medicinal use in skin medicines and induces vomiting for those who take in poisons. Sweetened with honey, seawater (V. 12) is made more moderate.

Vinegar (V. 13) has numerous medicinal usages internally and externally. Its property was to cool and to bind, whereas wines were warming and binding. We recognize some of his usages as utilizing the mild antiseptic quality and its quality to induce vomiting for poisonings. Four following chapters (14–17) are devoted to various additives to vinegar: honey, salt, thyme, and squill. Following squill vinegar, Dioscorides discussed squill wine (V. 18) because now that the subject was introduced one could compare the relative values of squill vinegar and squill wine.[49] Dioscorides elaborated the preparation directions for squill wine, which involved manufacture in a large quantity with Italian wine as base, three months of maceration, forty days of sunshine while it was bottled, and aging (six months in one recipe). Squill (*Urginea maritima* [L.] Baker) was discussed earlier by Dioscorides (II. 171) and, as a modern drug, it has recognized cardiotonic and diuretical properties.[50] Dioscorides recommended it for dropsy and as a digestive aid, much the same as he outlined its use for the herb alone in the earlier chapter. Squill wine ought not be given to those with fever or internal ulcers, he cautioned. Since he had not given this precaution in the earlier chapter on the herb alone, it can be assumed that he saw an abused employment of squill wine for those with a fever and ulcers. Squill wine must have had a degree of popularity.

The first section on wines concludes with "sea wine" (V. 19), a mixture of wines with seawater in varying quantities. Wine merchants added seawater to improve and regulate clarity.[51] Dioscorides wanted people to know that the practice was not without its medical consequences. Seawine has a number of usages but it is fundamentally bad for the stomach, he asserted.

Prepared Medicinal Wine Drinks

Section Two, "Wines and Things Metallic," has to do with various herbs and mineral additives that flavored the wines and gave them various medicinal usages. It was not particularly clear how Dioscorides decided on this arrangement, because, after having already discussed squill wine (V. 18), he introduced Chapters 20–73 by the following caustic remark:"I believe that it would not be useless to amplify to its fullness this inquiry for those persons who would be amateur physicians [φιλιατροῦσι, -έω], namely the preparation of more varied wines—not that many of them are necessary or useful, but that I would appear to omit none of them." Dioscorides apparently considered it superfluous to append this section, but he felt compelled because "amateur physicians" would not know enough to calculate the usages of well-known medicinal wines on the basis of composites of each ingredient's medicinal quality. This comment is of interest for a couple of reasons, albeit all inferred: (*a*) since he disparagingly referred to amateur doctors, his principal objective in writing *De materia medica* was for professional medical people; (*b*) in theory, he did not consider a compound medicine as anything more than the sum of its constituent parts.

The medicated wines were arranged in accordance with Dioscorides' method for classifying drugs. He began with the relatively mild fruit and honey wines, which were, we suspect, as much for flavor as for a medicine: quince wines (20–22) in three recipes, the last one with honey; *omphacomeltis* (23), a grape-and-soured-honey drink with a repressing-cooling property; pear wine (24); flowers of the wild vine (25); and pomegranate wine (26). Various resins (e.g., 30, 33–38) were added—Dioscorides cited their medicinal values and we learn from other sources that merchants added resins in order to prevent any after-fermentation. Familiar herbs flavored wines and made them medicinal, for example, germander (41), lavender (42), betony (44), thyme (49), marjoram (51), and such combinations as fennel-dill-parsley (65). An aromatic wine with balsam, myrrh, pepper, and iris (55) was given for coughs.

As the chapters progress, they recite harsher remedies. One wine with white hellebore (veratrum), wild cucumber, and scammony was aptly named "abortion wine" (67, φϑόριος ἐμβρύων). The last three chapters were very strong, indeed. A *kotulē* (½ pint) of mandrake wine (71) brings on a heavy and deep sleep and three *kotulai* are fatal. Wines of black hellebore (72) and scammony (73) complete the section. In these chapters Dioscorides gave preparation instructions, but one could have known their medicinal effects simply by reading his previous discussions of mandrake, black hellebore, and scammony (IV. 76, 162, 170). These wines must have been as familiar to the ancients as many patent medicines are to moderns. Dioscorides felt compelled to include them here despite the redundancy.

MINERALS

Rocks, metals, and minerals are important sources for pharmaceuticals, but, with the concentration on herbs and the quixotic fascination with animal drugs, minerals are often overlooked. Dioscorides' genius was to include them and to organize them by his scheme: (*a*) he grouped classes by the categories of experience with nature, as he had done with plants (trees, aromatics, sharp herbs, etc.) and with animals (shell animals, organs, etc.); (*b*) within these classes, he arranged his individual drug items by the physiological effect on the body. Again, it will not be surprising to learn that this method arranged many minerals by familiar, modern ways, principally by elements, although it included apparent incongruities. The incongruities are often resolved when a closer examination uncovers a rationale.

If he had told us, we would have seen the purpose, but he proceeded with his scheme with the silence of a quill's scratch on papyrus. A mineralogist today who reads the Greek and explores the secondary literature will observe that Chapters 76–79, 89–90, and 99–103 described copper compounds, both natural and manufactured. Why, one would ask, if Dioscorides could recognize copper, would he have not put the three sequences together as one? The modern mineralogist could observe the sequences because he would recognize copper as an element and the dominant, operative factor in determining its medicinal usages. Dioscorides' method was, of course, not determined by elements, but his observations were so good that he came close to a classification by elements.

The following (using modern terminology) is his scheme for minerals as grouped together in Book V:

- Metallic ores and products, 74–90
  - Zinc, 74–75
  - Copper, 76–79, 89–90 (99–103)
  - Iron, 80 (93, 96–97)
  - Lead/silver, 81–83, 85–88
  - Antimony, 84
- Pigments (including metallic ores), 88–105
  - White
  - Green
  - Blue
  - Red
  - Green
  - Yellow
- Miscellaneous Minerals, 106–117
  - Sulfur compounds, 106–107
  - Pumice, 108
  - Sodium, 109–114
  - Calcium, 114–122

Stones, 123–150
Earths, 151–160
Carbon, 161–162

Although the above content organization may seem matter-of-fact, it is not as clear as it appears. Dioscorides did not mark the divisions; one reading through the material would be apt to think the minerals were placed at random. Between the first two divisions, metals and pigments, he did not say, "Now that I have discussed metallic ores, I shall next take up pigments." Indeed, there is nothing explicit to indicate that the minerals in the second section were pigments, because his interest was in their pharmaceutical effects. Were it not for other ancient writers and chemical analyses of archaeological artifacts, we would not know that the substances in this section were used as pigments. Dioscorides assumed that the readers of his time already knew them to be pigments and, therefore, he need not waste words and could deal directly with their pharmacy.

"White lead," a synthetic product of lead carbonate, called in Greek ψιμύθιον (*cerussa* in Latin), is the last in the series on metallic ores and products (Chapter 88 by Wellmann's count). Dioscorides gave instructions for its manufacture and its medicinal qualities, but he omitted that it was a source for white pigments.[52] The next two chapters (89–90) are on copper ores, including our malachite and chrysocolla. Dioscorides described their mining locations and compared their qualities, but he did not say that they were green pigments widely used in paints, just as he had neglected to say that white lead was a white pigment.[53] The next chapter is κύανος, which is lazurite and possibly also a preparation of sand, alkali, and copper salts.[54] Again Dioscorides gave the same information as before but he omitted that it was a blue-to-purple pigment. According to Wellmann's text, the next chapter is ἴνδικος, or indigo, the plant dye for blue. Dioscorides did not confuse minerals and vegetables here but Max Wellmann confused his chapters. The word for indigo is not in the nominative form but genitive and was meant to follow the unit of the description of the blue mineral *kuanos*. Dioscorides' scheme was "now that one is reading about blue pigments, one should know that indigo has medicinal qualities as well." This would follow his method for assisting one's memory. Following indigo is a series of chapters on red pigments (93–97), beginning with ὤχρα, an iron oxide.[55]

The grouping of the same metals in different classes is the reason why one finds iron ore and products discussed in one chapter in the section on metals, then again other iron ores (Chapter 93) in the section on pigments, and still other iron ores (hematites and magnetite,

Chapters 126–127, 130) among stones. Metallic ores, pigments, and stones were the categories for human memory that Dioscorides accepted as the place to begin his physiological associations for the arrangement of medical materials.

Dioscorides may have been a better mineralogist than he was a botanist. His detailed manufacturing instructions are cause to place his work among the pioneer works on minerals. As Theophrastus wrote on plants from a theoretical standpoint, so did he also do with minerals.[56] Dioscorides' observations were practical, not theoretical, but the structural organization of his observations could have (but did not) provided the skeleton for fleshing out the elements—not the ones of Empedocles but our own elements.

Zinc

The first mineral in *De materia medica* is καδμεία, which is a composite for various zinc ores:

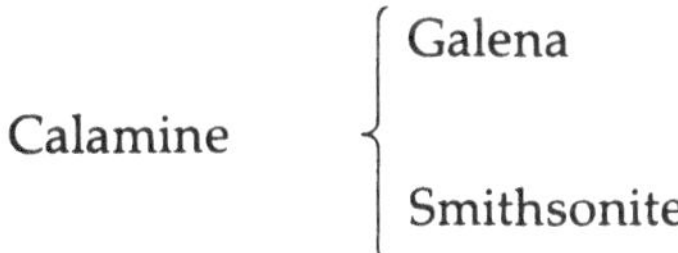

Hemimorphite

A pure zinc metal was not known to the ancients. Zinc melts at a relatively low temperature of 419°C, boils at 918°C, and must be processed in a retort and distilled. Dioscorides' *cadmeia* was zinc oxide, because, even when gasified, the zinc combines with oxygen and condenses in the form that Dioscorides knew it.[57] The various natural ores are well described, with the best kind, called *botryites*, coming from a mine in Cyprus. Other deposits, he said, occur in Macedonia, Thrace, and Spain, confirming what we know from other sources.[58] *Botryites* ore, Dioscorides said, is "thick, moderately heavy, and somewhat inclined toward lightness, having the outside appearance of bunching in clusters, ash colored [σποδοειδής], broken into the inside, ash [ἔντεφρος] and rust colored." This description is what a modern mineralogist would express in more quantified ways with terms of specific gravity, crystallography, cleavage, color, and luster.[59]

Dioscorides gave a description of different furnace processes and compared different ores based on their locations. The purpose of the information was to explain how to produce not brass but medicine. Two types of zinc oxide (i.e., *cadmeia*) are usually put in eye medicines but one should not use as medicines the zinc oxide from Spain, Macedonia, and Thrace. In general, zinc oxide has a binding quality, Dioscorides said. Specifically, it fills up the hollowness of sores, cleans dirt, stops up the pores, dries and draws (wounds and sores) to a scab, represses excrescencies of the flesh, cicatrizes malignant ulcers (κακοήθη τῶν ἕκῶν), and is put in skin medicines. The modern use of zinc oxide is given by the official U.S. *Dispensatory* as follows: "Zinc oxide finds its most important use in medicine as a dermatologic therapeutic application in a wide variety of cutaneous diseases. It is a component of most dermatologic powders, and of many ointments, pastes and lotions. Zinc oxide has no well-defined and specific pharmacologic action on the skin; its popularity may be attributed to a combination of four qualities: it is protective, mildly astringent, possibly weakly antiseptic, and non-toxic."[60] The ancient and the modern uses seem to coincide about as much as the differing concepts for afflictions allow.[61] The connection between the ages can be seen by the use of the name "calamine lotion," a name derived from the Greek, of a well-known, over-the-counter zinc oxide remedy sold in all drugstores today.

Another kind of zinc (discussed in the immediately following chapter, 75) is formed in the process of refining the ores of zinc and copper.[62] Dioscorides called it πομφόλυξ, *pompholyx*, and later alchemists referred to it as *lana philosophica*.[63] Dioscorides described it as follows: "*Pompholyx* differs from *spodos* [zinc ashes] specifically, but not generically. For *spodos* is blackish and generally heavier, being full of stalks, hairs, and soil as though it were a scraping and flaking of the floors and furnaces of the brassworkers . . ." His description of the manufacturing process served as the means for Helmut Wilsdorf to reconstruct a picture of it (see Fig. 3).[64] Dioscorides wrote:

> A furnace is placed in a two-storied building and in it toward the upper chamber is a symmetrical aperture that opens to the sky overhead. The wall of the building next to the furnace is perforated, with a small hole near the crucible itself for the admission of the draft. It has a door for the entry and departure prepared by the workman. Attached to this building is another one, in which the bellows and the blower work. The rest of the fuel is put on the furnace and ignited; then the craftsman stands by and sprinkles in the finely broken *cadmeia* [impure zinc oxide] from the room over the top of the draft; and the craftsman's assistant does the same, immediately casting on the charcoal until the amount that has been added on is consumed. While the *cadmeia* goes up in smoke, the fine and light small particles, carried off to the upper part, cling to the walls [of the furnace] and deposit themselves on the side and on the furnace top. In appearance the part, made up of that which went upward, is at first similar to bubbles that stand upon the water. Later it

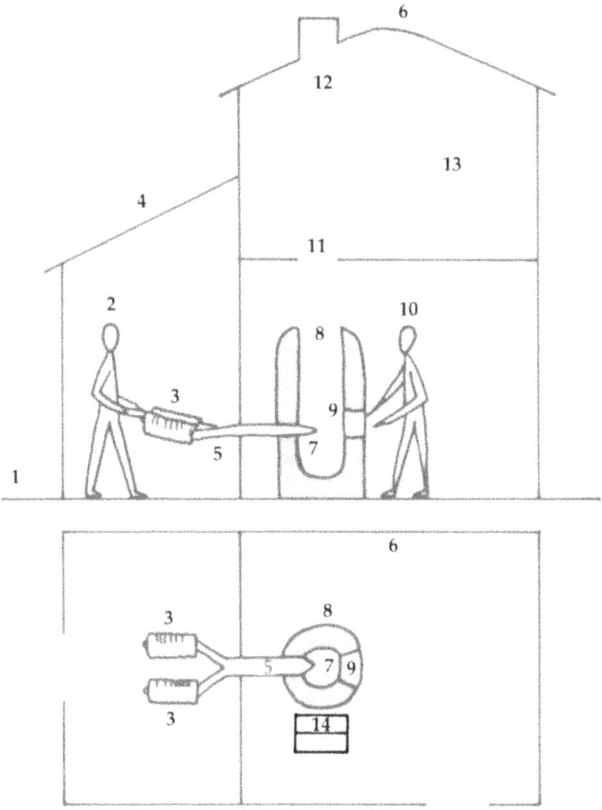

1. Ground floor (ἔδαφος)
2. Operator of bellows (φυσητής)
3. Bellows (φῦσαι)
4. Annex (συνῆπται ἕτεροσ οἶκος)
5. Tuyeres (τρῆμα)
6. Two-storied house (οἶκος διστέγος)
7. Nozzle (χωνη)
8. Furnace chamber (κάμινος)
9. Door (θύρα)
10. Craftsman (τεχνίτης)
11. Cutting through ceiling of first floor (ἐκτομη)
12. Vent for outside passage (ἐκτομή συμμετρή)
13. Upper part of house (ὑπερῷον)
14. Charging stairs (τόπος)

Fig. 3. Pompholyx (zinc-copper ore) manufacture, drawn from Dioscorides' description (*Klio* 59 [1977]: 17; courtesy Akademie-Verlag, East Berlin).

> resembles a little ball of wool as gradually more and more it comes together. The material left standing from the heavier part spreads itself on the floor of the furnace, some of it going as circles around the furnace, some over the pavement of the building. The latter part must be considered a little less valuable than that of the small parts because of the earth component and the mixing in of impure material.[65]

Factories with this same floor plan remained in England until about 1860.[66] Because of the nature of zinc, only zinc oxide and brass could be produced in such a furnace. Any pure zinc would have been small in amount, accidentally produced, and never on a commercial scale.[67]

Dioscorides must have been personally acquainted with mining and with metallurgical and mineral alchemical processes because of the quality and specificity of his descriptions. For instance, with the smelting of *pompholyx,* he described the color and smell of the Cyprian ore and, as we learned with the habitat descriptions for plants, Cyprus was undoubtedly on his itinerary. He related more details about the minerals than he did for plants, perhaps because of his interest or perhaps because the identification could hardly be conveyed through pictures, as plants could be drawn. Minerals also received more details about their manufacture.

Using his method of classification of materials by their physiological effects, Dioscorides came close to grouping minerals by what we recognize as elements. More important for medicine, his therapeutic usages of metallic ores and products closely, even uncannily, resemble modern usages. Even more than he did with plants, Dioscorides emphasized the medicinal properties of inorganic materials with less attention to specific usages. Almost all the properties listed for metals were the binding, drying, extenuating, cicatrizing, and repressing of the excrescencies of the flesh. Almost all metals were employed for these properties as dermatologic therapeutic agents in topical applicants, such as salves and ointments—much the way metals are presently employed. Another wide usage was in eye medicines (*collyria*).

Copper

Copper ores and products are together in Chapters 76–79, immediately following the zinc chapters. "Burnt copper," or copper oxide (76, χαλκός, κεκαυμένος), Dioscorides said, is binding, drying, extenuating, repressing, cleansing, and cicatrizing. Modern medicine collapses the adjectives by stating that copper "owes its therapeutic value chiefly to its irritant, astringent, and antiseptic properties."[68] "Flowers of copper" (77), which is a copper product from the furnace, has much the same property action, but in a list of specific usages, mostly dermatologic, Dioscorides said that it consumes excrescencies of the flesh in the nostrils. Copper is presently used for its dermatologic effects and for various chronic conditions of the mucous membranes.[69]

Like many heavy metals, copper is vital to the human body. Some diets or environmental conditions result in a deprivation of some essential metals, noticeable even in trace amounts, with accompanying physiological disruptions. Even so, copper seems adequately supplied in modern diets to the extent that it could not be regarded either prophylactically or therapeutically as an internal diet drug.[70] The ancients would have had no means of determining small amounts of metals in plants and there is no indication in Dioscorides that he saw metals in mineral form as ingested drugs. A possible exception is his prescription of the red earth of Sinope (V. 96), probably an iron oxide, which he prescribed for those with liver illness. Since ancient medicine associated the liver with blood, Dioscorides possibly recognized the modern knowledge of the connection of iron with hemoglobin.

Lead and Antimony

Following the chapters on copper ores and products, there is a long series of chapters on lead, Chapters 81–88, with the perplexing interruption of antimony for Chapter 84. Lead and its compounds have had a long history, moving from *materia medica grata* to *materia non grata*.[71] Its toxicity was long recognized. Dioscorides prescribed no internal usages and specifically observed that in smelting lead one should not breathe its harmful vapors (81). In fact, those moderns who frequently attribute the fall of the Roman Empire to lead poisoning of the upper classes[72] give little or no recognition to the fact that the ancients recognized lead poisoning acquired through their drinking water.[73] Some regional waters more readily absorb lead, but even in those regions where exposure to lead would be high, skeletal examinations reveal little differential in lead.[74] Water was not the only source for lead ingestion. The Romans employed lead cooking utensils and, probably most important, they added a lead compound, called *sapa*, to wine to sweeten and preserve it.[75] Recent X-ray fluorescence analysis of Roman skeletons reveals exposure to lead at the same level as that found in workers who have had a high lead exposure.[76] Dioscorides did not include lead in his list of wine additives.

Lead has about the same medicinal properties as zinc and copper, according to Dioscorides: cooling, binding, stopping the pores, and filling the hollows of the eyes and the fleshy excrescencies of ulcers, wounds, and sores. Specific usages were for dermatologic afflictions as an astringent and for various swellings, tumors, and sores. Because of salts, lead compounds do have astringent qualities, we know, and they are helpful as a skin applicant. Dioscorides' breadth of usage probably included carcinoma (*kondulōmata* and "sores hard to cicatrize"); lead was employed well into the twentieth century for cancer therapy.[77]

Dioscorides was economical in the way he discussed medicinal usages for lead. For the first lead product (81, "washed lead"), he gave an elaborate description, but for other lead products and ores he stated only what the properties were in comparison with "washed lead." "Burnt lead," he said, had the same properties (medical usages) as "washed lead," save only it was stronger. It would be because it was processed ore and therefore purer. Lead stone (83) had the same property as burnt lead and so did lead dross (82), but the latter was more binding. The natural ore of antimony to Dioscorides was *stibi* (84), which we recognize as antimony sulfide.[78] Dioscorides placed it between lead stone (83), a lead ore, and *molubdaina* (85), which is, interestingly enough, lead sulfate.[79] Dioscorides attributed about the same medicinal properties to *stibi* (antimony sulfide) as he did to other lead compounds but, he said, in general *stibi* acted like burnt lead and in particular it prevented burns from forming scabs and cicatrized scabby sores. Antimony is no longer therapeutically employed because of its toxicity.[80]

Mercury

Metallic compounds were discussed also by Dioscorides in the section on pigments. Two chapters, at least one of which is on mercury, are among the most confusing chapters in Dioscorides' entire work. For almost two millennia people have incorrectly taken mercury as a drug, sometimes with deleterious results, according to the present state of knowledge.[81] This harm was at least partially because of Dioscorides' confusion. One problem is that we cannot be certain whether his mistake arose from a complete misunderstanding about mercury or his failure to express himself clearly. He certainly was confused about terms. Cinnabar (HgS) is a natural ore of mercury sulfide. Seemingly, Dioscorides' word, κιννάβαρι (*kinnabari*), did not apply to mercury, contrary to usage before and after him. The chapter on *kinnabari* (94) begins with the statement that *kinnabari* is not *minion* (μίνιον), as some people think it is. *Minion*, he asserted, is a stone from Iberia and a product of the furnace whose vapors are so dangerous that workmen put bladders about their faces to prevent breathing its deadly vapor. His *minion* clearly is our cinnabar (mercury sulfide),[82] and this conclusion is confirmed when he reported that painters used it. Cinnabar, a mineral ore processed in a furnace, is found in Iberia and was employed in ancient paints.[83] Dioscorides said that *kinnabari* was an expensive, scarce product of Africa and was thought to be dragon's blood. We have to look to Pliny for an explanation for Dioscorides' *kinnabari*. When Pliny discussed *cinnabarus* as a red pigment, he said the Greeks' terms led to a confusion with "Indian cinnabar," which was the blood of various snakes crushed by elephants.[84] We identify his "Indian cinnabar" and Dioscorides' *minion* as the exudation from the oriental plant *Dracaena* in its several species.[85] Today the plant species is still called "Dragon's blood." The plant product (animal, to Pliny) was useful in medicine, Pliny said, "but our doctors, I swear, because they give the name cinnabar [i.e., Dragon's blood] to *minium* [i.e., cinnabar] also, employ this *minium*, which as we shall soon show is a poison."[86] Dioscorides gave medicinal usages for *minion*, as we shall also see.

Following the chapter on *kinnabari*, the next chapter is on ὑδράργυρος (95, *hudrarguros*). Dioscorides' description of *hudrarguros* clearly defines it as our mercury (or quicksilver), the metal manufactured from cinnabar. Dioscorides' words are very confusing: "And *hudrarguros* is prepared out of what is called *minion*, misapplied as being called *kinnabari*." By this statement *hudrarguros* is a product of *minion* and we learn from the next statement that *minion* yields *hudrarguros* in a furnace. In this chapter, Dioscorides reversed his terms, now *minion* equals *kinnabari*. In some mines, he said, *hudrarguros* is found in a pure enough state that it needs no furnace to purify it. Theophrastus said that the *kinnabari* (κιννάβαρι) from Spanish mines needed no preparation.[87] Dioscorides was completely confused when he wrote that the first step in the manufacture is to put *kinnabari* in an iron spoon and that into a covered earthen pot and finally the pot into the hot coals. Certainly this was not the plant dye "Dragon's blood," because, if this process were followed, all one would have is the evaporated liquid with a little residue, mostly carbon.

Dioscorides attributed various medical usages for *minion*: it has the same usages as hematite (an iron oxide ore), being good in eye medicines but even more binding and staunching of blood, and it heals burns and eruptions of pustules (ἐξανθήματα). In the chapter on *hudrarguros* (which we can unmistakenly label as the mercury ore, cinnabar), Dioscorides said that it was very poisonous and, if eaten, would eat through the internal organs by its weight.

Mercury has had a long history in medicine since Dioscorides' day. Careless readers of Dioscorides' text would note the medicinal usages for *kinnabari* and deem it cinnabar. Careful readers would note that in the following chapter *kinnabari* was a mineral ore (despite what was said before) and such readers might well conclude that the medical usages for *kinnabari,* the plant, applied to the mineral by that name.

Today we believe that the alleged medicinal use of mercury in ointments is largely because of the persistence of medical tradition and not on the basis of clinical evaluation.[88] Supposed benefits of mercury ointments, marginal at best, for skin lesions and eye problems are in juxtaposition with the risk of life because of mercurial toxicity.[89]

Dioscorides' chapter on mercury (*hudrarguros*) had more than one muddle. While he correctly described its manufacture and toxicity, he erred when he attributed the toxicity to its weight, although this theory would persist until the eighteenth century.[90] Such an error in postulating its action is understandable, but Dioscorides' observation about a physical characteristic merely shows that he had not observed its behavior. He said that mercury is kept in glass, lead, tin, or silver containers because it eats through all others and runs out. Had he seen mercury in these vessels, he would have seen that it will readily dissolve lead, tin, and silver, leaving only the glass vessel intact.[91]

More distressing, however, was his lack of clarity about *kinnabari.* What did he mean when he said that *kinnabari* was a plant product with its attendant medicinal usages? As stated above, he compared *kinnabari's* medicinal property to hematite, an iron ore, which he discussed later in the section on stones. In the chapter on hematite (V. 126), the specific medicinal usages are not the same as those for *kinnabari* (V. 94), although they resemble one another in general as being dermatologic aids similar to other metallic compounds. At best, Dioscorides was at his worst in failing to write clearly about *kinnabari* and *hudrarguros.* At worst, Dioscorides confused a plant's medicinal usages with those of mercury ore and, if he was not solely responsible, he contributed significantly to what we believe were gross misapplications of a metallic toxin with unfortunate consequences through the centuries.[92]

More Pigments

While grouping the mineral pigments, Dioscorides associated a number of elements as we know them. The chapters following mercury (95) are red hues: red earth of Sinope (96)—probably an iron oxide with sulfide of mercury from the Black Sea city of Sinope,[93] and Lemnian earth (97)—probably an iron ore from Lemnos; green and blue hues: *kalkanthes* (98)—copper sulfate[94] plus impurities; green hues: *kalkitis* (99)—a copper ore, *misu* (100)—a copper ore,[95] *melanteria* (101)—

a copper product, *sori* (102)—a copper (or iron) ore, and *dipsruges* (103)—a copper-and-zinc-oxide product of furnaces;[96] yellow hues: *arsenikon* (104)—an arsenic sulfide,[97] and *sundaraken* (105)—also an arsenic sulfide.[98]

To avoid redundancy, Dioscorides often gave comparisons rather than repeat medicinal usages. *Misu* (100, a copper ore) had the same properties as *kalkitis* (99); *melanteria* (101) and *sori* (102) had the same caustic quality as *misu*. All four are copper ores.

The arsenic sulfides (104–105), he said, were styptic, binding, and incrustating with a burning, strong biting property and were used in medicines that repress excrescencies (i.e., dermatologic aids), but they made the hair fall out. Only the advent of penicillin eclipsed the use of arsenical medicines in modern times.[99] Dioscorides recognized some of the benefits of arsenical medicines and some of their limitations.

Miscellaneous Minerals

Dioscorides put a number of minerals that did not readily fall into categories of metallic ores, pigments, and stones in another sequence, beginning with *στυπτηρία* (106), a sulfate of potassium, aluminum, and/or ammonium, *θεῖον* (107), sulfur, and *κίσηριν* (108), a pumice stone found near volcanoes.[100] The common theme in this first sequence is sulfur, the medical uses of which Dioscorides discussed in detail.

Nowhere, at least among the minerals, is the detail more elaborate than for salt (109, sodium chloride), for which he gave thirty-six medical usages. He listed binding, dissolving, and others as properties for salt but inexplicably and curiously omitted drying. Following salt are chapters devoted to sea-foam (110), brine (?, 111), soda (112), sodium carbonate or saltpeter (113), and lees of wine (114). The series shows that Dioscorides discerned a common theme of sodium compounds as they acted on the body.

Lees of wine (114) is the dense liquid at the bottom of a wine barrel. Dioscorides said that it was boiled until only a white dry substance, which burned the tongue, remained. This would be sodium ammonium, double salts from which racemic or paratartaric acid was obtained and explained in the famous experiments by Louis Pasteur in the 1870s.[101] Dioscorides said that some people burn shells with the lees of wine in a very hot fire when reducing it to a solid. The calcium from the shells would combine and result in a precipitation of calcium tartrate, anticipating the experiment by Carl Wilhelm Scheele in 1770 when he went on to liberate the tartaric acid by adding sulfuric acid.[102]

Without the chemical knowledge, Dioscorides knew that he was dealing with two preparations having the characteristics as a drug of sodium, on one hand, and calcium sodium, on the other, which caused him to place lees of wine at the end of the series on sodium and at the beginning of the one on calcium.

The last sequence in the miscellaneous minerals section is quite remarkable. The common theme is calcium for Chapters 115–122 as it occurs in inorganic and organic materials. Chapter 115 is calcium carbonate, or quicklime (*ἄσβεστος*), which Dioscorides said was found as a mineral and was produced from shell animals by burning them. Other chapters in the sequence are *γύψος*, or gypsum (116), which is calcium sulfate; *ἀλκυονία* (118), or various species of zoophytes;[103] *ἀδάρκης* (119), or a salty efflorence on the herbage of marshes (probably calcium chloride and other salts;[104] *σπόγγος* (120), or sponges; *κουράλιον* (121), or coral; and a type of "black coral" (122). Sponges secrete supporting spicules of calcium carbonate, and coral is mostly calcium. I cannot identify one chapter: *τέφρα κληματίνη* (117), or "Sarmentian ashes."

Calcium compounds are a very important part of pharmacopoeias. It is nothing more than astounding that Dioscorides saw the common element of calcium by observing its physiological actions in varying compounds found in such diverse things as limestone, gypsum, oysters, crabs, sponges, coral, and marble. Within each chapter variations were recorded. Sponges (120) are good for restraining bleeding and staunching new wounds. One reading their usages would not necessarily know that Dioscorides was probably using sponges here two ways. Burned and prepared as a medicine, sponges probably helped to increase coagulation time, but when simply put on a blood flow they absorbed the liquid in a way that surgeons today use sponges.

Stones

Thirty-eight stones are grouped together in a straightforward manner with a description of where they were found as well as their physical appearances, properties, and medicinal usages. Some I cannot identify. A few are organic fossils having a stonelike appearance. The chapters, all in Book V, are as shown in Table 9.

Dioscorides' use of stones ran counter to a tradition established in the early Hellenistic period, which regarded psychosomatic powers in stones as a means for humans to control all kinds of forces affecting their destiny. With the exception of three stones (141–143: selenite, jasper, and serpentine), which he said could be used as amulets, Dioscorides eschewed these qualities in favor of their physical effects on the body when employed as a regular drug. Since his work did not provide the expected information about stones, this section of his work would be the most emended by subsequent ages.

Rocks, mostly in the form of semiprecious stones, were thought to exercise mysterious and specific powers for those who carried them. If one wanted to win a business contract or a lawsuit, one should carry a chalcedony stone; to be protected from fraud, one ought to have a sapphire; to make one indomitable, the hard stone adamant is superior; and one who has a proclivity for bad thoughts can be cured of them if he or she has a jasper.[105] These are examples of traditions recorded in treatises called "lapidaries." They have information about stones for physical and mental therapies. We sometimes use the word "lithotherapy" to describe this tradition. Dioscorides put little store in such things. Galen and Pliny, on the other hand, were more willing to accept the claims.[106] We in the modern world can treat lithotherapy more sympathetically because we recognize that the stones were devices employed to build self-confidence, an objective of psychiatric therapy.

Amulets. Among the many stones, only three were listed by Dioscorides for use as amulets and these three he grouped together. Selenite (141) is a form of almost pure gypsum (calcium sulfate). In his inimitable way of disassociating himself directly with a supernatural claim, he said that women hung selenite about them as an amulet, without saying for what purpose. Also, "it is thought" that, if it is hung on trees, it causes them to increase their fruit. In his usual direct way of stating medical information, Dioscorides said that selenite, powdered and drunk, is given for epilepsy. An epileptic has an acidosis condition, which is an imbalance in high acidity and low alkalinity. Our modern therapy includes a ketogenic diet, thereby producing ketone bodies. Calcium sulfate, although not presently used, could possibly, in theory at least, have a beneficial effect on an epiletic.[107] In contrast, jasper (142) had no internal medicinal usages but was entirely used as an amulet—tied to the thigh, it sped delivery in childbirth.

The last amulet is serpentine (143), a magnesium silicate with varying impurities. Dioscorides gave its use both as an amulet and as a drug. As an amulet, it is good for those bitten by a snake or for those who have a headache. The streaks in it, he said, are good for lethargy and headaches. Today, magnesium silicate has been used for convulsions of tetanus or of puerperal eclampsia.[108] One can speculate that the lines of ores through the natural rock resembled snakes, hence the use as an amulet against snakebites. Dioscorides may have noted the

TABLE 9. *Stones*

Book V Chapter	*Greek*	*Translation/ID*
123	λίθος φρύγιος	"Phrygian stone"
124	Ἄσσιον δὲ λίθον	"Asian stone"
125	πυρίτης	Copper pyrite
126	αἱματίτης δὲ λίθος ἄριστός	Hematite
127	σχιστός	Hematite
128	γαγάτης	Lignite
129	θρακίας (ι)	Lignite (?)
130	μαγνήτος λίθος	Lodestone
131	Ἀραβικὸς λίθος	"Arabian stone"
132	γαλακτίτης	Chalk
133	μελιτίτης	"Honey stone"
134	μόροχθος λίθος	Soapstone or steatite (?)[a]
135	ἀλαβαστρὶτης λίθος	Alabaster
136	καλούμενος	Turquoise
137	Ἰουδαικὸς λίθος	"Jew stone"[b]
138	ἀμίαντος	Asbestos
139	σάπφειρος	Lapis lazuli
140	Μεμφὶτης λίθος	"Memphis stone"
141	σεληνίτης	Selenite
142	ἴασπις	Jasper
143	ὀφίτης	Serpentine
144	λίθοι οἱ ἐν τοῖς σπόγγοις	"Stones found in sponges"
145	λιθοκόλλα	"Beautiful stone"[e]
146	ὀστρακίτης	Fossil oysters
147	σμύρις λίθος	Emery
148	ἄμμος	Sand
149	ἀκόνης Νάξιας	"Naxian whetstone"
150	γεώδης λίθος	Geodes

[a]Paulus Aegina, *Seven Books*, 3:223.
[b]See "General Medical Values of Stones," below.
[c]D. E. Eichholz, Pliny, N.H., X: 15, but F. Adams (Paulus Aegina, *Seven Books*, 3:226) said that they were mostly morinte of lime.
[d]Dioscorides said that they were a mixture of marble and Parian stone.
[e]Margarite occurs on the island of Naxos with corundum and would seem likely to be the "Naxian Whetstone" (Cornelius S. Hulbert, *Dana's Manual of Minerals*, p. 355).
[f]Paulus Aegina, *Seven Books*, 3:226; cf. Pliny, *N.H.*, XXXVI. 31. 140.

Comments
Pumice with alum (?)
Alum, nitre, and salt
An iron oxide ore
An iron oxide ore
Organic fossil
Organic fossil
Magnetite
White marble
Possibly borax
Possibly talc
A form of gypsum
Fossil spines of sea urchins
No medical usages given
Identified as retinasphaltum and dolomite[c] [?]
A form of gypsum
As amulet
Any stone caught up by sponge[d]
Mixed stones used for mosaics
Organic
Silicon is not normally a stone
Margarite
Contains iron, argil, and silicon[f]

effect of magnesium silicate on the central nervous system and included it in his work rather than exclude this stone as he did numerous other ones having amulet powers.

General Medical Values of Stones. Dioscorides did not make great claims about the therapeutic uses of stones. The copper and iron ore stones (125–127) had medical usages similar to other physical forms of these heavy metals.[109] Lignite (128–129) was employed entirely as a fumigant. The "Arabian stone," perhaps white marble, is powdered and put on hemorrhoids to dry them and in dentifrices to act as an abrasive for cleaning teeth. Magnetite, or the lodestone (130), was observed to have magnetic qualities and perhaps this led Dioscorides to list its only medicinal use as drawing out humors. Two stones, the "Jew stone" (137) and stones found in sponges (144), were used internally as lithotriptic agents; that is, they broke up stones in the bladder.

Two stones had no medical usages given but had other uses. Asbestos (138), Dioscorides said, was made into cloth and used by workmen to protect them from burns. The "beautiful stone" (145) was heated and used as an iron to turn back wild eyelashes.

The Memphis stone (140) was used as an anesthesia in surgical operations. Pliny gave us the same story with more detail: "Memphis stone . . . is like a gem. The method of using this is to grind it to powder and to smear it mixed with vinegar on places which need to be cauterized or lanced; thus the body is numbed and feels no severe pain."[110] The Memphis stone is one of only two explicit anesthetics for surgical operations in *De materia medica*. The mandrake plant (IV. 75) is the other, apparently used as a general anesthetic because of its atrophine content. We would like to know the identity of the "Memphis stone," but, alas, we do not.[111]

Near the end of the stone sequence is sand (148), but it is difficult to understand why it was thought to belong here since it is not normally considered a stone. Sand had only two medical uses: it dried the moisture of gout when used as an applicant and it was used as a substitute for salt to dry things.

Earths

Taking dirt as a medicine appears at first to be "dirty, ignorant medicine." Any soil scientist and a few historians of pharmacy will know that *dirt* is a word that describes a variety of minerals, some of which have medicinal use. Chapters 151–159 are about different "earths." In the short chapter (151), Dioscorides said that earth (γῆ) has general cooling and stopping-of-the-pores properties but that there are many kinds, each with its own usage.

The first particular earth is "Eretrian earth" from the city of Eretria. Rackham and Forbes believe that it was heavily laden with magnesite,[112] and the medical usages given by Dioscorides roughly correspond with current usages for this inorganic compound.

On the island of Samos there was an important commercial product—earth. The Samian earth (153–154) came from a mine described by Theophrastus.[113] Samian earth was principally kaolin, a hydrated aluminum silicate. In a purer form kaolin is sold today as an over-the-counter remedy for mild diarrhea.[114] Americans recognize one of its brand names, Kaopectate (Upjohn). Since "Samian earth" (153) and the "Samian earth stone" (154) were probably the same chemically, we have difficulty in justifying the distinctions Dioscorides gave.[115] For each ore he gave slightly different usages, each one including some of the modern usages. He said that Samian earth is an astringent, assuages inflammations of the testicles and breasts as an applicant with water, represses perspiration, and counters various poisons when taken internally with water. Modern usages are somewhat similar but they do not precisely coincide.[116] We do employ kaolin as an excellent absorptive in the stomach for toxins. Strangely omitted from Dioscorides' list is any use for the digestive tract.

The Samian earth stone, on the other hand, Dioscorides said was good for those sick in the upper tract (στομαχικός) by counteracting things drunk. Also he said that the drug from the stone is good as an ophthalmological agent and as an amulet for childbearing.

With Samian earth, we have once again the perplexing and intriguing mixture of the familiar and the bizarre. Even allowing for different ways to explain the same phenomenon, we cannot make Dioscorides' usages coincide with our own knowledge of the material,[117] but there is enough similarity for us to know that he was observing the actions of drugs and not merely placebos. We cannot arrive at a full understanding but we can develop a respect and an appreciation for his science.

Carbon

The last two chapters in *De materia medica* are on carbon. Soot (161, ἀσβόλη) has a putrifying and sharp property and is used as an application to help form scabs. Soot is used, he said, by painters, but the best kind for a medicine comes from the glassmakers. The last chapter is on black ink (162), which consists of one part gum to three parts soot. The ink is good in septic medicines. Since soot was used by painters,[118] one would like to know why Dioscorides did not complete his series of pigments (88–105) by placing these chapters on carbon there as black pigments? He chose not to do it and further speculation seems fruitless. Vexing though these inconsistencies are to us, we should not lose sight of the magnificent achievement of Dioscorides in organizing the materials of medicine in a rational order by their physiological effects according to natural categories.

End of De materia medica

Dioscorides ended with a postscript to Areios, his mentor from Tarsus, to whom he had dedicated his work: "And now, dear Areios, concerning the size of this work in respect to both the mass of materials and how they are used, we believe that this is sufficient."

DE MATERIA MEDICA IN PERSPECTIVE

In the Preface, Dioscorides claimed that his predecessors' contributions suffered from a number of faults: noncomprehensiveness, mistakes of information, confusions of drug identities, too little attention to drug properties, insufficient emphasis on experimental testing of drugs, and poor organization, such as arrangement by incompatible properties and by the alphabet. His work, he explicitly stated (Pref. 5), differed from that of his predecessors in the following ways: direct and personal observation of "most" drugs; clinical observation that he verified in the written authorities "in checking what was universally accepted";[119] personal field inquiries of folk practices "in each botanical region"; a new and different arrangement of "classes according to the properties of the individual drugs,"[120] an arrangement that linked pharmacology with medicine; and provision for an orderly, regular means for placement of future knowledge within this organizational scheme so as "to extend its range of preparations and mixtures and its trials on patients."[121] He inferred that his system would be easier to learn and retain. Finally, he pointed to the comprehensive coverage of his work, which included drugs from all kingdoms—herbs, rocks, and animal parts.

Today most physicians employ the *Physicians' Desk Reference* as a principal guide to drugs. It contains about 10,000 medicaments, or slightly more than twice the 4,740 medical uses in Dioscorides' *De materia medica.* As important as the scale of his work was, the quality of his information and his organization by drug affinities were potentially of greater significance. It seems relatively clear how he could accomplish this: he obtained most of his information through direct clinical observation. He asked his readers not to criticize his style of writing but to consider "my careful practical experience" (Pref. 5).

The ability to synthesize so much empirical data almost certainly would have been based on experience. Thomas Edison's claim that genius is mostly perspiration with inspiration only a small part seems to apply. Dioscorides must have made his observations in clinical situations, because it is highly unlikely that he could have acquired the knowledge in any other way. He must have been a practicing physician, trained in the Hippocratic way of Hellenistic physicians. His mentor, Areios, stressed drug therapy in his practice in Tarsus, a pharmacology center. As a physician, military or not, Dioscorides traveled considerably, mostly in the eastern Mediterranean provinces; he talked with local people about their remedies; he read the authorities; he observed the effects of drugs on patients' bodies; he saw relationships in how different drugs affected the patients; and he identified drug affinities. Above all, he had the ability to observe nature and then to base his working postulates on empirical data.

Much has been written about the thought processes of the Greeks in relation to their empirical observations and theoretical formulations. Classical Greek and Hellenistic philosopher-scientists developed logical schema to relate their arguments and they supported the logic by appealing to the observations of the physical world. But as G. E. R. Lloyd suggests, empirical data were used to undermine and refute one's opponents' views or common assumptions.[122] The results were deductive sciences. The rigor was applied to the logic of the argument and not to the method of determining the observational support for facts.

Coming as he did at the end of the era of Hellenistic science, Dioscorides seems to have perceived that there was no need to begin yet another theoretical argument. The various competing schools of thought had shown him enough of the results when theoretical argumentation was presented to advance medical theory. Standing aside from polemics would give his inductive science a better chance of being accepted.

I noted that other Greeks argued using demonstration through observable physical appearances. This is different from an attempt to reduce nature (φύσις) to an orderly explanation adduced through a concerted, rigorous, and procedural method for obtaining observation. The postulate necessary for the existence of science is that nature acts in orderly ways.[123] The historian's task is to determine not only whether and to what degree pronouncements on that order are descriptive of order perceived by ourselves (truth as we know it) but also whether they are a product of the individual and/or his or her culture separated from natural phenomena being explained. Dioscorides' understanding of drug properties is close to the order that we perceive in the behavior of natural-product drugs. We cannot be disinterested in this anticipation of modern ideas, but an understanding of Dioscorides' world and the reaction it gave his work tells us far more about early science.

Dioscorides saw patterns in how various materials reacted on and in the body, and he recorded them without seeking to condense them to the more comprehensive systems his ancestors and colleagues were wont to form and defend. The Asclepiadeans, Methodists, Dogmatists, Herophilists, Empiricists, Skeptics, and others attempted either to explain too much too simply or to give up the search for order too quickly and thereby accept that the world was disorderly and capable of only crude, empirical manipulations in the darkness. The historian can acknowledge that Dioscorides probably described a part of nature as did no other person before him and, moreover, he knew the limits of what he saw. Those who followed him understood neither his method nor the order he identified because his system did not relate to the age's paradigm. Nature was left to be scrutinized by the authority of Aristotle and Galen, whose great intellects grasped more than their eyes could see and whose profound words described more than there was to explain based on what they learned directly from nature. In contrast, Dioscorides organized complex data into empirically derived patterns, but he did not seek to frame his organization within a cosmology. Dioscorides did not offer an alternative to the paradigms established by classical Greek thought because his scheme was too limited. He did propose an alternative method to the contemporary paradigms. He hoped, he said, to provide the framework around which new knowledge could be organized.

Let the evidence speak for itself, Dioscorides said. But the evidence did not speak to those who came after him. Medicine and science did not follow the unique direction in which he pointed. They saw him point and described the end of his finger. They used, corrected, and elaborated on information in *De materia medica* but they did not follow his system.

Successors to Dioscorides took simples and mixed them to control multiple results. For a long time after Dioscorides, the tendency was to develop medicines containing many natural drugs, that is, polypharmacy. Not until the sixteenth century was the direction reversed; the reversal came about partly with the observation by Paracelsus (ca. 1493–1541) that a simple, that is, a single natural-product drug, was itself a mixture of compounds. If Dioscorides' method had been followed, his successors would have looked within each simple for those active ingredients which caused similar reactions regardless of their natural home, just as Dioscorides did when he saw calcium oxide as the common substance shared by shell aquatic animals and the mineral limestone. Inobtrusively, Dioscorides offered science a direction, but it took fifteen hundred years to catch up with him. Explaining why it took so long is as important as understanding Dioscorides' achievement.

5. DONE AND UNDONE

PUBLISHED AND MISREAD

In 1847 in Alexandria, Egypt, in the garden of the house of Laurin, then the home of the Prussian consulate, an empty stone box was found, which had on one side the words "Three Books of Dioscorides."[1] We do not know positively if this was Dioscorides of Anazarbus, but this is likely a tangible link between Dioscorides' *De materia medica* and the great depository of ancient learning in the famed Alexandrian Library. The missing scrolls, of course, are more important than the finding of the box. The reaction to Dioscorides' publication is not known, nor can it likely ever be known, but the earliest scrolls, while not surviving, left a fertile legacy not confined to a consulate garden where once a mighty library stood.

The first recognition of Dioscorides in surviving works occurs in the *Glossary to Hippocrates*, written by Erotian, who lived sometime in the second half of the first century; in other words, he was a contemporary or near contemporary of Dioscorides. While discussing the synonyms for *akonitum*, Erotian correctly cited a passage from Book IV, Chapter 76, of *De materia medica* and he named Dioscorides as his source.[2] This meager evidence is all that we have for an initial reaction to Dioscorides' work. When the sources are as few as they are in ancient history, it is not unusual that we cannot measure reactions to written works.

Around a century later, Galen provided testimony to Dioscorides' impact. In writing his prolific medical works, Galen often asserted his authority by degrading his predecessors and medical contemporaries. Like Pompey and Caesar, Galen could have neither equal nor rival. Nonetheless, when he came to a judgment of Dioscorides, his negative criticisms were uncharacteristically muted:

> Dioscorides the Anazarbian brought together in five books all useful materials, not only herbs, but trees, fruits, saps, and liquids, while discussing in addition all metals [minerals] and animal parts. To me this work appears to be the most perfect of all treatises on materia medica. This judgment is believed by most of those who concern themselves with these matters; a few speak otherwise, like Tanitros the Ascelpedean, but these critics, it is thought, being beyond rationality, speak above causes. Lesser writers ought to be read and studied for their experiences with materia medica, lest one omit the works of Heraclides of Tarentinum, Crateuas and Mantias. They did not all write the same things nor do they agree in all things. Dioscorides, whose five book work was titled, "Concerning the Materials of Medicine," truly on his own wrote about the preparation (δοκιμασία) and the testing (σκευασία) of drugs, just as Heraclides, the Tarentine, did about purgatives, as drinks and clysters, just as Mantias about household remedies, and just as Apollonius did about where they are found as Mantias did also.[3]

True to his high opinion of Dioscorides, Galen referred to him by name many times throughout his numerous works and, even when he was not named, much of the information about drugs came from Dioscorides.[4] Once—in confusion, we presume—Galen said "Dioscorides of Tarsus," no doubt making the connection between him and his mentor, Areios of Tarsus.[5]

Ironically, despite Galen's approval of Dioscorides' work, Galen more than anyone else destroyed what Dioscorides considered to be his greatest claim to fame, namely his arrangement and classification of materials. It is an open question whether Galen was even cognizant of what Dioscorides' accomplished because Galen ignored it. Galen wrote much on pharmacy, specifically, *Properties and Mixtures of Simple Drugs, Compound Drugs Arranged by Location of Ailment, Compound Drugs Arranged by Kind, Antidotes, Theriac by Piso, Theriac by Pamphilus, Household Remedies,* plus others. Galen neither discussed more drugs than Dioscorides—473 plant drugs by one count and about 438 by another,[6] compared to Dioscorides' 1,000 plus—nor delivered the botanical and preparation information that Dioscorides had in *De materia medica.*

In his arrangement in *Simple Drugs,* Galen partially employed what Dioscorides decried, alphabetical order, but this arrangement did not harm Dioscorides' contribution. Galen's treatises on drugs and medicine were eventually harmful to Dioscorides' hard work in arranging drugs by affinities because Galen supplied a theory as an explanation for pharmaceutical behavior. His pharmaceutical theory was accompanied by a comprehensive medical theory, which was philosophically based and rationally appealing. Each drug then re-

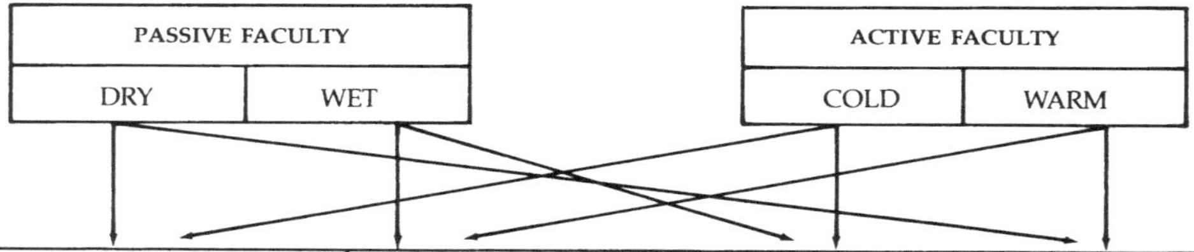

PASSIVE FACULTY		ACTIVE FACULTY	
DRY	WET	COLD	WARM

Elements	Earth	Air	Water	Fire
Season	Fall	Spring	Winter	Summer
Period of Life	Adulthood	Childhood	Old Age	Youth
Humors	Black Bile	Blood	Phlegm	Yellow Bile
Sense Perception	Black—Sour (Sharp)	Red—Sweet	White—Salty	Yellow—Bitter
Temperament	Melancholia	Sanguine	Phlegmatic	Choleric
Principal Organ	Spleen	Heart	Brain	Liver

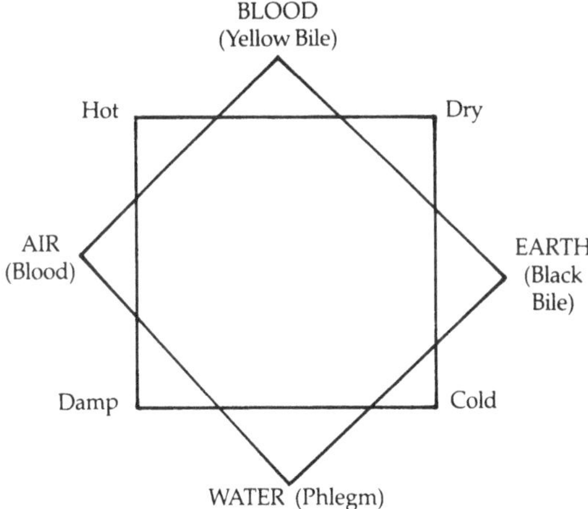

Fig. 4 (left and above). Galenic pharmacology.

lated to a comprehensive theory and not directly to another drug. The theory had greater appeal than Dioscorides' attempt to associate physiological behaviors of drugs by their affinities on the basis of "what works."

Galen reduced all primary drug properties (Dioscorides' *dynameis*) to four: warm, cold, wet, and dry; these four properties related to the four humors, thereby supplying an explanation for both illness and mental condition.[7] In turn the four humors related to the four elements: earth, air, fire, and water (see Fig. 4).[8] Humors are formed of elements with a combination of an active faculty (cold, warm) and a passive faculty (dry, wet). Earth, for instance, has a dry and cold faculty; therefore, potentially, it is actively cooling and passively drying. Neither an element nor a humor has only one faculty; it must have both an active and a passive one. A drug is but a mixture (*krasis*) of elements and differs from a food insofar as a drug acts on the body whereas the body acts on a food. But, being composed of elements, a drug potentially has two types of action on the body: either a warming or a cooling and either a drying or a moistening action. The only exception is when the particular combination of elements results in a temperate state for one property (and potential action). Even when this occurs, there is an action as a drug because the other faculty would have a property due to its mixture, such that a drug may be temperate between warm and cold but at the same time be drying or moistening in its action. In accounting for the fact that some drugs appear stronger than others, Galen asserted that each drug has its actions (properties) determinable through experience to four degrees of

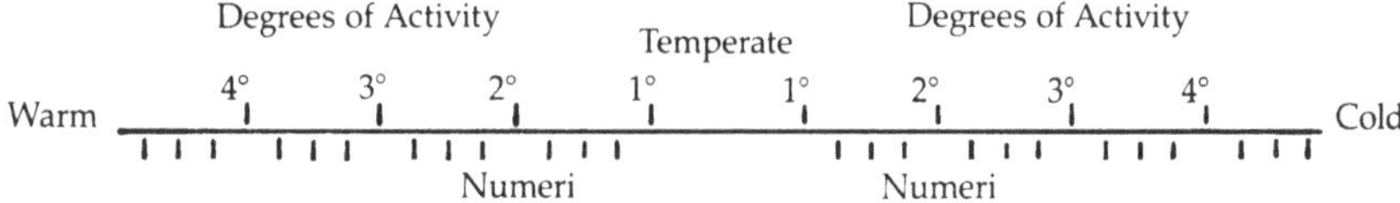

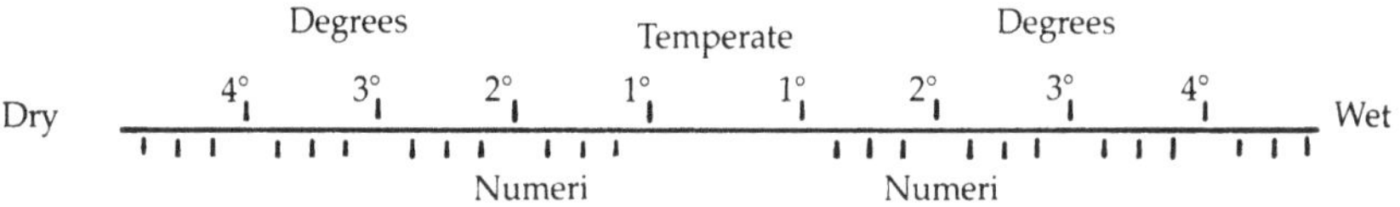

Fig. 5. Galenic drug intensities.

intensity (see Fig. 5).[9] Thus, a drug could have such a mild cooling action, say 1°, that it would be virtually imperceptible to the senses but nonetheless register a slight cooling action on the body. Or a drug could be as much as 4° cooling, in which case it would be so intensively cooling as to be life threatening. No one way, save experience, can be trusted to determine a drug's primary property.[10] Seawater, Galen said, is wet to the sense of touch but to the body its property is drying.[11] On the other hand, pepper does not feel warm but it tastes hot and imparts a warming quality.[12] Having a warm property, pepper theoretically could be tested for things varying from a simple chill to a trauma, such as shock. Since warming has a dispersing quality, the secondary qualities (such as dilating, dissolving, and diuretical) would be related and pepper thus might be good for such things as boils or internal poisons. Only the testing of drug on patients could confirm the theoretical hypothesis.

A drug's property, although related in a fashion to its quantity, is a qualitative distinction. This is important: since it is a quality, it would not follow that when doubling a dosage the drug's action is increased twofold. Experience, Galen underscored, is the only means of determining various drugs' properties—qualitatively and quantitatively.

The action of a drug's properties was not absolute but it was relative to the individual. Each person has his or her own temperament (*krasis*, "mixture"). Whereas certain general rules determine a person's temperament, the particular individual has his or her unique temperament. As a general rule, a boy of four years requires a strong cooling medicine, should he have a fever, because by nature a child is of a sanguine temperament. An old man of eighty, who has a naturally phlegmatic temperament, needs only a mildly cooling drug for a fever of the same intensity as that of the boy of four. Similarly, a girl of four requires a less strong cooling remedy because females are by nature of a colder temperament (although there was disagreement about this among ancient authorities).[13] Personality, race, and climate are some of the other variables that only the experienced, wise physician could know through examination. Not only is the nature of the disease important in a diagnosis but also the condition, background, and personality of the patient are critical.

Whereas Dioscorides had numerous possible properties for each drug, Galen divided them into the four primary properties (warm-cold, wet-dry) and secondary ones (e.g., sharpness, sour, cutting), with the effect of reducing the secondary properties to relative obscurity. Although Galen would argue for the importance of secondary qualities for therapeutical precision, the legacy of his theory reduced their importance.[14] Dioscorides said that henbane (IV. 68) had a soporific property and Galen said that it was cooling to the third degree.[15] The principal organ ("member") of coldness was the brain; thus, when he observed henbane's strong, cooling action, he was imparting that its action was likely to affect that organ. There are other cold "members," such as hair, skin, bones, nerves, and fat. Each property had its list of members or organs.

One could not know through theory that a cold remedy's action would be for one or a combination of the cold organs. Such knowledge came through empirical observation. The theory can neatly explain many observable medical effects of drugs. Take the strong, cytotoxic alkaloids in Dioscorides (IV. 147–150), which have a strong warming effect by Galenic theory and one or more of which were given by Dioscorides for antitumoral activity. These cytotoxins will cause hair to fall out as a side effect of chemotherapy. Since, in Galenic terminology, hair is a cold member, there is an explanation: the drug resulted in an imbalance of heat and therefore could predictably be a depilatory. According to this theory, then, when one administered an extreme drug for a particular therapy, one should be alert to counter the unwelcomed side effects by giving a drug whose action is the opposite. For the example of an antitumoral, extremely warming drug, one would want to add to the therapy a suitable cooling remedy, one known to promote the vitality of hair but known through experience not to counter antitumoral activity. Galen's theory has empirical and theoretical attractions.

Galen's pharmacology was not complete; he neither harmonized all inferences nor brought all his ideas together in one work. He scattered them, sometimes contradictorily. When discussing specific drugs, he often even omitted a drug's property, as he omitted whether henbane's passive quality was drying or moistening and to what degree. He tried not to force his theory into a position divorced from experience such that would jeopardize a patient's life. Sometimes things appear muddled as when he had rose oil as being moderately warming and then elsewhere as cooling to the first degree.[16] For one herb, he said, "Orache [*Artriplex hortensis* L.] is moistening and its coldness is temperate, the moistening to the second degree from the middle, its cooling to the first degree, but it can be tepid towards warmness."[17] Here he was not contradictory. In theory, a mild drug like rose oil could be cooling to a cold-temperament person and warming to one with the opposite temperament. Cool to Peter, warm to Paul. What Galen possibly intended was more empirical; that is, he wanted to list those mild drugs which normally can be expected to have a warming or cooling action to the first degree of intensity so that an experienced, wise physician could make critical judgments in planning the therapy. In effect, he may have intended what we would call a mathematical mean whereby a drug would have a range of action, but he was, of course, no mathematician and was not thinking in precise mathematical logic of our era.[18] He was attempting consciously to formulate experience with drugs into a rational system of explanation.

Galen's effort to correct Dioscorides' designation for coriander as a cold remedy affords an opportunity to see the method and some of the consequences of Galen's pharmacology.[19] Dioscorides said that coriander (III. 63) had a cooling property and was employed as an applicant with bread or polenta (pearl barley) to cure erysipelas and herpes. Galen said that Dioscorides was in error about the cooling quality as the cure for erysipelas. For both Galen's and Dioscorides' discussion, it is necessary for us to know that we do not know whether either one's use of the term referred to erysipelas as we now define it, nor do we know whether Galen's use of the term was the same as Dioscorides'. Erysipelas in antiquity seemed to have a broader meaning and it is likely that Dioscorides' erysipelas was broader in meaning than Galen's. By the Middle Ages (when it was sometimes also called Saint Anthony's Fire), erysipelas had come to have our modern meaning. Dioscorides' use of the word suggests conditions due to mortification and putrefaction of tissues on or near the skin. Pliny's use of the Latin equivalent (*ignis sacer*) suggests that at times it meant lupus or shingles.[20]

Be erysipelas as it may, Galen used this "error" in Dioscorides not only as a correction to the Master of Pharmacy but also as an example of his own superior method for therapy. "Certainly I will explain the causation of these particular actions," Galen said, "just so that the proposition will be in the future associated with me."[21] In a lengthy discourse, Galen explained that the skin eruptions called *erysipelata* arose out of a condition whose etiology was an excess of watery humors, thus producing a phlegmatic condition. One must proceed from the theory of drug administration by opposite actions to restore humoral balance, thus a cooling remedy given to a cold-temperament disease would exacerbate the condition, not relieve it. Dioscorides' error was not in giving coriander for erysipelas, but his mistake was in its action. Actually, Galen said, coriander has a slightly sweetening and astringent effect and it was really mildly warming, whereas Dioscorides should have been more alert to these (secondary) properties and known that it was not cooling. To be sure, many physicians make this error, Galen acknowledged, and he was willing to set the record straight by his demonstration through experiences with erysipelas. The danger—and this he only implied—was that one might substitute a cooling remedy for coriander in the mistaken notion that a cooling action was the proper therapy.

Galen's point, from our standpoint, is well taken. The essential fact, however, is that, for all intents and purposes notwithstanding, Galen shifted the question away from the underlying logic of the procedure Dioscorides sought to establish. Later writers, for example, ibn Māsawaih, Sarābiyun, ibn Sīnā, Al-Kindi, Matthaeus Platearius, and Rufinus, debated whether coriander's action is warming or cooling and not the nature of its actions shared with affinity drugs having similar effects.[22] The drug's "properties," not their usages, received a focus of attention. Certainly, almost all physicians of all ages were concerned about the usages because they wanted beneficial results for their patients. Galenic theory, however, directed attention to the identification of properties, to the degrees of intensity of action, and to the counterbalance of unwanted properties. If generations following Dioscorides had concentrated on the qualities within each simple, and if they had associated simples by their affinities, chemistry would have developed much faster than it did, because, in identifying properties, attention would be directed to the causes for the properties. The cause for the drug action lay within each simple drug just as Paracelsus proposed much later. Galen's method resulted in directing attention toward compounding medicines.

In fact, Galen's theory was much more central to the thought of the ancient world than was Dioscorides' work. The primacy of two pairs of opposites (warm-cold, wet-dry) went back to the pre-Socratics, at least back to Alcmaeon,[23] and possibly to antecedent Chinese thought. It was held by a number of philosophers and students of natural science in a continuous and increasingly elaborate chain down to Galen. With most of their works lost, we cannot know the degree to which

Galen was synthesizing, codifying, and regularizing thought or the degree to which he was original. Still Galen left medical gaps of inexplicable behavior and many factual data were unexplained about specific properties for specific drugs. Other generations would find Galenic theory as the basis of which to build and to make their contributions based on their medical experiences. Dioscorides' method, unexplained, was unperceived. His method was almost purely empirical. Not only did Galen's theory rest on a comprehensive explanation in the form of humoral theory for health and disease, physical and mental, but it also carried with it an entire cosmology based on the elements. Such a cosmology became not simply compatible with the Christian and Islamic world views but integral to the core of their thought.

COPYISTS' PENS AND ARTISTS' BRUSHES

Although Galen's theory was in the long run decisive in the failure to accept Dioscorides' method, it was the copyists of Dioscorides' manuscripts who, shortly after his writing, did not understand or appreciate his contribution. Consequently, some of them rearranged his chapters and put them in alphabetical order. That way one could easily find a given entry—provided, of course, one knew what to look for.

When Dioscorides wrote, his age was on the verge of one of the greatest revolutions in information storage and retrieval (as we now say) since writing had begun about three thousand years prior to Dioscorides. The codex, or book, as we now know, was invented around A.D. 100 (some would put it slightly earlier) while I dated Dioscorides' writing as being around A.D. 60–78.[24] (The next revolution was printing in 1450 and the last, electronics in our age.) Dioscorides wrote on papyrus rolls, that is, single sheets of papyrus paper glued together at each end so as to make a continuous roll wrapped around two sticks, called a scroll. The Greeks wrote in vertical columns, usually narrow for prose, wider for poetry.

From the very early second millennium B.C. the Egyptians had illustrated papyrus scrolls. Starting at least in the fifth century B.C. the Greeks illustrated literary works, such as Homer, and diagrammed scientific works, such as a mathematical treatise by Hippocrates of Chios.[25] Herbals, as Pliny observed, were illustrated: ". . . Crateuas, Dionysius and Metrodorus adopted a most attractive method, though one which makes clear little else except the difficulty of employing it. For they painted likenesses of the plants and then wrote under them their properties."[26]

It is my belief, without much doubt—though it has been expressed[27]—that Dioscorides' *De materia medica* was illustrated at the time of composition, for the following reasons: (*a*) The requirements of the text necessitated an accompanying picture; for instance, in his chapter on laurel (I. 78), Dioscorides gave no verbal description of the chief "kind" (our species, *Laurus nobilis* L.), but he described in words another "kind" with smaller leaves. Unless there was a picture with the text, neither this chapter nor many similar ones would make sense. (*b*) Although there are no papyrus fragments of a Dioscorides' text that is illustrated, there are papyri of a portion that would not be illustrated in any circumstances. Also there are illustrated herbal papyrus fragments that resemble his text. (More on this subject below.) (*c*) There are various manuscript families with differing families of illustrations. We can conjecture that one particular family has evidence that puts its illustrations back to a papyrus tradition. (More on this subject as well.) Even though Pliny said that some herbals just gave the bare name and medicinal properties, we can be reasonably sure that Dioscorides' *De materia medica* had pictures.

The dry sands of Egypt preserved papyri thrown away as garbage by their ancient owners. Most of the surviving remains are but fragments of such things as letters and business records—ancient equivalents of grocery and laundry lists. Occasionally, a piece of a literary work is uncovered. At Umm el Baragât in the Fayum region of Egypt,[28] there were fragments (6.5 × 6.4 cm) of a rolled, illustrated herbal in a second-century A.D. handwriting, the earliest herbal ever discovered, and it has a broken text related to Dioscorides' work. It is neither an exact copy nor a sloppy condensation, but an independent work.

The first fragment (a) appears to be Dioscorides' *chondrillē* (II. 133, *Chondrilla* spp.). Where Dioscorides wrote that its root "glues hair back [τρίχας ἀνακολλᾷν]," the papyrus reads "holds hair fast [τρίχας . . . κατέχει]." The illustration of the chondrilla plant is crudely drawn above the text, just as Pliny had stated that Crateuas, Dionysius, and Metrodorus had depicted their herbals. Another fragment (d), this one on the herb *arktēon*, mentions poulticing (καταπλάττω), presumably of the leaves, and crushing (τρίβω) of the root, neither preparation being so specified in Dioscorides (III. 90) for *arktēon*. The text, judging on what little is extant, generally seems to be a shorter version of Dioscorides' full entry. Still another fragment (e) of the same papyrus codex claimed that the herb *pseudodiktamnos* was good for nasal discharge, a remedy unlisted by Dioscorides (III. 32) for the same plant.

The Umm el Baragât papyrus is possibly from a source Dioscorides employed, but this seems unlikely. The additional information to Dioscorides' text is also not found in Pliny's *Natural History*, which used much the same sources as Dioscorides. Probably, then, the herbal was composed by an author who used Dioscorides, who perhaps added his own experiences, and who seemed to be more interested in medicine than botany.[29] The differences in the text are not sloppy copying errors nor are they mere condensations. What we seem to have is the first evidence of a pattern that repeated itself many times in the centuries afterward. Future users of Dioscorides' text contributed their experiences with plant, animal, and mineral drugs by adding to and subtracting from the text as they made their own copies. Dioscorides' *De materia medica* was no literary work that had a unity, nor a religious work that testified to divinity. It was a work of science. If one believed a plant to look different, whether because of incorrect identification or other reasons, then he or she might make emendations according to personal understanding of reality. Similarly, he or she added new remedies, dropped some (fewer than added), or modified the text according to rational grounds. One can overstate this phenomenon because it is still possible to combine most of the manuscript texts and arrive at some reasonable judgments about what must have been in the original. The next papyrus fragment discussed will help to show this. Even so, this papyrus is the first of many examples of a classical work that has so many emendations in its various copies, and the complexities of establishing a critical text are so immense that one can seldom be certain about the authorship of innumerable passages.

Another papyrus, now at the University of Michigan, was written by someone who knew Greek poorly.[30] Because of his mistakes, we can learn more certainly what Dioscorides wrote than in those by smarter copyists whose changes were grammatical and rational. The Michigan papyrus was by one who copied Dioscorides so sloppily that it is replete with errors, such as mistaken letters, dropped words, and repeated phrases. This writer was copying a text of Dioscorides without the kind of variation found in the Umm el Baragât text. A note on the back is dated in the year 190 by the Roman method for the emperor, but this note was added later. Judged by its handwriting, the papyrus may have been written as early as A.D. 150. It has parts of three columns in 87 lines, more writing than the other papyrus.[31] The misfortune comes in the fact that it is on animal fats (II. 76), one of the largest chapters in *De materia medica*. By its nature, it would not be illustrated. Had fortune have been otherwise and preserved a fragment on herbs that bridged chapters, we could know about the early illustrations in a pure Dioscoridean text and learn whether Dioscorides' original order had been retained. This being our earliest textual fragment, it is important that its text is closest to a manuscript family Max Wellmann distrusted, so he chose to favor another family when he decided on his critical text. This raises some important questions, which we shall postpone.

Other papyri are of minor assistance. None indicate an alphabetical order. One small section from Book III, Chapters 130–131, dates from the second or third century and is now in the Aberdeen Museum.[32] The others are from codices, no longer in scrolls. The first of these is an excerpt from Book V and dates from the third or fourth century. The order of presentation of chapters is neither Dioscorides' original order nor alphabetical. The papyrus writer rearranged the material to suit his or her own need. Its importance also lies in the fact that the codex was not on *materia medica* as such but on alchemy, thus showing the breadth of appeal of Dioscorides as an authority.[33] A fragment of an illustrated herbal in color, dated around A.D. 400, was found at Antinoe.[34] The meager portion of text is beneath a picture of the plant *symphyton* but it cannot be matched to Dioscorides' chapter for *symphyton* (I. 28). The style of illustration resembles that found in the illustrated herbals of Pseudo-Apuleius and Pseudo-Dioscorides and the style differs from that found in the principal Dioscoridean illustrated manuscripts. The most recently found papyrus is also the youngest, dating from the sixth century. It is a *materia medica*, but it too is badly fragmented. It contains excerpts from the first three books of Dioscorides but adds information about plant and animal drugs, including an excerpt from Diocles, whom Dioscorides did not quote—at least not directly by name.[35]

All in all, the papyri demonstrate an abiding tradition in transmitting pharmaceutical information in the form Dioscorides prescribed. Notably, none contain herbs he did not discuss. They reflect that he had an established position as a leading authority. They also reveal what Pliny had told us explicitly: some herbals were illustrated, some not. The papyri are important for what they do not contain, specifically whether Dioscorides' work had been rearranged by alphabetical order.

The oldest, best preserved, most beautifully illustrated manuscripts of Dioscorides' *De materia medica* have plants arranged in alphabetical order. The oldest dates from about A.D. 512 but its survival does not tell us when alphabetization first occurred. Instead we look for evidence in the fourth century when Oribasius, physician and friend to the emperor Julian (A.D. 361–363), authored a large medical encyclopedia. Books XI–XIII are a condensation of Dioscorides so faithfully done that since the sixteenth century scholars have employed these books to help interpret Dioscorides' text. Max Wellmann frequently drew upon this resource. In Oribasius' Books XI–XIII, the drugs are discussed in alphabetical order.[36] Certainly, Oribasius himself could have rearranged Dioscorides, but Max Wellmann did not think that he did. Wellmann noted that certain chapters interpolated into Dioscorides' text by the Alphabetical Dioscorides Manuscript Group were also in Oribasius' condensation. This suggested that Oribasius used a text of an alphabetical Dioscorides. Since the interpolated chapters were not in Galen's *Simple Drugs*, Wellmann concluded that alphabetization occurred sometime between Galen (ca. 129–post 210) and Oribasius (ca. 325–ca. 400).[37] Wellmann apparently did not observe that, in his section on wines, Oribasius preserved the original order of Dioscorides' Book V.[38] I am not sure what this means. It might bring into question Wellmann's entire premise about the date for alphabetization. It is also possible that Oribasius either had two versions of Dioscorides or had a version that alphabetized the plants and left the material on animal parts, wines, and minerals in its original order.

In conclusion, the evidence of neither the papyri nor Oribasius demonstrates when Dioscorides' work was rearranged in such a radical way as to destroy his method for grouping drugs by their physiological effects.

MANUSCRIPT ILLUMINATIONS AND DIOSCORIDES' ORIGINAL VERSION

A picture of a plant or animal is better than one thousand words—even when they are Dioscorides' concise Greek. As we saw, the study of papyrus fragments yields some information but it is to the manuscripts that we must turn in order to learn better what Dioscorides' work was like when he wrote it. The manuscripts range in dates from the early sixth century to the sixteenth century. Less than half are illustrated. Most are in Greek, but one illuminated Latin manuscript and another in Arabic provide supplementary evidence. All of them contain variations and we shall look to these variations to discover new contributions to science and medicine that each age made when they copied, corrected, and interpreted his text. The illustrations also reflect a continuity with Dioscorides' original work. The manuscript illuminators preferred to copy the picture from the codex rather than go to the garden and field. In this final section, the manuscript illustrations of Dioscorides' *De materia medica* are used to reconstruct, as best I can, the scrolls as Dioscorides' wrote them.

Illustrations are essential to the understanding of the text. The illustrations in the extant manuscripts are stylized and most of them are substitutes for those in the original. Even with these limitations these manuscript pictures offer indications about the quality of illustrations in Dioscorides' original version as well as other ancient archetypes. The understanding of what the earliest pictures might have been like is assisted by studying pictures of herbs and animals in ancient mosaics, frescoes, and vases.

The Anicia Manuscript

The oldest and most famous Dioscorides codex is an elaborately illuminated manuscript produced around A.D. 512 for Anicia Juliana, who was the daughter of the West Roman Emperor Clavius Anicius Olybrius and a member of the prominent noble Anicii family at Constantinople.[39] In it Dioscorides' herbs are rearranged in alphabetical order and his animal and mineral drugs are omitted. Missing also from the text is Dioscorides' Preface but added to it are emendations including synonyms (which will be discussed later) and sections by Crateuas and Galen (which are clearly designated). These changes are important, because this manuscript served as a model for many later works. The fame of the Anicia manuscript depends on its magnificent depictions of herbs. The parchment codex has 984 large pages (310 × 380 mm) with 392 full-page illuminations and another 87 illuminations in the text. The colored illustrations display the artists' ability to render nature with exactness and sensitivity. Photography still cannot duplicate the "reality" of a well-painted herb. Folios 2–387 are devoted to Dioscorides.[40] Normally, on one side of the folio is a fully colored picture of the complete plant showing flowers, buds, stemmation, fruits, and root systems. The illumination is so detailed that often the venation system of leaves is depicted. Because of the artistry, the Anicia is the center for art displays in Vienna, where it has had a home since it left Constantinople in the sixteenth century. Because of the artistry and its early date for a text, the manuscript has received much scholarly attention.[41] The history of its text will be discussed in Volume II. Despite the extraordinary attention this manuscript has received, fundamental questions about the manuscript remain unanswered. Among them, what is the relationship between the herbal pictures in the Anicia manuscript and the pictures in Dioscorides' original version?

Frontispieces in the Anicia. The Anicia Codex begins with a series of full-page frontispieces. One (fol. 6v; Fig. 6) shows Princess Anicia Juliana seated in court flanked by two ladies personifying Magnanimity and Prudence, the latter holding an illustrated codex on her

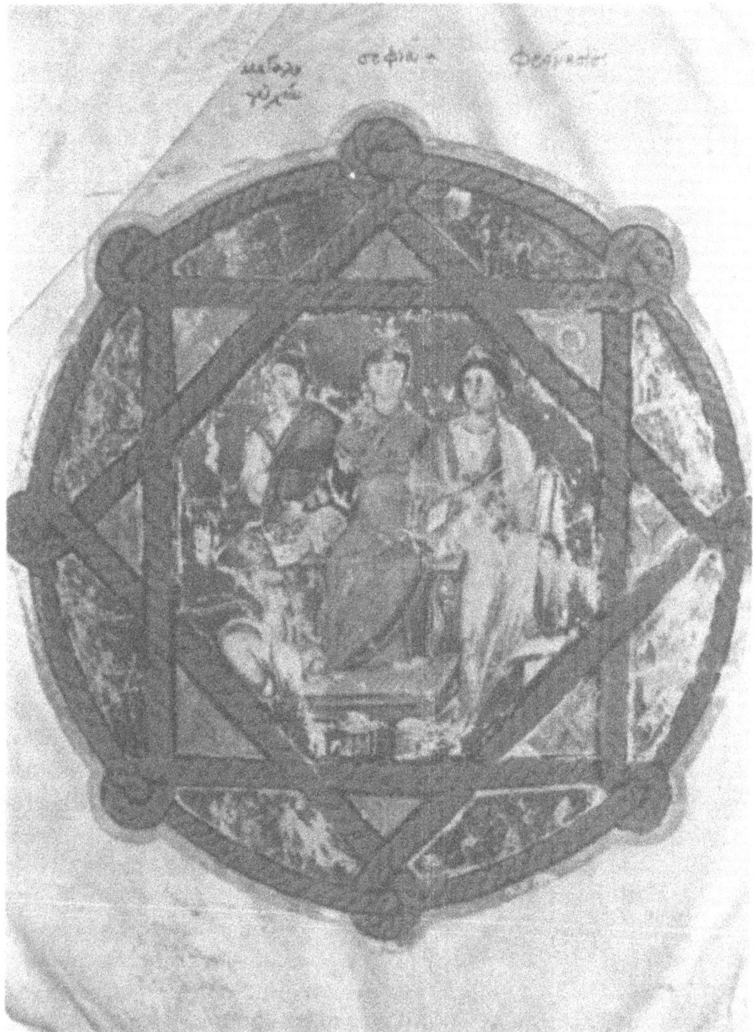

Fig. 6. Anicia Juliana flanked by Magnanimity and Prudence (dedicatory frontispiece, Vienna MS med. gr. 1, fol. 6v; courtesy Österreichische Nationalbibliothek).

lap. From the picture and dedicatory text we learn that the princess had founded a church in Constantinople, built in A.D. 512–513, and the citizens in gratitude presented her with the gift of this manuscript.

Three folios contain portraits of Dioscorides, each of which poses questions. Two portraits, folios 3v and 5v, are identified as Dioscorides by inscriptions. In these two, he appears middle-aged, with brown hair and a pointed beard. A third portrait (fol. 4v), also assumed by some scholars to be Dioscorides, depicts a man slightly rounder of face with a darker beard and a full moustache.

The portrait on folio 5v shows Dioscorides seated and writing a codex while an artist with a painter's easel draws a mandrake plant held aloft by a woman (Fig. 7). The lady is identified as the personification of Epinoia, "Power of Thought," by her inscription. The painter, who is not labeled, is assumed by a modern scholar, Charles Singer, to be Crateuas.[42] Singer interprets this painting to signify that, while Dioscorides wrote the text, the paintings were done by someone else. Inescapably, the artist is drawing from real life, as Epinoia holds the actual plant. Because of the quality of the herbal drawings, one might assume that they were drawings from nature. This, however, was not the case. The pictures were taken from an earlier model and not directly from nature.

Modern scholars believe that Crateuas' root herbal indirectly supplied the model for many of the pictures.[43] They assert that Crateuas' pictures and others from unknown sources were appended to Dioscorides' text. Beneath Dioscorides' text for some eleven herbs are quotations designated as being by Crateuas. The drawings for these eleven herbs are of very high quality,[44] which leads some modern scholars to conclude that these eleven pictures, at least, are in a direct linear descent from Crateuas' illustrated root herbal[45] (see Fig. 8*a*). Further, some plants in the Anicia manuscript are not in Dioscorides (e.g., ἀδρακτυλλίς, fols. 62v–63) and some have the same text as in other Dioscorides manuscripts but the plants have different names (e.g., φυλλοις, fols. 359v–360; cf. IV. 71, Wellmann ed.). Moreover, the plants in the Anicia are in alphabetical order, just as Wellmann postulates the order of Crateuas' root herbal.[46] Pliny inferred that Crateuas himself had drawn the plants in his work from real life.[47]

Since the picture on folio 5v shows the writing and painting as separate operations by two different people, it is hypothesized that the compilers and artists of the Anicia herbal's archetype substituted some of Crateuas' pictures for those in Dioscorides' *De materia medica*. This hypothesis receives more support when the picture of some herbs seem not to match the textual descriptions,[48] as if someone had confused the plant being discussed. This conclusion receives added

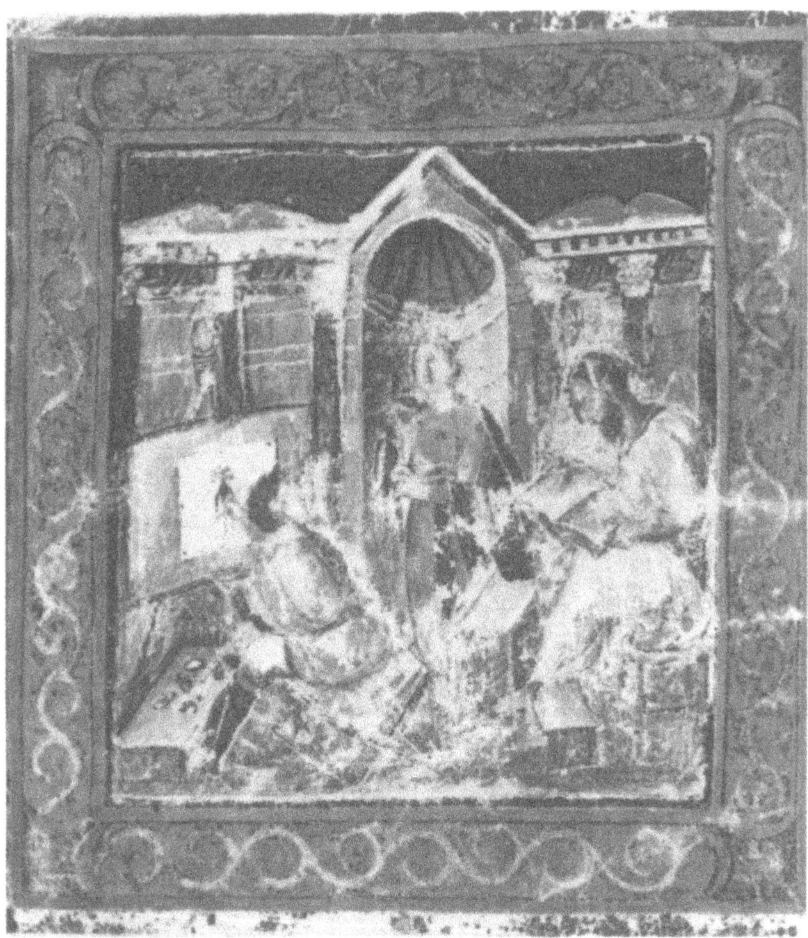

Fig. 7. Dioscorides seated and writing while young artist on left draws a picture of the mandrake held by Epinoia, "Power of Thought" (Vienna MS med. gr. 1, fol. 5v; courtesy Österreichische Nationalbibliothek).

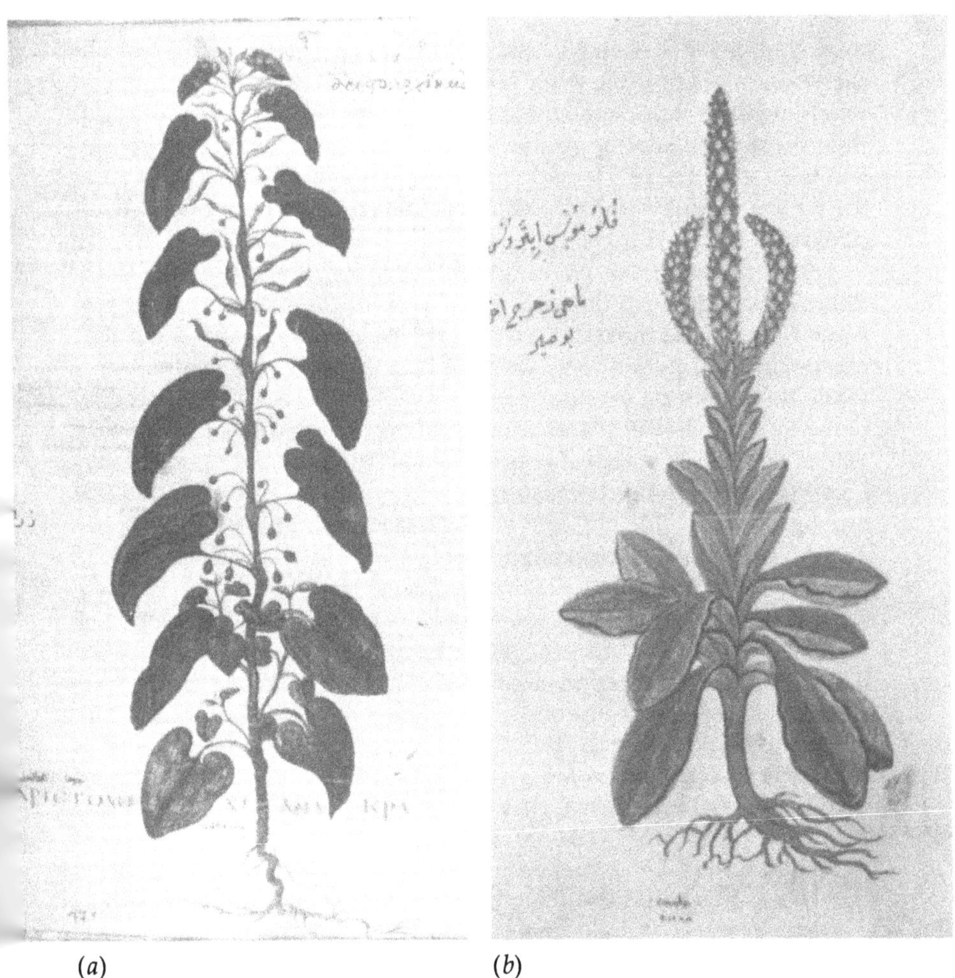

(*a*) (*b*)

Fig. 8. (*a*) Drawing of the climbing birthwort (*Aristolochia sempervirens* L., III. 4, Wellmann ed.), believed by Charles Singer and others to be based on original by Crataeus (Vienna MS med. gr. 1, fol. 17v), and (*b*) mullein (*Verbascum sinuatum* L., IV. 109, Wellmann ed.) depicted in the Anicia—note stylized symmetry of flower stalks at top (Vienna MS med. gr. 1, fol. 361; courtesy Österreichische Nationalbibliothek).

weight when one observes that the quality of some herbal drawings is distinctly lower than that of the majority (see Fig. 8*b*).[49] This last observation might indicate that Crateuas' paintings were often employed when available but, if they were not available for a particular plant, then those from another source were substituted. The picture of mullein is an example of a lesser-quality drawing. (Compare Fig. 8*b* from the Anicia manuscript to the same plant in Fig. 12*b* from the Johnson papyrus.)

Another frontispiece painting (fol. 3v) shows the Seven Physician-Pharmacists, in much the same motif as some Pompeian frescoes and some Roman villa mosaics (see Fig. 9).[50] Galen was awarded the central position of honor—and only he had the easy chair with a back while the others sat on stools. Like Crateuas, Galen also is quoted by name in a number of places from his work, *Properties and Mixtures of Simple Drugs*.[51] The appearance of equality between Dioscorides and Crateuas is deceiving because in the iconography of the period the one on the right side of Galen would be favored. Marcus Varro (116–27 B.C.) published a work called *Hebdomades*, which contained the pictures of seven hundred illustrious Greeks and Romans.[52] Possibly some of the pictures in Figure 9 were taken from Varro's lost work and were likenesses of Andreas, Nicander, and Crateuas.[53] Because he lived after Varro, Dioscorides' portrait could not have been in the *Hebdomades*. Nonetheless, the picture could actually be Dioscorides. The portrait on folio 3v with the other six physician-pharmacists shows the same likeness as on folio 5v: middle-aged, brown hair, pointed beard. Paul Buberl believes that the depiction of Dioscorides may derive from Dioscorides' original scrolls.[54]

The picture of Dioscorides on folio 4v of the Anicia manuscript is that of a different person (Fig. 10). Like the picture on fol. 5v, it too centers on the mandrake plant. A man labeled Dioscorides is seen seated while a lady named Euresis ("Discovery") holds the plant aloft with its root in the likeness of a man. Nearby is a dead dog, which has expired because of pulling the root up, according to the legend recorded by Josephus. Anthony de Premerstein proposed that, since this likeness of the man labeled Dioscorides is different from the other two, this could be a portrait of Crateuas derived from a frontispiece of Crateuas' root herbal.[55] Paul Buberl accepted this thesis, but he wondered about the fact that the mandrake legend only went back in the extant sources to Josephus (late 1st c. A.D.) while Crateuas lived in the early first century B.C.[56] Kurt Weitzmann objected to elements of the thesis by noting that the picture as it appears in the Anicia manuscript is framed and has an illusionistic background. Weitzmann associates such illuminations with codices; he connects simpler im-

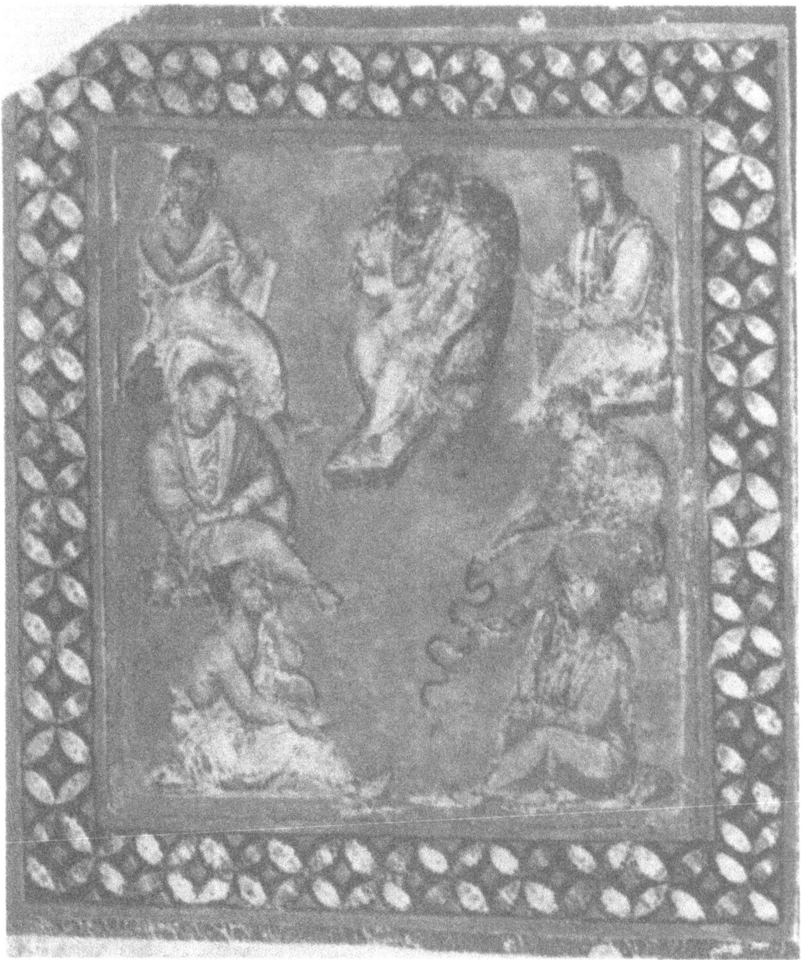

Fig. 9. The Seven Physician-Pharmacists: *clockwise from top left*, Crateuas, Galen, Dioscorides, Nicander, Rufos, Andreas, and Apollonius Mus (Vienna MS med. gr. 1, fol. 3v; courtesy Österreichische Nationalbibliothek).

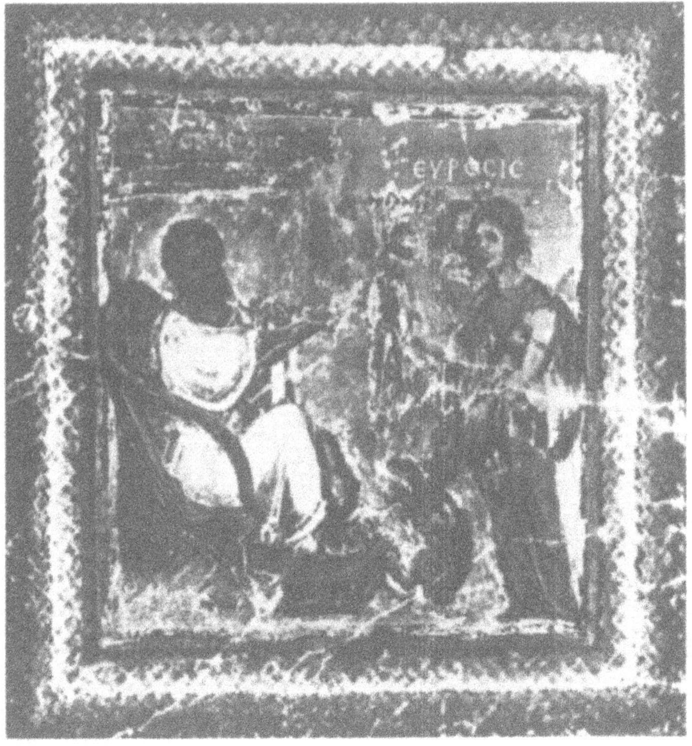

(*a*)

ages, without frames or backdrops, with papyrus for reasons to be explained later. Crateuas' root herbal was certainly a rolled papyrus scroll in its original form, and, accepting Weitzmann's thesis, Crateuas' frontispiece did not have a representation of the same picture as appears in the Anicia manuscript, folio 4v. Rather than to break completely with Premerstein's thesis that the herbalist is actually Crateuas, not Dioscorides, Weitzmann allowed that the picture of the man and woman could have been free standing in a papyrus roll drawing and that the dog, the background, and the framing could have been added later.[57]

Evidence against Crateuas as Source. Not all evidence supports the contention that many of the paintings are traceable to Crateuas. The painter of the mandrake on folio 5v (Fig. 7) is a youth and Dioscorides is in the prime of life. The Emperor Justinian in the Ravenna mosaics and Jesus in the period's favorite representation of him are shown as stern, middle-aged men, such as those at St. Catherine's. In earlier pic-

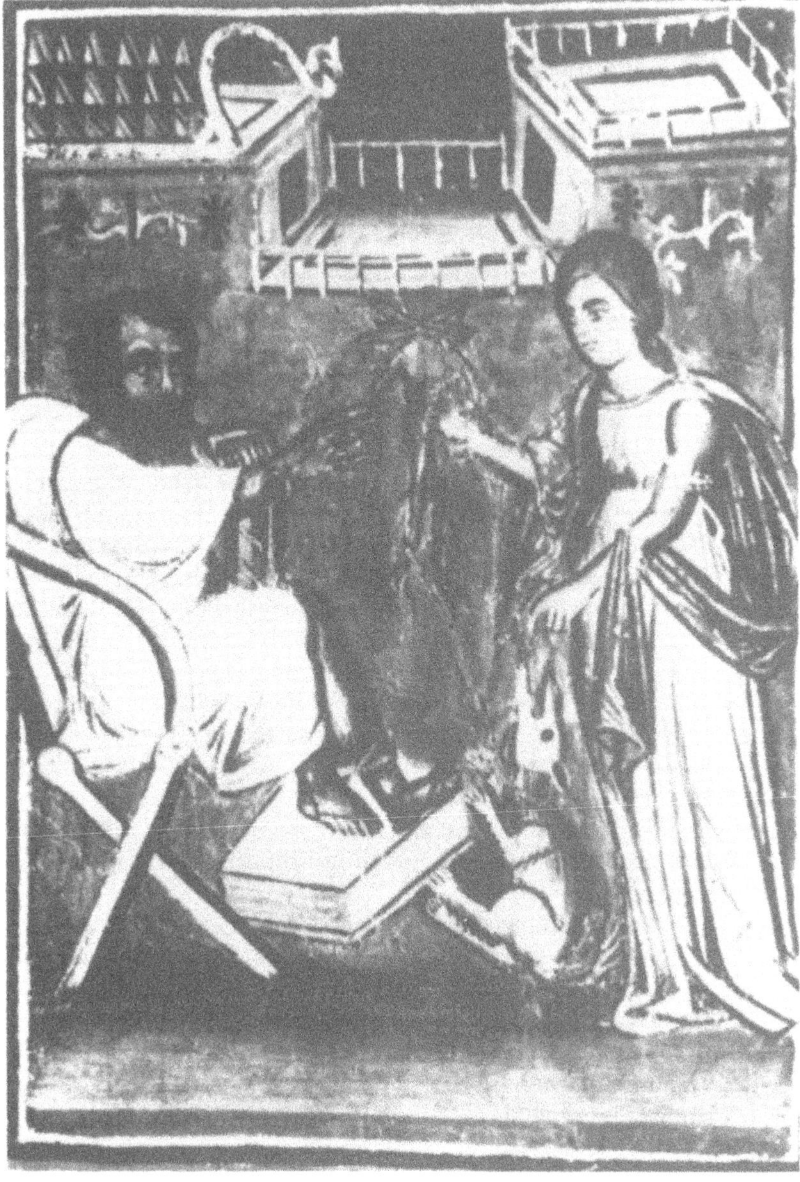

(*b*)

Fig. 10. (*a*) Dioscorides (or Crateuas?) pointing to mandrake held by Euresis, "Discovery" (Vienna MS med. gr. 1, fol. 4v; courtesy Österreichische Nationalbibliothek); (*b*) fifteenth-century copy (Vatican Chigi MS 53 [F. VII. 159], fol. 221v; courtesy Biblioteca Vaticana).

tures, Jesus was as an Apollo-like youthful shepherd. The painter in Figure 7 is unlabeled while Dioscorides and Epinoia have their names above them, which indicates that the painter had a less prestigious, anonymous position in contrast to Dioscorides' status. Crateuas' position at the top right on the folio of the Seven Physician-Pharmacists (3v; Fig. 9) would obviate a more prestigious portrait while working beside Dioscorides.

Papyrus Roll and Parchment Codex. The depictions in the Anicia manuscript reveal a close stylistic parallel to the Pompeian paintings, but this would not necessarily mean that the painters of the Anicia manuscript were slavishly copying drawings from an archetype that looked just like the original herbals by Crateuas, Dioscorides, and their contemporaries. By all our available information, both Dioscorides' work and Crateuas' earlier root herbal were originally on papyrus rolls. Drawings on papyrus were only wash drawings because papyrus has a rough surface and is short-lived. If gouache were used, the rolling would cause paints to break and chip away quickly. Moreover, with a roll's short, albeit useful, existence, talented painters would be reluctant to invest the time in the medium. On the other hand, parchment has a smooth surface and, when its individual leaves are sewn at one end to form a codex, it would not be bent the way of a roll. Gradually replacing papyrus in the second century A.D., parchment was found to be very durable, thus giving a talented artist a medium to display his talents for the attention of many years.[58] The details of the parchment paintings in the Anicia manuscript are so intricate, so fine in depicting nature's smallest veins in leaf structure or stamens in flowers, that it is almost inconceivable for an original papyrus painting to have closely resembled Anicia drawings.

The argument that the best herbal drawings in the Anicia came from Crateuas' root herbal is too simplistic a formula. Charles Singer had no evidence that Crateuas' drawings were those on the same folio that contained the Crateuas quotations. The handwriting for the Crateuas quotations are in smaller uncial and at the bottom of Dioscorides' text. Crateuas' quotations are often accompanied by similarly written quotations from Galen, which we have no reason to suppose was ever illustrated. Other drawings of plants in the Anicia are also of fine quality and include plants that one would not consider root herbs. Just because Pliny said that Crateuas and Dionysius and Metrodorus painted herbs from real life themselves and just because Dioscorides thought highly of Crateuas, it does not follow necessarily that the archetype from which the Anicia modeled its pictures had in turn taken the best pictures from Crateuas' work. There were surely other herbals, not mentioned by Pliny.

Anicia Seen as Composite. In summary, the archetype for the Anicia undoubtedly borrowed drawings from a variety of sources in addition to Dioscorides and one of them may have been Crateuas. On the other hand, since papyrus roll illustrations were of relatively poor quality when compared to the realism in Anicia's pictures, I cannot be persuaded that the best pictures descended directly from Crateuas' original work.

The postulated existence of an archetype for the Anicia is made certain by other manuscripts, which have paintings in the same style as the Anicia manuscript but include important variations, such as additional drawings and text. This excludes the possibility that they derived their lineage directly from the Anicia. Instead, they also may be traced to an archetype related to the Anicia's source.

Neapolitan Dioscorides Codex

If the Anicia had not survived, more attention would be directed toward a seventh-century herbal of the Alphabetical Dioscorides in lavishly colored illuminations (see Fig. 11). The manuscript now in Naples had 409 illustrations on 172 folios, and, as one can see from the arithmetic, the economy of space resulted in two or three plants per page.[59] The drawings are iconographically so similar to those in the Anicia manuscript that one might suppose, as some have,[60] that the Neapolitan manuscript was copied directly from the Anicia. Stylistically, however, the pictures are different and a closer examination shows that the Neapolitan parchment codex has some drawings that the Anicia does not and its text has some differences not attributable to a seventh-century recension.[61] Later, the same things also will be said when the tenth- and eleventh-century illustrated manuscripts of Dioscorides are described as being derived from a source earlier than the Anicia manuscript.

Egyptian Recension and Papyrus Style

Professor Weitzmann observed that the requirements of a roll, where writing was in columns, were to have the illustration in the margins with the writing indented so as to provide space for the picture. The earliest papyrus drawings were in the left margin. Later they were also found in the right margin (see Fig. 12*a*) and still later they interrupted the text, thereby permitting a picture to fill an entire column from left

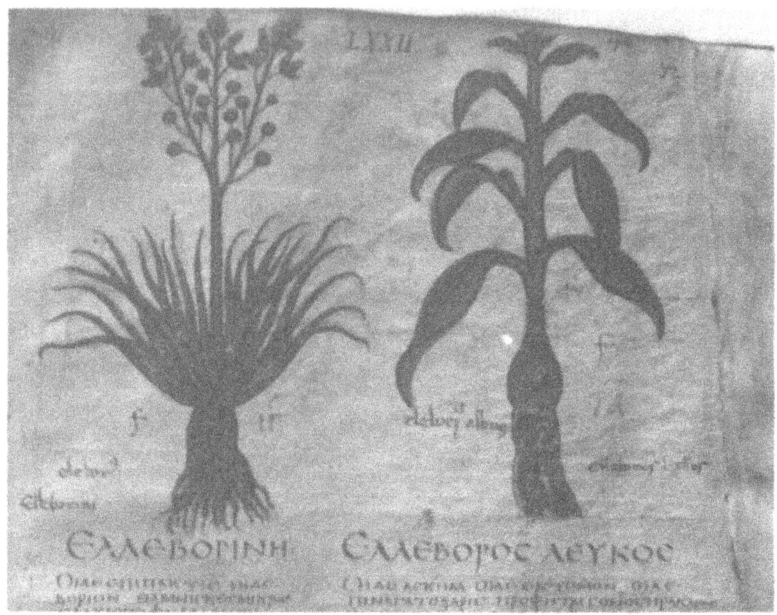

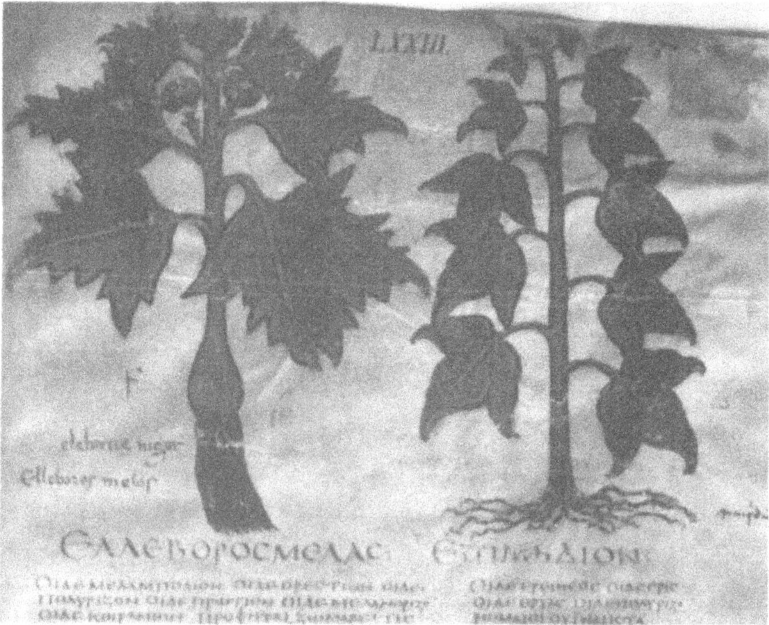

Fig. 11. Elleborine (*Herniaria glabra* L.), *elleboros leukos* (*Veratrum album* L.), *elleboros melas* (*Helleborus officinalis* L.), and *epimedion* (*Ephimedium alphinum* L.) (Naples MS gr. 1, pp. 72–73; courtesy Biblioteca Nazionale).

to right margins.[62] The illustrated Johnson papyrus herbal—though it is in a codex—is an example of the last stage of papyrus-style illustration (Fig. 12*b*).

Whereas the Anicia manuscript has entire pages devoted to a single illustration and the Neapolitan manuscript had drawings at the top and bottom of texts, some Dioscorides manuscripts have marginal illustrations. The oldest of these is from the ninth century, now in Paris (B.N. MS gr. 2179) and probably of Egyptian origin.[63] Wellmann calls this "the best manuscript of Dioscorides."[64] Weitzmann believes that this Paris manuscript copy descends from the roll format, the "papyrus tradition," because of such evidence as columned writing and illustrations mostly within the column indented on the right side (Fig. 12*a*).[65] Some of its illustrations are so similar to those in the Anicia that the Paris and Anicia manuscripts could not fail but to have descended from one common source (see Fig. 13). Just the same, many of the pictures are very different.[66] An important distinction between these manuscripts is that the drawings in the Paris copy are relatively poorer in quality, although they are colored. The Paris manuscript preserves Dioscorides' regular order, but it is in a poor state of preservation and many of its leaves are missing. A sizable portion remains from Book II. 101 through Book V. 123 in 171 folios, a large enough segment that Wellmann used the manuscript as his primary textual reading. Where portions were missing, he employed later manuscript texts closest to the extant text in the Paris manuscript as best preserving Dioscorides' original text. I shall discuss later a problem with Wellmann's method for determining a critical text, but, for now, let us concentrate on the illustrations.

Since the archetypes for both recensions are lost, let us refer to these two traditions as the Byzantine/Anicia (Vienna MS gr. Med. 1, s. VI) and the Egyptian (Paris B.N. MS gr. 2179, s. IX) based on the fact that these two manuscripts are the oldest surviving representatives and the probability that the Viennese and Parisian manuscripts were produced in Constantinople and Egypt, respectively.

Other manuscripts, all but one dating later than the Paris manuscript, reveal the existence of these two or more traditions and how they related to one another. Two pages of an illustrated Dioscorides manuscript are preserved as the flyleaf to an Armenian manuscript. The hand is ninth century and the text is Book III, Chapters 156 and 158 and the drawing for Chapter 157, thereby showing that the textual order was in Dioscorides' original, as in the Egyptian tradition.[67] Its one illustration, crudely drawn, of *κόρις* precedes the textual description (Fig. 14). The format is the third stage of Weitzmann's papyrus style and the same as the Johnson papyrus.

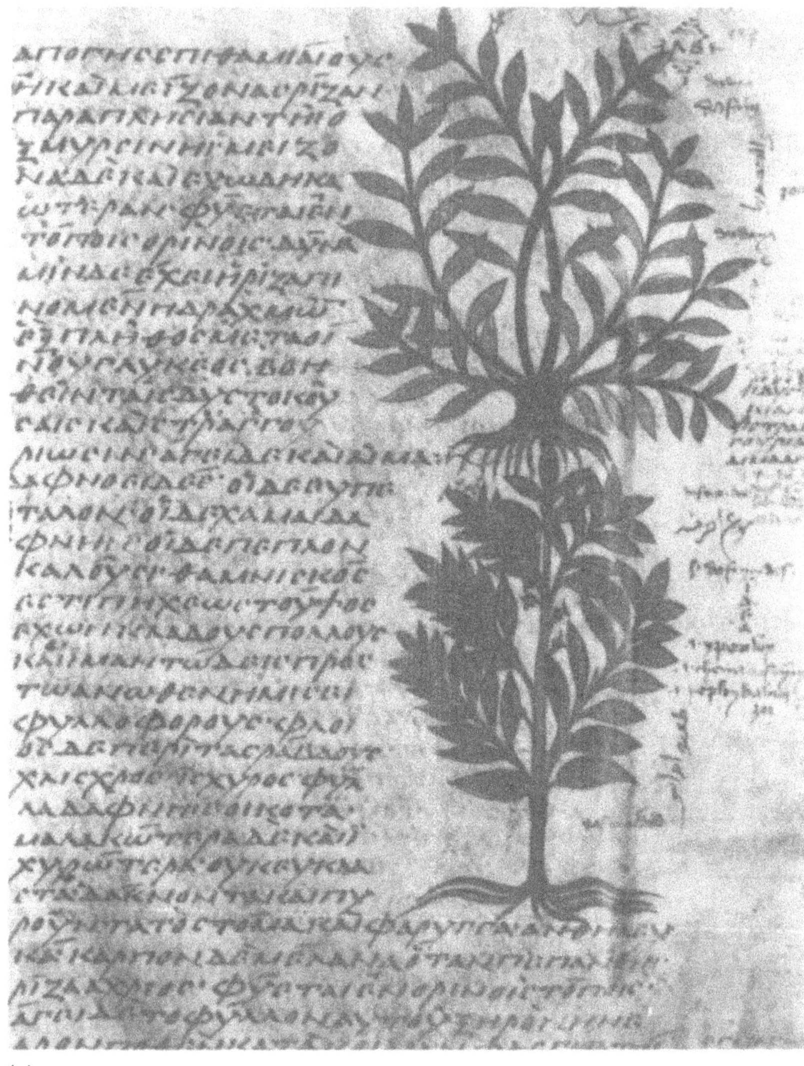

(*a*)

Fig. 12. (*a*) Ninth-century Paris codex showing second stage of papyrus style with drawings of two kinds of daphne, probably *Daphne laureola* L. and *D. mezereum* L., in the right margin—the pictures are not in the same iconographical tradition as those equivalent ones of daphne in the Anicia tradition (Paris MS gr. 2179, fol. 124; courtesy Bibliothèque Nationale); (*b*) picture of mullein (*Verbascum* sp.) above the text as found in the Johnson papyrus, ca. A.D. 400; compare with the drawing of mullein in Fig. 8*b* (Johnson papyrus in the Wellcome Institute for the History of Medicine, London; courtesy Wellcome Trustees).

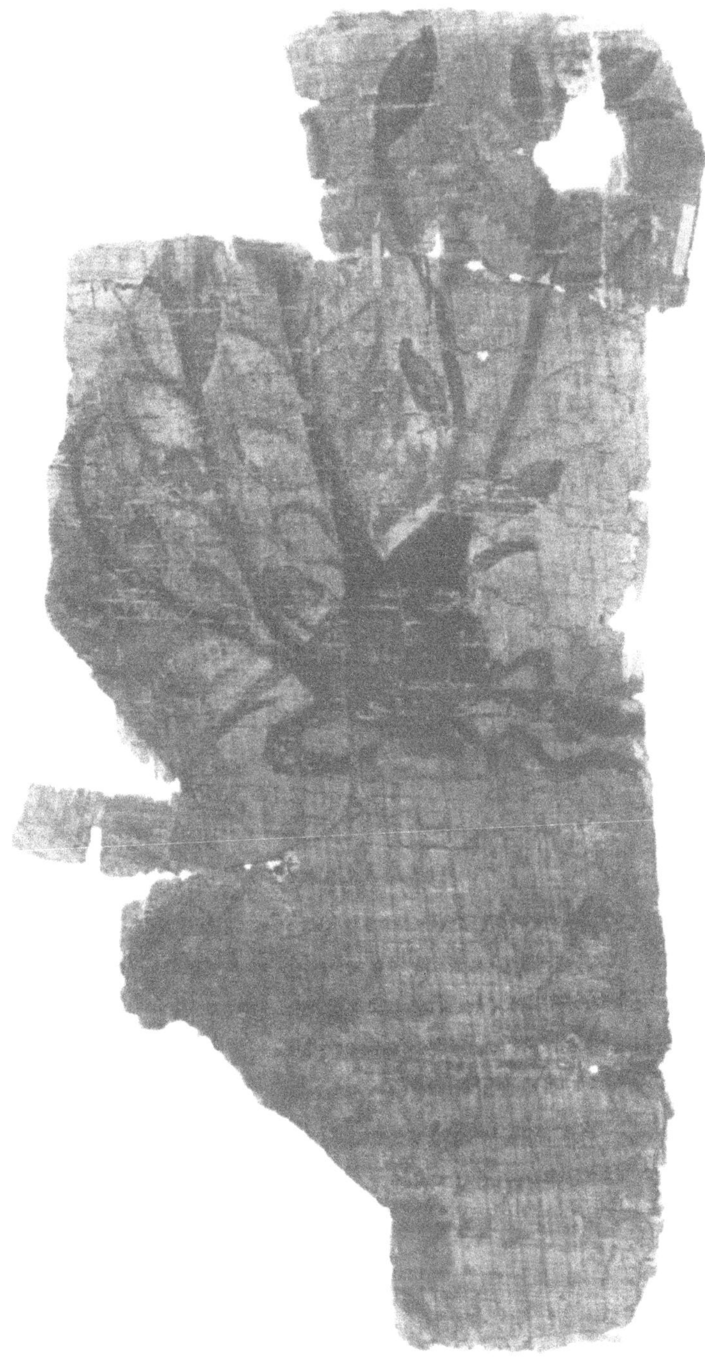

(*b*)

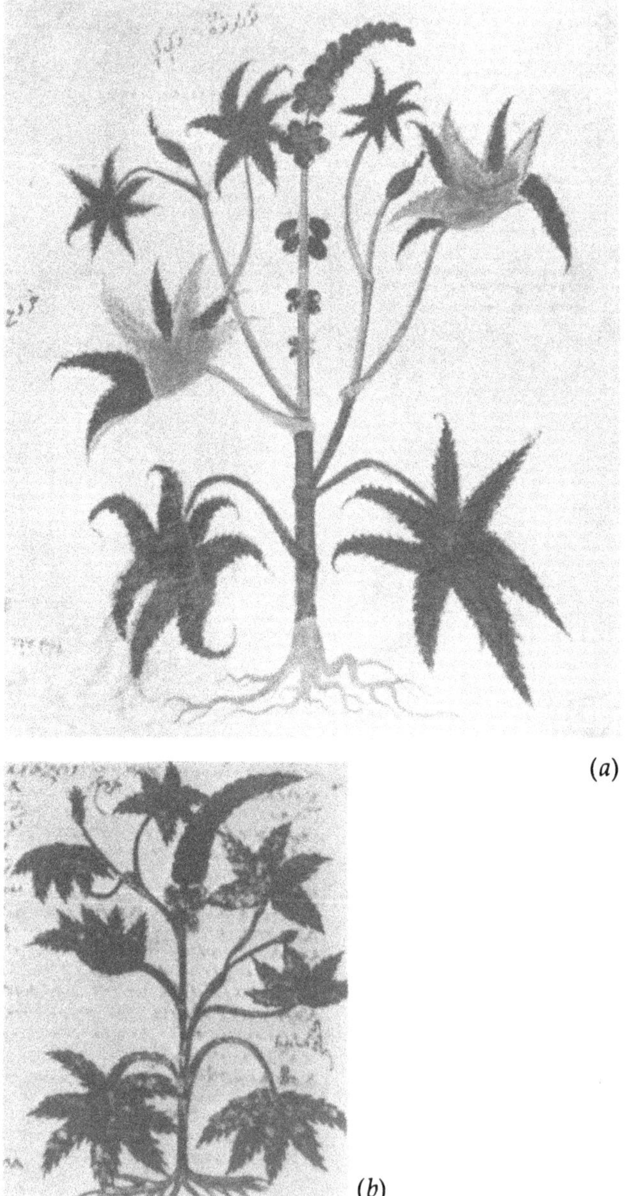

Fig. 13. (*a*) Castor oil plant (*Ricinus communis* L., IV. 164) (Vienna MS med. gr. 1, fol. 170v; courtesy Österreichische Nationalbibliothek); (*b*) castor oil plant employing the same model as the drawing in the Anicia (Paris MS gr. 2179, fol. 131v; courtesy Bibliothèque Nationale).

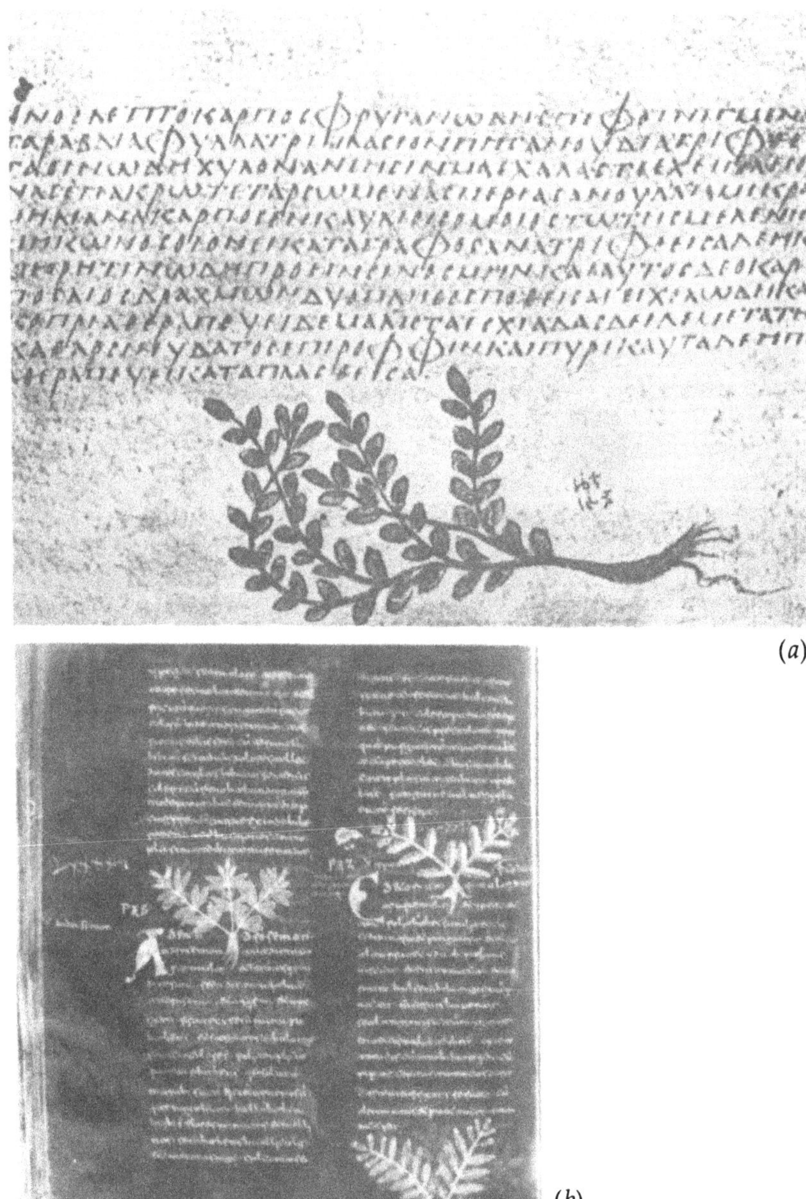

Fig. 14. (*a*) *Koris*, from Yrevan, Edschmiadzin Library, Dioscorides fragment preserved in a manuscript with a ninth-century hand (photocopy made by F. C. Conybeare now in Oxford, Bodleian Library MS gr. class. e. 19; courtesy Bodleian Library); cf. (*b*) *koris*, top plant in right column (Munich MS lat. 337, fol. 108v, 10th c.; courtesy Bayerische Staatsbibliothek).

The later manuscripts have crude marginal illustrations but, by then, the convention of indentation had gone. The later illustrations are in the left and right marginal space and the drawings are clearly subordinate to the text. Quite possibly they were added to the text later. Salamanca manuscript 2659 of the fifteenth century has Dioscorides' order with colored pictures in the margin but, like others in the Egyptian tradition, crudely drawn.[68] Even Dioscorides' Preface (which was omitted in the Anicia and Neapolitan) has five illustrations of plants mentioned in the text. The drawing of the iris in the right margin (I. 1, fol. 19) has a red-colored flower while another iris is drawn at the bottom with a white flower, perhaps intended to represent a Florentine iris (*Iris florentina* L.) or fleur-de-lis. The iris drawing in the Anicia and Neapolitan manuscripts is unmistakably the common iris (*I. germanica* L.). Dioscorides' herbal description of iris is insufficient to identify what species of iris was or were intended. On folio 22 of the Salamanca manuscript, there are two drawings, one for *malabathron* (I. 12) and the other for *kassia* (I. 13), which were plants not illustrated in the Anicia and Neapolitan manuscripts. These two plants were imperfectly known and were described by Dioscorides because they were known as plant products brought by long-distance trade, but he probably did not know them directly as whole plants. The picture of the "cassia" plant is totally unrecognizable as either cassia or cinnamon. If one wanted to draw "plant," it might look like this—a stick with leaves on it.

Human Figures Illustrating Medicinal Usages

In some Greek, Latin, and Arabic manuscripts of *De materia medica* humans are drawn beside the plants. To demonstrate this aspect of the illustrations, we shall examine pictures of the "mouse-ear" plant (II. 183, *μυὸς ὦτα*) in Paris MS gr. 2179; a wild carrot (IV. 153, *θαψία*, *Thapsia garganica* L.) and the white hellebore (IV 148) in a Latin translation in Munich MS lat. 337; and *malabathron* (I. 12) in an Arabic translation now in Leiden. The purpose of the persons beside the plants is clearly to demonstrate medicinal use for the plants. Even if one were not literate, one might use the herbal by identifying both the plant and its medicinal usage from the pictures. The question that the human figures pose is whether they are based on ancient archetypes and traceable to Dioscorides' original or whether they represent iconographical innovations in herbals.

Kurt Weitzmann, a modern scholar who has explored this question, shows an ambiguity in his various writings. In a ninth-century Greek manuscript (Paris MS gr. 2179; Fig. 15) a young man in a golden tunic

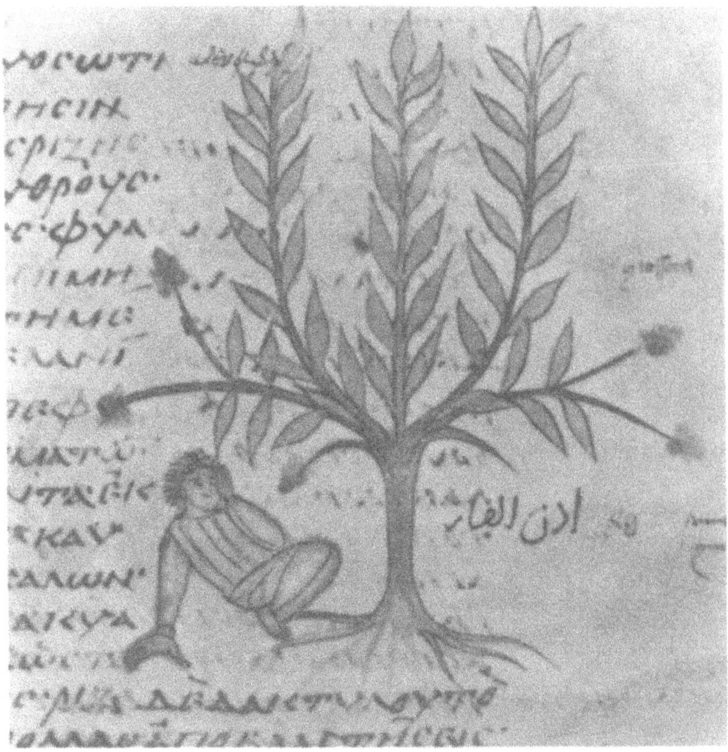

Fig. 15. "Mouse-ear" plant with man beside it demonstrating the plant's use for treating eye ulcers (Paris MS gr. 2179, fol. 5; courtesy Bibliothèque Nationale).

holds his left hand to his eye while the text explains that the "mouse-ear" plant, presently unidentified,[69] heals eye ulcers. Kurt Weitzmann says of this picture: "Significantly, the Anicia codex in Vienna and the Neapolitan are both devoid of any such human figures, and the fact that in the Greek miniature . . . the scale of the human figure is incongruous to that of the plant serves, on the formalistic side, to strengthen our thesis that human figures like these were added later."[70] Human figures are seen in the first seven folios of the Anicia manuscript. Book I and most of Book II are missing from Paris MS gr. 2179 and so there is no way to compare whether this later Paris manuscript had the equivalent frontispieces.

A figure of thapsia[71] is found in the Latin translation of Dioscorides written in Beneventan script in the tenth century, now Munich Ms. 337 (see Fig. 16).[72] The text preserves Dioscorides' order and the

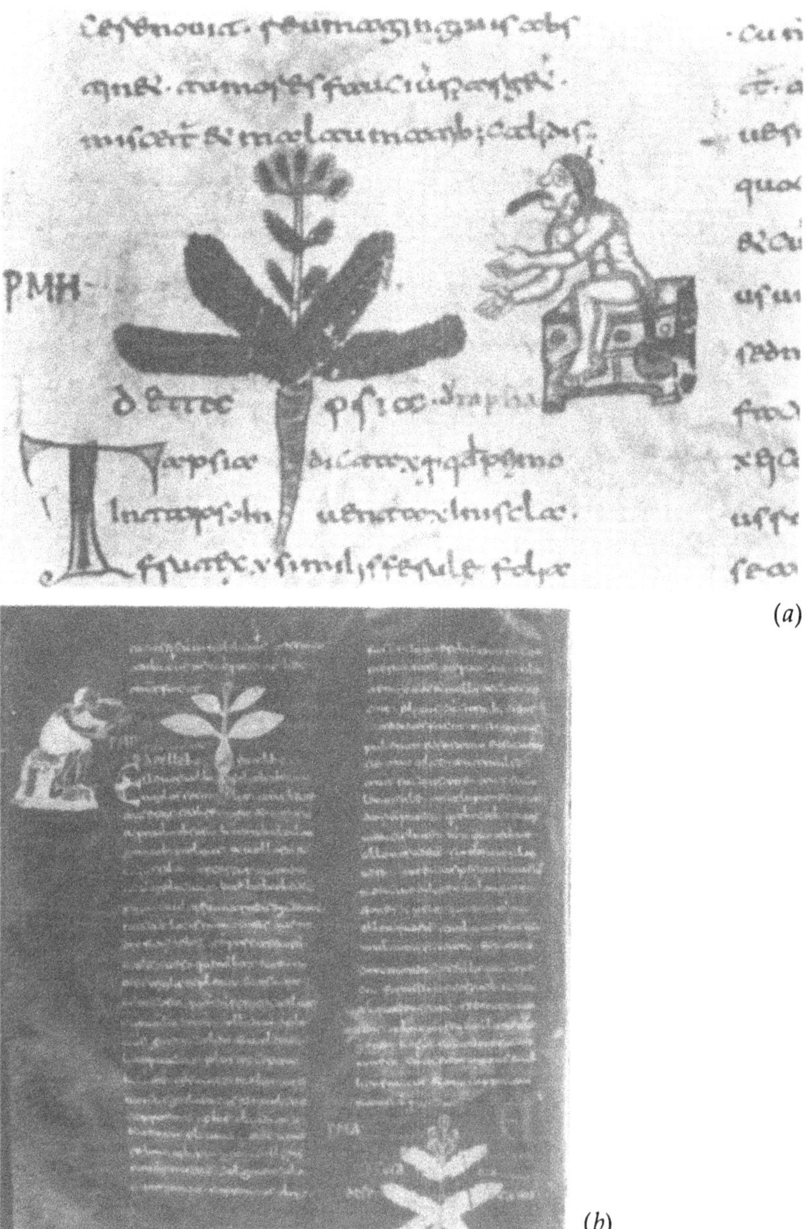

(a)

(b)

Fig. 16. (*a*) Man demonstrates thapsia's emetic and drastic purgative qualities (Munich MS lat. 337, fol. 123v), and (*b*) demonstration at top of left column of emetic quality of white hellebore, or *Veratrum album* L. (Munich MS lat. 337, fol. 108v; courtesy Bayerische Staatsbibliothek).

chapters are numbered by Greek letters.[73] It has colored plant figures throughout but, like many of the drawings in Paris MS gr. 2179, the pictures are not iconographically related to the Anicia and Neapolitan manuscripts. The drawing of thapsia here does not even appear to be the same plant as in the Anicia (fol. 140), which is a good likeness of *Thapsia garganica* L.[74] Hermann Stadler believes that the plant pictures in Munich MS 337 might have derived from a textual description since the artist was not relying on the Anicia tradition.[75] His suggestion cannot be allowed, however, because there is not enough textual description to yield the details of the drawings. Still viable is an alternate suggestion by Weitzmann, who thought the figures represented an artistic desire to supplement scientific drawings and that this development "does not become discernible to us before the ninth century."[76] The accompanying text for thapsia in Munich MS 337, fol. 125, says, ". . . it [thapsia] is warm and cathartic; if taken mixed [with honey] it purges a man upward and downward." From this description an artist could easily arrive at the drawing's message, just as he equally could have done the same from the "mouse-ear" plant.

The first human figure demonstrating a medical use to appear in an extant Arabic translation of Dioscorides is found in a drawing in a Leiden manuscript, dated A.D. February 1083 (Fig. 17). Since the Arabs were more precise in identifying their manuscripts, the colophon says that the Leiden manuscript was copied from one of the year A.D. 990,[77] but this does not necessarily mean that the drawing of the man was also in the A.D. 990 model. In an indented left margin, leaves of *malabathrum*, possibly a species of cinnamon,[78] are depicted as floating on top of water while a man sits beside the pond, as it were, holds one hand in the water, as if picking a leaf, and with the right hand holds leaves to his eye. Dioscorides' text has the explanation that the leaf "reportedly" grows without roots on the surface of Indian marshes. The leaves are harvested, he said, by being strung on a linen thread for sun drying. Boiled in wine, perforated, and placed on the eyes, the leaves are good for ophthalmological inflammations. Therefore, the details of the text here are sufficient to provide an artist, one who quite apparently may have had no knowledge of what the plant looked like, with the information to draw the picture.

In apparent contrast to his conclusions on pictures in Paris MS gr. 2179, Professor Weitzmann ended his discussion of the human figures in the Leiden Arabic Dioscorides as follows: "Was this a fancy of the illustrator of the Leiden codex or, perhaps, of its Arabic model, or was there a precedent for it in earlier Greek Dioscorides manuscripts? Intrinsic probability as well as the fragmentary, extant material supports the latter alternative."[79] Unfortunately, Weitzmann was not more

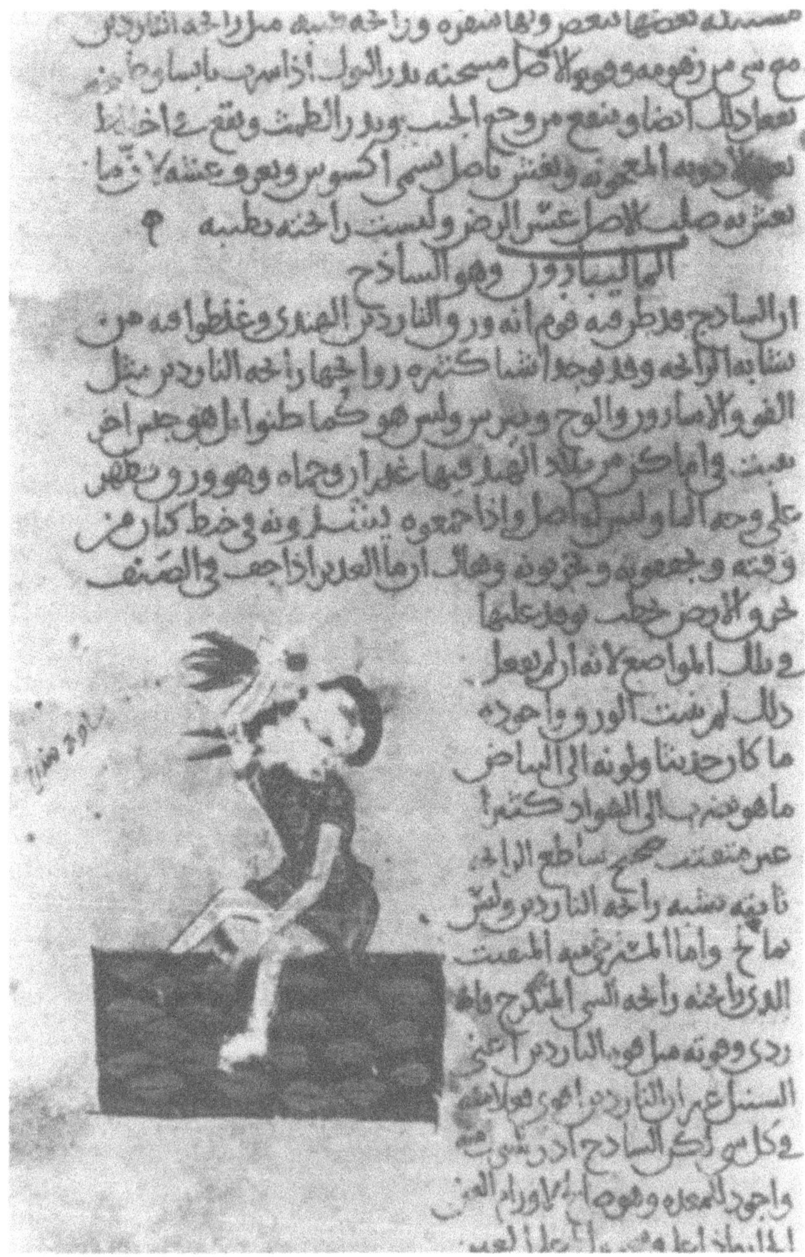

Fig. 17. Arabic manuscript, A.D. 1083, drawing of man demonstrating ophthalmologic use of *malabathrum* (Leiden MS Or. 289, fol. 8; courtesy Bibliotheek der Rijksuniversiteit).

explicit in discussing the details of his "fragmentary, extant material." Unless he was restricting his earlier observations entirely to the Byzantine tradition, in different writings Professor Weitzmann is on both sides of the issue of human figures in prototypes of classical herbals.

The Leiden picture of *malabathrum* is in sharp contrast to the equivalent picture in the Salamanca Greek Dioscorides (MS 2659, fol. 22). *Malabathrum* is seen here as an entire plant with fernlike leaves and what appears as fruit opposite some leaves coming from a single node. The Salamanca picture clearly does not follow Dioscorides' text. The same is true with the *malabathrum* picture in the Munich Latin Dioscorides of the ninth century (fol. 7v), where still a third plant is depicted with three large, symmetrical leaves coming from a root bulb out of which roots branch. The leaf shape is similar to water lily leaves. The following picture of a cassia plant (fol. 8) is entirely different from that in the Salamanca manuscript. The Munich picture is a rough likeness of the cassia plant. To the right of the plant is drawn a scorpion, alluding, we presume, to cassia's antidotal qualities, although the text does not specify a scorpion per se. For the section on perfumes (fols. 12c–13v), there are representations of alchemical equipment for perfume manufacture. From the evidence of the illustrations in Dioscorides manuscripts, the use of human and other figures to supplement the herbal pictures was an innovation of around the ninth century and derives from textual description and contemporary experience, not from ancient archetypes. Dioscorides' original work was probably devoid of these embellishments.

Continuation of Papyrus Style

Two more manuscripts have marginal drawings in the "papyrus tradition," like those in Paris MS gr. 2179 and similar to the Paris and Salamanca manuscripts. Both of them are now in Paris, Bibliothèque Nationale, where they sit side by side on the shelf as MSS gr. 2182 and gr. 2183. Both date from the fifteenth century, have colored illustrations in the margins, and preserve Dioscorides' original order. There are some dissimilarities, however. Manuscript gr. 2182 has only eleven drawings, iris (I. 1) through *malabathrum* (I. 12). Paris MS gr. 2183 has a more complete set of illuminations of both plants and animals. For example, the picture of the black hellebore (fol. 113v) bears no iconographical relation to the drawing in the Anicia and Neapolitan manuscripts for black hellebore.

Union of Byzantine and Egyptian Traditions

A beautifully illustrated manuscript of Dioscorides in alphabetical order now at Padua provides clues to the double, Byzantine and Egyptian, tradition of illustrations. Dating from the fourteenth century, it has 477 pictures of plants in all colors except gold, often one picture to a full page.[80] Its uniqueness is in its two parts. The Padua manuscript discusses the herbs from Alpha to Omega and then back again from Alpha to Omega, this second time with mostly different drugs. Unquestionably, the copyist-artist was aware that not all of Dioscorides' plants had been served, so he began another section for Part Two (fols. 180–200v) with the text borrowed from the same tradition as Salamanca MS 2659 and Paris MSS gr. 2179, 2182, and 2183.

As we now have come to expect, the pictures in Part Two are more crude but, unlike in the other manuscripts, they are not confined to the margins. Part Two begins with *amomon* (I. 15, Wellmann), a text and picture not in the Anicia manuscript. Part Two concludes the end of the manuscript with basil (II. 141, ὤκιμον), the same plant with which the first part concluded, save only the pictures of the basil plant are different. The first picture (fol. 179) shows basil's broad leaves in an opposite arrangement (i.e., two leaves at a node on opposite sides of the stem) with green flowers arising from the leaf axils. The second picture (fol. 200v) has basil with smaller leaves in the same opposite arrangement but with stalk flowers at the termini of the stems. Each picture chose to depict two different aspects of the same natural arrangement. Basil has flowers arising from both a terminal whorl globular and an axillary whorl. Neither picture was entirely right or wrong, but neither was complete. The pictures clearly arose from differing iconographical traditions.

From the pictures alone in the Dioscorides manuscripts the evidence indicates that there are at least two principal traditions in the transmission. The sixth-century Anicia and seventh-century Neapolitan manuscripts used as a model an iconographical tradition that employed non-Dioscoridean herbals, one of which was possibly Crateuas' root herbal. The date for the archetype could have been any time between the development of the codex in the second century and the end of the fifth century. Given the lower level of artistic tradition in the late empire, an earlier date, perhaps the second century, seems more likely. Accepting Weitzmann's thesis that the ninth-century Paris Dioscorides derived from a papyrus roll tradition, I tentatively suggest that Paris MSS gr. 2179, 2182, and 2183, Salamanca MS 2659, and Padua, Seminario MS 194, Part Two, derived from a tradition that was inspired by more of Dioscorides' original illustrations. The source for the Anicia-Neapolitan manuscripts also borrowed from the Dioscoridean illustrations but to a lesser extent, which would explain the iconographical similarities in some illustrations even though most pictures are dissimilar and do not derive from the same source.

Zoological Drawings and Second Alphabetical Group

Pictures of animals in *De materia medica* manuscripts are helpful in evaluating Dioscorides' illustrations, but in order to conduct the examination we must look to still another group of manuscripts. As we observed, both the Anicia and the Neapolitan manuscripts deal only with herbs[81] and Paris MS gr. 2179 is not extant for the Book Two animal section.[82] Two families of manuscripts bear witness to animal drawings. The first is the so-called Second Alphabetical Group (SAG), which, as the name suggests, has the rearranged alphabetical text.[83] Although the illustrations in this class bear a strong relationship to the Byzantine Anicia-Neapolitan family, nonetheless the source for SAG is neither the Anicia nor the Neapolitan but an earlier mutual source, the same for the Anicia-Neapolitan manuscripts. For one thing, the representatives of the SAG have more plants in them than do the Anicia and Neapolitan and, for another, SAG manuscripts have a more complete text, supplemented with illustrations of animals and even minerals.

The earliest surviving copy of the SAG is now in New York's Pierpont Morgan Library, MS 652, which dates about A.D. 890 and was probably written and drawn in the Palace at Constantinople (Fig. 18).[84] The next earliest is Vatican Library MS Pal. gr. 284, tenth century, which, for the herbal section, is similar to the New York manuscript but illustrates only a small number of the animals.[85] A twelfth-century manuscript at Mount Athos, Grand Laura Monastery, MS Ω 75, is next in the chronological line.[86] All three are beautifully illustrated with colors but the New York and Mount Athos codices are closest to one another, have the same order of treatises, and have similar illustrations. *De materia medica* in both of them is divided into five books, each with the items in alphabetical order: I, plants; II, animals; III, oils; IV, trees; and V, wines, stones, and metals (minerals). Unfortunately, the zoological illustrations are missing from the Mount Athos manuscript. The Vatican manuscript is similar in text and pictures of plants but it has a different arrangement for the other books, including pseudo-Dioscorides' *On Poisons*. Its seventy-four animal pictures are in the margin and J. Théodoridès observed that the copy-

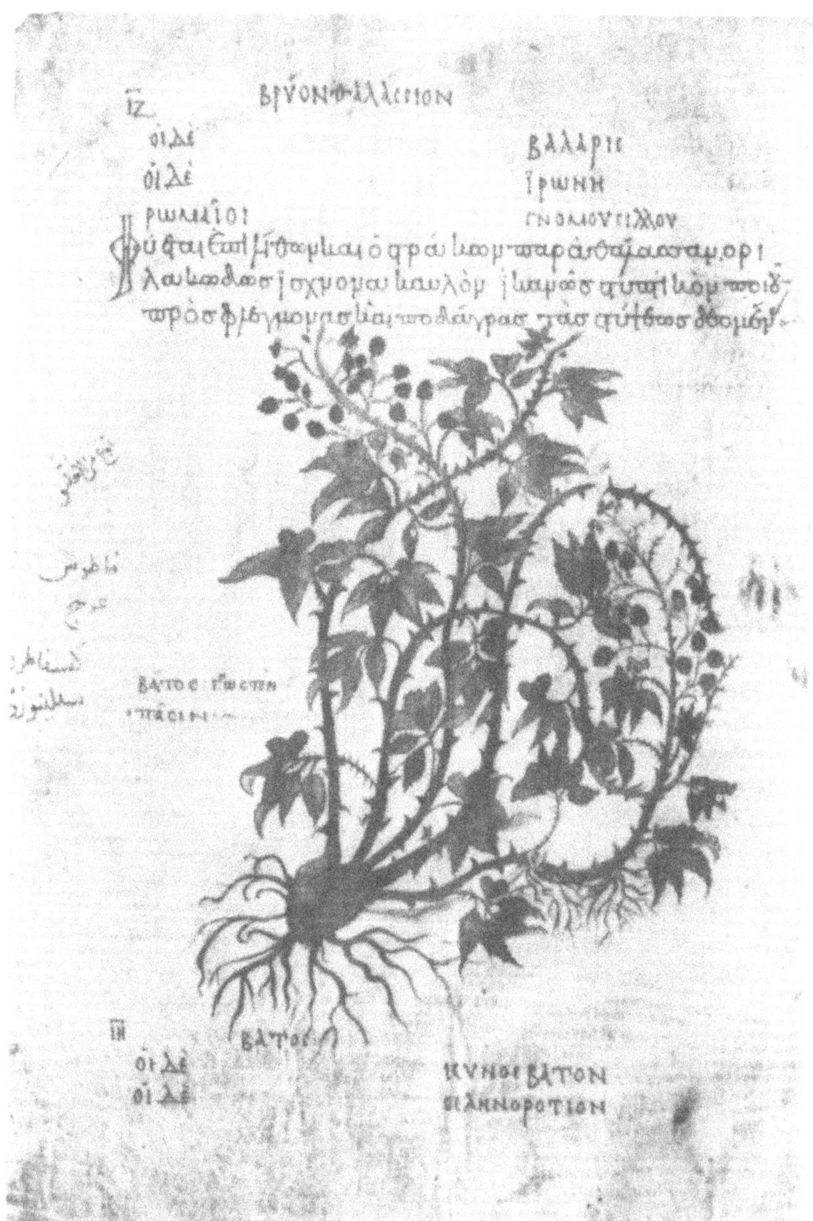

Fig. 18. Bramble (*Rubus ulmifolius*) from colored manuscript of A.D. 890, which closely resembles drawing in the Anicia (Pierpont Morgan MS 652, fol. 25v; courtesy Pierpont Morgan Library).

ists did not appear to have intended illustration. Paleographic evidence establishes that the animal pictures were added much later, in the late Byzantine period.[87]

Another group of Dioscorides manuscripts having animal pictures consists of two fourteenth-century codices, which have the illustrations and chapter headings but not Dioscorides' text: Vatican, Chigi MS 53 (F. VII. 159)[88] and Bologna, Bibl. Univ. MS gr. 3632.[89] The Vatican manuscript is more complete—the Bologna one being a mélange from various other sources. The Vatican Chigi manuscript has the plants and animals in alphabetical order and, in Otto Penzig's opinion, the plants are a direct copy of the Anicia manuscript, complete with several frontispieces, which the Chigi puts at the back.[90] The source for the animal pictures in Book Two of the Chigi escaped detection by Penzig but Kurt Weitzmann said there is no doubt that the Pierpont Morgan manuscript directly supplied the model for the animal pictures.[91] I shall shortly propose an alternative possibility that the Chigi came from the same mutual source as did the Pierpont Morgan.

The picture of the sea urchin (II. 1, Wellmann ed.), our familiar sea creature, helps resolve some problems with Dioscorides' illustrations. The sea urchin is shown in three pictures: top, bottom, and side views (Fig. 19*a*).[92] J. Théodoridès observed that the pictures in the New York Pierpont Morgan manuscript could only have been meant to illustrate the anatomy of the sea urchin. Dioscorides' text has no such description.[93] It is conjectured that these three pictures derived from Aristotle's lost *Anatomai*, supposedly once illustrated. In a brilliant study of Byzantine zoological illuminations, Zoltán Kádár said of Théodoridès' observations: "It appears, therefore, that the prototype of the time of Dioscorides for the Byzantine codices cannot have been produced after the original Aristotelian illustrations, and it is more likely that Dioscorides' illustrator would have been familiar with the pictures of the Master's treatise from later, revised and even coloured versions in the works of his pupils. . . . It is possible, therefore, that the illustrator of Dioscorides also took over the pictorial material of the *Anatomai* from this source."[94]

While I am skeptical that the lost *Anatomai* was necessarily the source, Théodoridès' and Kádár's suppositions are well taken that the pictures were not in Dioscorides' original. On the other hand, the picture of the sea urchin is entirely different in Munich manuscript 337, and this manuscript apparently has a descent different from those in both alphabetical groups (see Fig. 19*b*). Here the sea urchin appears as a mythical, bifurcated creature with the lower body of an eel with a triple-blade tail and the head of a dog or horse. This, of course, does match Dioscorides' verbal description, as the Pierpont Morgan manu-

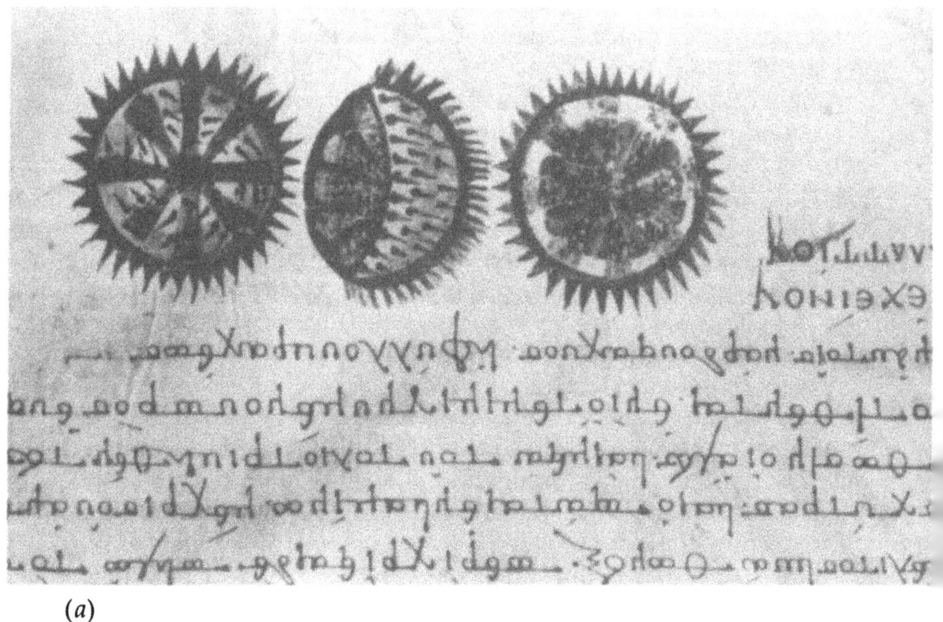

(*a*)

script did not. Similarly, the Pierpont Morgan manuscript depicts the hedgehog (II. 2, Fig. 19*c*) as what appears to be a porcupine (fol. 204), while the Munich manuscript (fol. 39) draws a running horse. Théodoridès and Kádár show how Dioscorides' chapter on the *silphe*, or cockroach (II. 36), was transformed by the Pierpont Morgan (fol. 211v) and the Chigi (fol. 210) into an aquatic animal similar to a jellyfish.[95]

In sharp contrast, the pictures of most vertebrate animals in the Second Alphabetical Group (excluding Vatican MS Pal. gr. 284) represent, Zoltán Kádár says, a "toxonomic precision and refinedness of artistic realism."[96] As an example, eight species of saltwater and one of freshwater fishes are drawn very well. The pictures of mammals and probably the testaceans as well are, according to Kádár, direct descendents likely "contemporaneous with the date of Dioscorides' treatise."[97] Kádár noted that the details for these pictures are compatible with the textual descriptions.

Because of the illuminators' propensities in the Greek-, Latin-, and Arabic-speaking areas to copy pictures of plants and animals rather than to model directly from nature, I am confident in claiming that most of the pictures are copies of ancient prototypes, whatever the language of the manuscript.

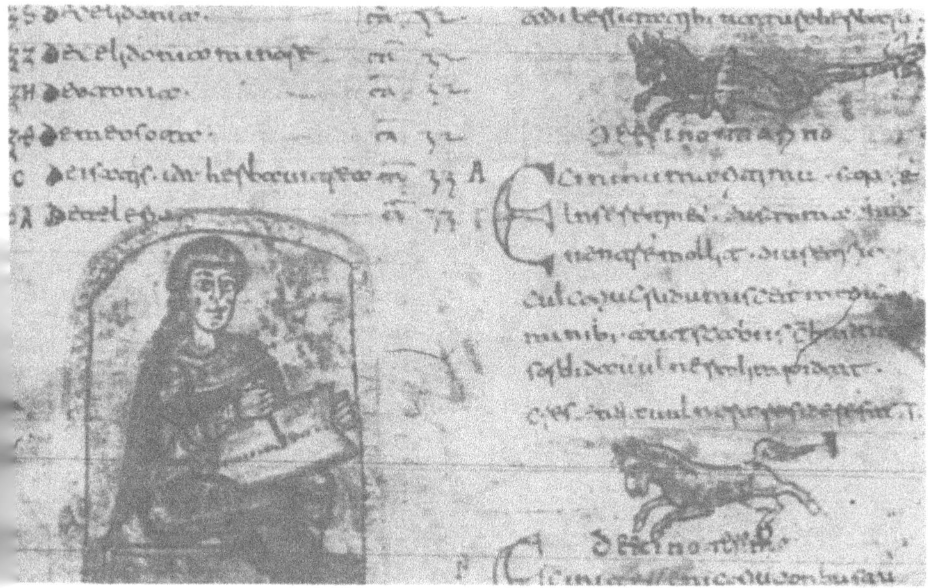

(*b*)

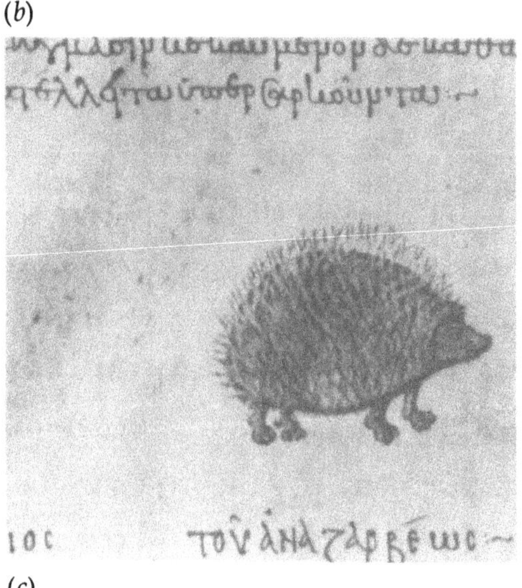

(*c*)

Fig. 19. (*a*) Anatomical views of sea urchin (Pierpont Morgan MS 652, fol. 214v); (*b*) mythical sea urchin with unrealistic "land urchin," or hedgehog, beneath; man on the left is Dioscorides (Munich MS lat. 337, fol. 39); (*c*) "land urchin," or hedgehog (Pierpont Morgan MS 652, fol. 204; courtesy Pierpont Morgan Library and Bayerische Staatsbibliothek).

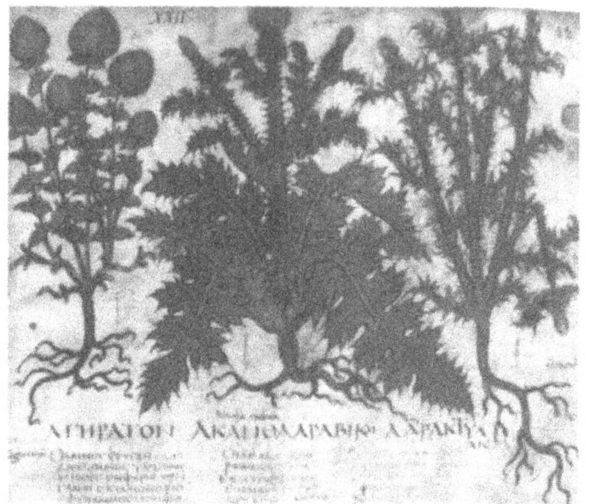

(*a*)

(*b*)

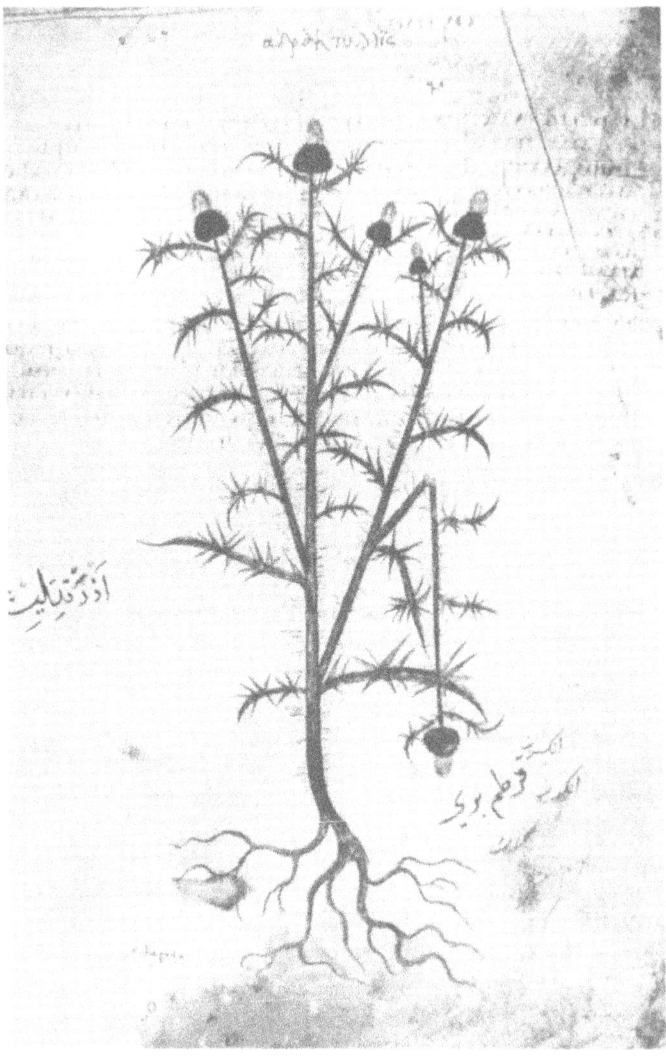

(*c*)

Fig. 20. (*a*) Thistle (*on right*) showing broken twig in seventh-century manuscript; plants shown are (*left to right*) ἀγήρατον (*Achillea viscosa*), ἄκανθα ἀράβικη (*?acanthus*), and an unidentified thistle (Naples MS gr. 1, fol. 22; courtesy Biblioteca Nazionale); (*b*) southernwood (*Artemisia abrotanus* L., III. 24, Wellmann ed.) showing broken twig on lower left (Vienna MS med. gr. 1, fol. 23v); and (*c*) thistle (Vienna MS med. gr. 1, fol. 62v; courtesy Österreichische Nationalbibliothek).

Innovations can be detected but substantially there is more continuity than interruption. A. de Premerstein, M. Diehl, H. Gerstinger, C. Singer, P. Burberl, K. Weitzmann, and Z. Kádár all affirm Hellenistic and Roman archetypes.[98] The question is how many archetypes and whether any are attributable to the original Dioscorides. The Anicia, Neapolitan, Pierpont Morgan, Mount Athos, and Chigi manuscripts are prominent examples of one direct descent, which went back no earlier than the codex, probably in the second century. The Paris MS gr. 2179 and Salamanca manuscript are examples of a second Hellenistic archetype, probably written on papyrus and earlier than the other archetype. The Latin Munich 337 and the ninth-century Armenian fragment seem to indicate possibly even a third or fourth archetype, although the evidence is less clear. Further, we had some evidence—perhaps no stronger than indications—that the Paris MS gr. 2179 line may have kept a papyrus style. Dioscorides' work probably served as a source for some, if not all, classical archetypes.

Naturalism and Phototropism

Let us return to the initial reaction that one has when seeing the beautifully illustrated herbs in the fabulous sixth-century Anicia manuscript. No scholarly attack can take away from its artistry and realism. If the Anicia artist(s) copied from manuscript models and not from real life, then someone with a keen eye, somewhere at some time, looked directly at nature and translated lines and colors onto parchment with genius. In exploring these questions, can we learn more about Dioscorides' pictures?

On folio 22 of the seventh-century Neapolitan manuscript, there is a picture of what appears to be a thistle, called ἀδρακτυλλίς, a name not appearing in Wellmann's critical edition of Dioscorides (see Fig. 20*a*). The right stem of the thistle is broken as sometimes stems were in other pictures to demonstrate something about the text or seasonal stages. For example, southernwood (III. 24) is drawn with a broken, leafless limb, thereby revealing the shrub's appearance when bare during the winter (see Fig. 20*b*). The thistle in the Neapolitan manuscript has two leaves on the brown branch that have turned upward. Depending upon the time lapse after the twig was broken, the upward leaves could be either because of a phototropic response or, if drawn immediately after breaking, because of a leaf's concavity in order to produce maximum light exposure. The artist of the Neapolitan manuscript has all leaves turned up except the leaf on the left, which turns downward, because there is an insect drawn on it. Although it is difficult to see in the photograph, the insect is clearly drawn with six legs.

Gravity pulls the left-side leaf downward, overcoming either phototropism or the concavity. The drawing of the same plant in the Anicia manuscript (Fig. 20c) is clearly copied from the same source as the Neapolitan, but there is an important difference: the lower leaf does not have an insect on it but still it turns downward. This is impossible in nature. We could suppose that the archetype had the broken stem with two leaves upward, one downward, as in the Anicia, and that the artists of the Neapolitan recognized that nature was being violated. This supposition is highly unlikely since no such innovation is reflected in the other 408 illustrations. I know of no ancient observation of phototropic action; but either for this reason or for the reason that the twig was immediately inverted, a good artist saw nature as it is. In near certainty, the ancient archetype had the insect on the downturned leaf, which the copyist artist of the Neapolitan dutifully put in his picture. On the other hand, the Anicia's illustrator excluded it, perhaps in compliance with the project's policy of dealing only with plants.

Two or More Recensions

Max Wellmann postulated that there was a second-century recension, which he called by the name of Joannine, after an obscure medical writer in the second century. Wellmann said the Joannine recension existed prior to the alphabetical recension.[99] From this recension allegedly stem all lines of extant Dioscorides' texts, be they in regular or alphabetical order. Eugen Oder challenged Wellmann's Joannine recension.[100] Campbell Bonner asserted that there were "two good but different forms of Dioscorides' text known within a generation or two after the author's death."[101] As evidence, Bonner cited the extant manuscript that is closest to the Michigan papyrus text. The postulated second recension of the second century is a nonillustrated eleventh-century manuscript in El Escorial Library (III, R 3), and its text, Bonner believes, is closest to Dioscorides' original.[102] This manuscript preserves Dioscorides' original order and comes closest textually to the Latin translation in Munich 337, which in turn is closer to the Paris MS gr. 2179 descent than to the Anicia family. Max Wellmann distrusted the Escorial manuscript reading and allowed its rendering to guide him only when confirmed by the Latin translation in Munich 337 and in a pseudo-Dioscoridean work, *Ex herbis femininis*.

If Bonner is correct—and I believe that he is—then there are serious faults with Wellmann's critical edition. We might employ the illustrations to supplement textual criticism and give us a better understanding of the early Dioscorides recensions. My analysis of the illustrations supports the hypothesis that in the Middle Ages the manuscripts—Greek, Latin, and Arabic—reveal at least two and probably three iconographical traditions that can be traced to the classical period, one of which may have been by Dioscorides' authorship. There can be little doubt that Dioscorides' manuscript was illustrated from the beginning and that those illustrations in Paris MS gr. 2179, Salamanca MS 2659, and, possibly, Munich 337 incorporated more of the artistic style of the original than did the Anicia family.

Mosaics, Frescoes, and Vases

The comparison of plant and animal drawings in mosaics, frescoes, and vase paintings introduces an additional element, one that helps us to deal with the question of the date when the artists were looking and copying directly from a natural model. The running brown rabbit in the Pierpont Morgan manuscript (fol. 213v; Fig. 21) resembles in artistic detail the depiction of a rabbit in monumental pictures, such as the hunting mosaic found at Roman Thysdrus and later in the Imperial Palace floor at Constantinople. In contrast, the Chigi manuscript (fol. 209v) portrays the rabbit seated, similar to the fresco at Herculaneum.[103] Since both the Pierpont Morgan and the Chigi have a common descent (although Weitzmann says Chigi directly used the Pierpont Morgan)[104] and since both contain rabbit pictures, one running and one seated, it is possible that these two manuscripts each took only one rabbit portrait from a common source. Nonetheless, the other pictures in the Chigi manuscript are so similar to those in the Pierpont Morgan that the weight of the evidence supports the thesis that the Chigi was a direct copy of the Pierpont Morgan manuscript.

The various birds in the Pierpont Morgan, in the words of Zoltán Kádár, "manifest a definite relationship with late Greek and Italian vase paintings of birds."[105] The murexes in the Pierpont Morgan (fol. 213), Vatican 284 (fol. 232v), and Chigi (fol. 209v) manuscripts are, Kádár wrote, "almost exact copies of the mollusc in the mosaic from Pompeii," now in Naples' museum.[106] Similarly, an *aspis* drawing in the Nicander portion of the Anicia manuscript appears to have had the same model as the Alexander mosaics from Pompeii.[107] Frescoes of plants from Pompeii and Herculaneum reveal a stylization in botanical representations, while, at the same time, some other plants were pictured in real-life representation. Wilhelmina F. Jashemski proposes that there was a new realism that was a distinctive Roman development. The garden paintings of the first century suggest that the realism innovations in naturalistic rendering existed with the traditional Hellenistic and Egyptian stylized botanical representations.[108]

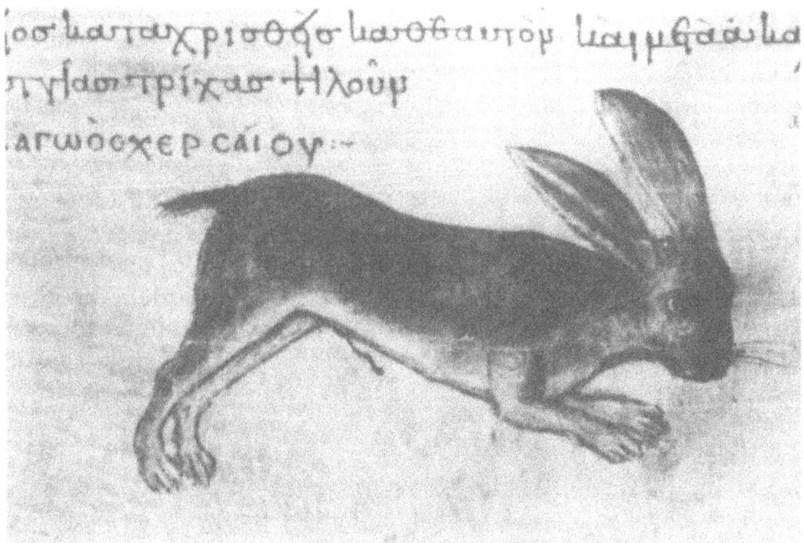

Fig. 21. Running rabbit (Pierpont Morgan MS gr. 652, fol. 213v; courtesy Pierpont Morgan Library).

The realistic fish portraits in the Pierpont Morgan resemble in artistic presentation the fish mosaics at Pompeii and Palestrina. Max Wellmann speculated that the fish pictures were based on a treatise of fishes by Dorion (1st c. B.C.), which has not survived.[109] Curiously, in 1961 at Anazarbus, Dioscorides' hometown, there was uncovered an animal mosaic with fishes whose artistic presentation varies from realism to fancy.[110] By no stretch of anyone's imagination could Dioscorides or his first illuminator have copied pictures of these natural things from mosaics, vases, or frescoes, certainly not those at Pompeii. Ancient artists-craftsmen likely consulted illustrated manuscripts when executing projects.[111]

Conclusions

At the time Dioscorides wrote, a stylized artistic presentation of nature's plants and animals was in operation, perhaps because stylization had always been a part of ancient art. Dioscorides' original manuscript may itself have been a composite, just as his later manuscripts were of drawings derived and modeled from many sources in rolled papyrus. There is no reason to suppose that his original drawings represented a pristine purity of artistic expression while modeling directly from nature.

On the contrary, if my thesis about the manuscripts closest to Dioscorides' original is correct, his drawings were not as good as those in the Anicia or the Byzantine recension. Dioscorides' originals were likely crude line drawings, such as appear in the Armenian fragment and the Umm el Baragât papyrus. When Pliny noted that Crateuas, Dionysius, and Metrodorus painted their own likenesses of medical plants and, for all artists, "the aim is to copy nature," Pliny was not delivering a compliment. Pliny belittled such efforts, perhaps because he believed nature was so diverse that no single plant can be captured so as to present the diversity of the same plant in various seasons or individual differences. Pliny did not think very highly of plant representations, I think, because they were not of the quality that we see in the Anicia.

The naturalism of the Anicia drawings cannot be pushed aside even though all evidence points to their being stylized copies of an earlier model. Wellmann, Premerstein, Singer, and others are undoubtedly correct in proposing a second- or third-century archetype for the Anicia and its family. The evidence as to when in classical times naturalism was strongest is not entirely clear. I believe on the available evidence that, from the time of Dioscorides, and probably before, the practice of drawing nature using as a model a prior picture of nature was routine. When artists began to draw the materials of medicine to illuminate Dioscorides' text, they sought various models. They fit the picture that they thought best among those available to the text. Probably, Dioscorides or his artist did this with the first five scrolls. Likely, with the development of the codex, naturalism and less stylization were more evident. Nonetheless, the copyist-artists would employ earlier pictures for their drawings to a greater or lesser degree until printing. Even with the printed books, the fifteenth- and sixteenth-century woodcutters followed the same procedure to illustrate the printed words. Mistakes were made about the identity of a particular plant or animal, but, in the same process, corrections were made in older manuscript copies.

Dioscorides' work became the vehicle to make adjustments in knowledge about nature. Even now, we cannot be certain about some aspects of his original presentation. The quality of his pictures was not as great as the quality of his written word. I presume that the quality of the pictures improved sometime before the early sixth century, largely because the medium changed. Parchment codex was superior to roll papyrus. From the time of the Byzantine recension (ca. A.D. 150–450), there was decline in the artistic quality—though there would be some few advances. Notably, the Arabs, a people whose culture was not known for naturalism in art, made some of the more significant changes in the drawings and, notably more so, in the interpretation of Dioscorides' text.

Life is short, the art long, Hippocrates said and Dioscorides demonstrated. Adorning the Anicia manuscript as a frontispiece is the picture of an artist who drew the mandrake from real life. When that artist lived is not known, nor can it be known. In a way he lived in all ages. Certainly, he was outnumbered for sixteen hundred years by those artists around him who drew nature from a book in front of them. Dioscorides' original pictures were the easel for following generations to draw their own interpretations of what he first discussed and drew.

NOTES

Introduction

1. The title is taken from the rubrics of most manuscript copies and Galen spoke of it as περὶ ὕλης (*De simplicium medicamentorum temperamentis ac facultatibus*, VI. pref., 11: 795). In the body of the text, the title is used by Dioscorides in the Preface to Book III. Max Wellmann ("Dioskurides," *P.W.* 5, pt. 1 [1903]: 1131–1142) said that Dioscorides may have taken his title from the title of Sextius Niger's lost work on drugs, but there is no reason to question that this was the correct title to Dioscorides' work nor is there any particular problem with the possibility of two works with similar titles, since scrolls had no easy way to be titled as a book format permits.

2. Since modern scientific names for individual plants do not correspond exactly with Dioscorides' "kinds" (εἴδα) of plants, exact quantification of the number of plants he described for their medicinal properties is impossible. It is also difficult, to a lesser extent, to quantify the minerals and animal products he discussed. For instance, in one chapter Dioscorides described the plant *tithumalos* (IV. 164) and said that there were nine kinds. We recognize *tithumalos* as spurge, or Euphorbiaceae, a *family* of plants of which there are about 280 genera and over 8,000 species (L. H. Bailey, *Manual of Cultivated Plants Most Commonly Grown in the Continental United States and Canada*, p. 616). Most modern scholars have listed *tithumalos* in Dioscorides as one plant and arrive at a rough figure of 500–600 plants they say Dioscorides discussed. In the case of spurge, one cannot list nine plants corresponding to Dioscorides' nine "kinds" of *tithumaloi* because his "kinds" are not always discernible. Hermolaus Barbarus in the 1480s counted 813 plants and plant products, 101 animal products, and 102 minerals in the entire five-book work. I believe Hermolaus Barbarus' counting procedures to be more accurate than Max Wellmann's in identifying the quantity of items.

3. Antonius Pinaeus or DuPinet, *Historia plantarum*.

4. Charles Singer, "The Herbal in Antiquity," *Journal of Hellenic Studies* 47

(1927): 21; cf. Johann Heinrich Dierback, *Die Arzneimittel des Hippokrates,* which has a higher count, but his classification scheme is dates, both too precise for the Hippocratic corpus and too imprecise for us today.

5. Arthur K. Shapiro, "The Placebo Effect in the History of Medical Treatment: Implications for Psychiatry," *American Journal of Psychiatry* 116 (1959): 298–301.

6. Herbert Benson and David P. McCallie, Jr., "Angina Pectoris and the Placebo Effect," *New England Journal of Medicine* 300, no. 25 (1979): 1424–1429; Henry R. Bourne, "Rational Use of Placebo," in *Clinical Pharmacology,* ed. Kenneth L. Melmon and Howard F. Morrelli, pp. 1052–1062; Jean Comaroff, "A Bitter Pill to Swallow: Placebo Therapy in General Practice," *Sociological Review* n.s. 24 (1976): 79–96.

7. Charles E. Rosenberg, "The Therapeutic Revolution: Medicine, Meaning, and Social Change in Nineteenth-Century America," *Perspectives in Biology and Medicine* 20 (1977): 491.

8. J. Worth Estes, "Making Therapeutic Decisions with Protopharmacologic Evidence," *Transactions and Studies of the College of Physicians of Philadelphia* 1, no. 2 (1979): 131.

9. Henry F. Dowling, *Medicines for Man,* p. 14.

10. E.g., Antonio Scarpa, "Pre-Scientific Medicines: Their Extent and Value," *Social Science and Medicine* A, 15A (1981): 317–326; Julia F. Morton, *Major Medicinal Plants;* Paul Schauenberg and Ferdinand Paris, *Guide des plantes médicinales;* Siri von Reis Altschul, *Drugs and Foods from Little Known Plants;* Tony Swain, ed., *Plants in the Development of Modern Medicine;* and the contributions in the *Journal of Ethnopharmacology* 1– (1979–), *Quarterly Journal of Crude Drug Research* 1– (1961–), and *Acta Phytotherapeutica* 1– (1954–).

11. Aristotle, *Physics,* VII. 25 (242B. 59 ff.).

12. Andrejus Korolkovas and Joseph H. Burchhater, *Essentials of Medicinal Chemistry,* pp. 7–8.

13. Kaspar von Sternberg, *Catalogus plantarum ad septem varias editiones commentariorum Matthioli in Dioscoridem.*

14. Curtius Sprengel, in *Medicorum Graecorum opera quae exstant.*

15. Janus Saracenus, *τὰ σωζόμενα ἅπαντα . . . Opera quae extant omnia.*

16. Julius Berendes, *Des Pedanios Dioskurides aus Anazarbos Arzneimittellehre in fünf Buchern.*

17. Robert T. Gunther, *The Greek Herbal of Dioscorides.*

18. Charles Daubeny, *Lectures on Roman Husbandry.*

19. For a brief history of the treatise, see John Riddle, "Dioscorides," *Catalogus Translationum et Commentariorum* 4 (1980): 134–139.

20. Joannes A. Fabricius, *Bibliotheca Graeca,* 4: 682–683.

21. Max Wellmann, "Dioskurides," p. 1140.

22. Max Wellmann, *Die Schrift des Dioskurides Περὶ ἁπλῶν φαρμάκων: Ein Beitrag zur Geschichte der Medizin.*

23. Ibid., p. 74.

1. *Dioscorides and the Materials of Medicine*

1. In addition to the fact that most manuscript copies include Anazarbus as part of Dioscorides' name, Galen (*De simpl. med.*, VI. pref., 11:794) gave his hometown.

2. David Magie, *Roman Rule in Asia Minor*, 1:275, 2:1151; A. H. M. Jones, *The Cities of the Eastern Roman Provinces*, pp. 195, 200, 204–207.

3. E.g., *De materia medica*, III. 68, cf. IV. 32. Unless otherwise noted, all citations are to Max Wellmann's edition, *Pedanii Dioscuridis Anazarbei De materia medica libri quinque*.

4. E.g., Wellmann, "Dioskurides," pp. 1131–1132; George Sarton, *Introduction to the History of Science*, 1:258–259; Lynn Thorndike, *A History of Magic and Experimental Science*, 1:605–611.

5. Petrus Lambecius, *Commentariorium de augustissima Bibliotheca Caesarea Vindobonensi*, 2:197.

6. Franz Susemihl, *Geschichte der griechischen Litteratur in der Alexandrinerzeit*, 2:443–444; Ernst H. F. Meyer, *Geschichte der Botanik*, 2:96–97; for a long list of those named Dioscorides, see Fabricius, *Bibliotheca Graeca*, 6:3.

7. John Scarborough and Vivian Nutton, "The Preface of Dioscorides' *Materia Medica*: Introduction, Translation, Commentary," *Transactions and Studies of the College of Physicians of Philadelphia* 4, no. 3 (1982): 197–198.

8. Max Wellmann, "Λεκάνιος Ἄρειος," p. 626, with references in Galen; Scarborough and Nutton, "Preface," pp. 198–199.

9. Dioscorides' expression, *φύσει μὲν πρὸς πάντας τοὺς ἀπὸ παιδείας ἀναγομένους οἰκειούμενος, μάλιστα δὲ πρὸς τοὺς ὁμοτέχνους* (*De materia medica*, Pref. 4, lines 21–23), seems at first to be referring to a close friendship between him and Areios (see translation by Scarborough and Nutton, "Preface," p. 196). The use of the word *οἰκειούμενος*, however, conveys a stronger sense than friendliness; instead, it denotes a direct physician-apprenticeship relationship. The Hellenistic expression (*ὁ ἀπὸ τῆς . . . φίλου οἰκίας*) "coming from the house of . . ." meant, in the opinion of Peter Marshal Fraser (*Ptolemaic Alexandria*, 1:357, 2:526–527n.), ". . . a particularly close relationship between master and pupil, and not merely to an adherent of this or that particular school"; cf. Erotian, *Erotani vocum Hippocraticarum collectio cum fragmentis*, Pref. 31 (p. 4), and Galen, *De venae sectione adversus Erasistratum*, 2, 11:196–197. Liddell and Scott, *Greek English Lexicon*, translate the expression in Erotian and Galen (17a:826) as "medical school." Fraser's study shows that the term is not employed when denoting indirect pupil-teacher relationships, such as Plotinus was a student of Plato.

10. Acts 21:39; W. M. Ramsay, *The Cities of St. Paul*, pp. 228–235; Strabo, *Geography*, XIV. 13.

11. The recognition of Tarsus as a pharmacy-pharmacology center is made by Scarborough and Nutton, "Preface," pp. 192–193.

12. Although *ἐκ πρώτης ἡλικίας* is translated here as "youth," it also may mean "the beginning of prime life," or "the first of manhood," or even "puberty." Berendes' German translation (p. 20) has "von der ersten reiferen

Jugendzeit." The context suggests the beginning of a medical apprenticeship.

13. Curtius Sprengel believed him to be a military physician. John Goodyer in 1655 (p. 2) translated the phrase as "I led a soldier's life" and Julius Berendes translated (p. 20) the phrase as "unsere militärische Laufbahn." Max Wellmann ("Dioskurides," p. 1131) said that he was a "Militärarzt wohl unter Claudius," or "a military physician probably under Claudius" (ruled A.D. 41–54). More recently, John Scarborough and Vivian Nutton proposed "my soldier's life."

14. The error is commonly made, as when T. Clifford Allbutt (*Greek Medicine in Rome*, p. 375) said that "he travelled in Italy as a military doctor." More recently, Ricardo Archila ("Pedacio Dioscorides," *Sociedad Mexicana de Historia y Filosofía de la Medicina Boletín* suppl. [1980]: 4–5) wrote ". . . que adquirió de derecho de ciudadania en Rome por haber survido en al ejército romano, sin duda en calidad de médico militar." And Chauncey D. Leake (*An Historical Account of Pharmacology to the 20th Century*, p. 60): ". . . Dioscorides, the surgeon who trampled all over the Empire with the armies of Nero."

15. For binding wounds: I. 102, 103; for binding bloody wounds: I. 68, 74, 84, 109, 110, 127; for cleaning dirty or festering wounds: I. 19; for prevention of wound infection: I. 69.

16. Pinaeus, *Historia plantarum*, nos. 239–249. Pinaeus sometimes listed usages from Andreas Mattheolus' commentary on Dioscorides, so these figures may be inflated.

17. From my own translation of Book I.

18. Pinaeus, *Historia plantarum*, nos. 183–200.

19. Although there is some inscriptionary evidence to indicate that military physicians may have treated civilian population in the camps around the legionary posts. See Gerhard Baader, "Ärzte auf pannonischen Inschriften," *Klio* 55 (1973): 273–279.

20. John Scarborough, "Roman Medicine and the Legions," *Medical History* 12 (1968): 254–261; Vivian Nutton, "Medicine and the Roman Army," *Medical History* 13 (1969): 260–270. There was one *medicus* by the name of Callimorphus mentioned by Lucianus (*How to Write History* 16. 24–25, 6:27, Kiburn ed.), but he wrote a history, not a medical work. R. W. Davies, "The Medici of the Roman Armed Forces," *Epigraphische Studien* 8 (1969): 97, and "Some More Military Medici," ibid. 9 (1972): 2–3. Graham Webster, *The Roman Imperial Army*, pp. 250–251.

21. In counting, I have excluded the first twenty-nine chapters in Book I, which are on aromatics, because they were mostly trade items from distant places that Dioscorides did not see.

22. *De materia medica*, I. 19, 67, 70; IV. 157.

23. Scarborough and Nutton, "Preface," pp. 213–217.

24. W. Morel, "Pharmakopoles," *P.W.* 19, pt. 2 (1938): 1840–1841.

25. Galen, *De fasciis liber*, 1, 18a, 770; Fridolf Kudlien, *Der griechische Ärzt im Zeitalter des Hellenismus*, p. 94, and "Medical Education in Classical Antiquity," in *The History of Medical Education*, ed. C. D. O'Malley, p. 9.

26. Diodorus, *Library*, XXXII. 11. 2–3; cf. Fridolf Kudlien. "Diodors Zwitter-

exkurs als Testimonium hellenistischer Medizin," *Clio Medica* 1 (1960): 319–324.

27. Kudlien, *Der griechische Ärzt*, p. 94.

28. For instance, Galen, *De compositione medicamentorum secundum locos libri X*, VIII. 7, 13:204. See also Julius Berendes, *Die Pharmazie bei den alten Kulturvölkern*, 1:253–254; Vivian Nutton, "The Chronology of Galen's Early Career," *Classical Quarterly* 23 (1973): 158–171, esp. 160–161.

29. Theophrastus, *Enquiry into Plants*, IX. 8. 5, 2:257, and IX. 8. 1, 2:250–251. A good discussion of the *rhizotomoi* is by G. E. R. Lloyd, *Science, Folklore, and Ideology*, pp. 119–135, esp. 120; Lloyd observes that Sophocles wrote a play entitled *Rhizotomoi*, about which we know little except that it related to the Medea legend.

30. In addition to Crateuas, Galen wrote of "Antonios, the Root-cutter," *De comp. med. secundum locos*, II. 1, 2, 12:557, 580.

31. Kudlien, *Der griechische Ärzt*, p. 94.

32. Pref. 1, p. 195, Scarborough-Nutton trans.

33. For the most thorough discussion, see Max Wellmann, *Krateuas*, and collected fragments by Wellmann in vol. 3 of *De materia medica*, pp. 139–146.

34. Galen, *De comp. med. secundum locos*, VII. 3, 13: 68: "*ἡ Παμφίλου μιγματοπώλου καλή*."

35. Galen, *De antidotis*, I. 2, 14:24: "*καὶ οὐκ ἂν εὐπορήσειεν* [in sense of household remedies] *ἐν ἄλλῳ χωρίῳ, καὶ διὰ τοῦτο ἐν Ῥώμῃ σκευάζουσι τὰς τοιαύτας ἀντιδότους οὐχ οἱ ἄριστοι μόνοι τῶν ἰατρῶν, ἀλλὰ καὶ οἱ μυροπῶλαι, πάντες μέντοι τῶν ἐν αὐταῖς ἁμαρτάνοντες ἔλαττον ἢ μεῖζον, ὅμως μὴ συντιθέντες ἄχρηστον φάρμακον*."

36. Dioscorides, *De materia medica*, I. 109 (4, 1:103, 6, Wellmann).

37. For a listing of Latin terms for various druggists, see Edward Kremers and George Urdang, *A History of Pharmacy*, p. 20, and more detailed discussions in Berendes, *Die Pharmazie*, passim.

38. Kudlien, "Medical Education in Classical Antiquity," pp. 8–9.

39. George M. Foster and Barbara Gallatin Anderson, *Medical Anthropology*, pp. 104–110.

40. Pref. 5, p. 196, Scarborough-Nutton trans. The words have a range of meaning, including "the same profession," "fellow workers," "fellow physicians," and "fellow craftsmen."

41. The phrase *οἶσθα γὰρ ἡμῖν στρατιωτικὸν τὸν βιόν* can also mean "for *we* as you know have lived a soldierlike life." If this were Dioscorides' meaning, Dioscorides would have included Areios as one who, like him, had a life resembling a soldier's, if not part of it.

42. Soranus, *Vita Hippocratis*, I. 252.

43. Galen, *De compositione medicamentorum per genera*, VI. 15, 13:857; cf. VI. 11, 13, VI. 13, 13:852, I. 1, 13:347, and *De comp. med. secundum locos*, VI. 3, 12:829; M. Wellmann, "Ἄρειος p. 626.

44. Jerry Stannard, "Asclepiades," in *Dictionary of Scientific Biography*, 1: 314–315, refs.; Scarborough and Nutton, "Preface," pp. 206–208; Elizabeth Rawson, "The Life and Death of Asclepiades of Bithynia," *Classical Quarterly*

32, no. 2 (1982): 358–370. Of particular interest is John Scarborough, "The Drug Lore of Asclepiades of Bithynia," *Pharmacy in History* 17 (1975): 43–57, esp. 55, where he shows that Dioscorides valued Asclepiades' drugs.

45. Celsus, *De medicina*, Prooemium, 8.

46. The Hippocratic Oath was influential to some degree in the first century on the testimony of Scribonius Largus (*Conpositiones*, Pref., pp. 2 ff.) and Soranus (*Gynaeciorum*, pp. 45, 8 ff.); cf. K. Deichgräber, *Professio medici—Zum Vorwort des Scribonius Largus*.

47. Kudlien, "Medical Education in Classical Antiquity," pp. 8, 19–20.

48. On the Oath, see "Contraception," below.

49. Especially good for connecting Hellenistic physicians with those of the Classical Age is P. M. Fraser, *Ptolemaic Alexandria*, 1:338–376, and Kudlien, *Der griechische Ärzt*.

50. Wesley Smith, "Galen on Coans versus Cnidians," *Bulletin of the History of Medicine* 47 (1973): 569–585, and incorporated in his book, *The Hippocratic Tradition*.

51. Kudlien, "Medical Education in Classical Antiquity," p. 3.

52. On the position of physicians and specializations, see Gerhard Baader, "Der Ärztliche Stand in der Antike," in *Jahrbuch der Universität Düsseldorf, 1977/8*, pp. 301–315. Celsus, *De medicine*, Prooemium, 9, divided medicine into two divisions, one of them being a tripartite subdivision: "one . . . which cures through diet, another through medicaments (*quae medicamentis*) and the third by the hand." The same tripartite division was made by Galen, *Hippocratis de acutorum morborum victu*, I. 5, 15:425.

53. Kudlien, "Medical Education in Classical Antiquity," pp. 16, 23.

54. Pref., 5, Scarborough-Nutton trans.

55. See "Wines, Waters, and Medicinal Drinks" in Chap. 4, below.

56. The question as to how a community acquired public physicians is examined by Louis Cohn-Haft, *The Public Physicians of Ancient Greece*, pp. 18, 65–67.

57. The literature on the subject of temple medicine is large, but a good start with references can be found in P. M. Fraser, *Ptolemaic Alexandria*, 1: 343–346, 2:497–503n, and E. J. Edelstein and L. Edelstein, *Asclepius*.

58. Kudlien, "Medical Education in Classical Antiquity, p. 9.

59. Cohn-Haft, *Public Physicians*, pp. 21–22; accepted by Kudlien, *Der griechische Ärzt*, p. 29.

60. Cohn-Haft, *Public Physicians*, p. 21.

61. There is a procedure in selecting a public physician in Athens by Plato (Georgias 455B, 456B, 514 D=E) and discussed by Cohn-Haft (*Public Physicians*, pp. 56–61), but the Athenian procedure was not typical and, even so, represented a procedural means of polling the community.

62. Cohn-Haft, *Public Physicians*, p. 67 and passim. An Oxyrhynchus papyrus of A.D. 182 (P. Oxy. 475) reveals that one function of the public physicians was to act as a coroner (see Naphtali Lewis, *Life in Egypt under Roman Rule*, p. 106).

63. A situation resented by the Hippocratic author of *The Art*, VIII.

64. John Riddle, *Marbode of Rennes' De lapidibus*, pp. 4–5.

65. See Hippocrates, *The Art*, VI.

66. P. M. Fraser, *Ptolemaic Alexandria*, 1:353.

67. For biographical information about each of the named writers, see Scarborough and Nutton, "Preface," pp. 205–260 refs.

68. Pref., 2, Scarborough-Nutton trans.

69. Stannard, "Asclepiades," pp. 314–315.

70. For an example, see criticisms made by Caelius Aurelianus (5th c. A.D.), *On Acute Diseases and on Chronic Diseases*, 1:15–17 and passim.

71. Ludwig Edelstein, "The Methodists," in *Ancient Medicine*, pp. 173–191; Kudlien, "Medical Education in Classical Antiquity," p. 17; Caelius Aurelianus, *On Acute Diseases*, p. xvii. Galen is an excellent but highly partisan source for these schools in his treatise "On Medical Sects: For Beginners," trans. by A. J. Brock, *Greek Medicine*, pp. 130–157.

72. Caelius Aurelianus, *On Acute Diseases*, pp. xvi–xvii; Edelstein, "The Methodists," pp. 190–191.

73. Galen, *De methodo medendi*, I. 1, 10:4–5. Hans Diller, "Thessalos," P.W. 6A, pt. 1 (1936): 169; cf. Kudlien, "Medical Education in Classical Antiquity," p. 17, who seems more skeptical.

74. Kudlien, "Medical Education in Classical Antiquity," p. 18; Cohn-Haft, *Public Physicians*, pp. 23–31.

75. The leading Skeptic writer on medicine is Sextus Empiricus (ca. A.D. 200), who devoted a concerted attack on the Dogmatists. See his work with an excellent introduction in *Sextus Empiricus*, ed. and trans. R. G. Bury. The link with the Methodists is discussed by Ludwig Edelstein, "Empiricism and Skepticism in the Teaching of the Greek Empiricist School," in *Ancient Medicine*, ed. Oswei and C. Lillian Temkins, pp. 195–203, esp. 197.

76. In general, see E. R. Dodds, *Pagan and Christian in an Age of Anxiety*.

77. The Dogmatists were sometimes called the Rationalists (see Galen, "On Medical Sects," 3). The Empiricists are thought by some to have separated from the Logicians (see L. Edelstein, "Empiricism and Skepticism," pp. 193–196).

78. The still-classic study is Karl Deichgräber, *Die griechische Empirikerschule*.

79. Celsus, *De medicina*, Prooemium, 65: ". . . according to Themison, knowledge of a disease is outside the Art, and medicine is confined to practice."

80. Ibid., pp. 23–24, 27, 40–45.

81. Kudlien, "Medical Education in Classical Antiquity," p. 15.

82. Max Wellmann, "Athenaios," *P.W.* 2 (1896): 2034–2036.

83. Philo Judaeus, *On Husbandry*, 13 (I. 302); cf. Liddell and Scott, *Greek English Lexicon*, and Kudlien, "Medical Education in Classical Antiquity," pp. 23–24.

84. K. Deichgräber, "Petronius," *P.W.*, 19, pt. 1 (1937): 1193–1194; idem, "Sextius Niger," *P.W.* 5 suppl. (1931): 971–972.

85. Max Wellmann, "Sextius Niger: Eine Quellenuntersuchung zu Dioscorides," *Hermes* 24 (1889): 546.

86. *De materia medica*, IV. 148.

87. Max Wellmann, "Zur Geschichte der Medicin im Alterthum," *Hermes* 23 (1888): 564; Ernst Bernert, "Philonides," *P.W.* 20, pt. 1 (1941): 73–74.

88. Pliny the Younger, *Letters*, III. 5.

89. Charles G. Nauert, Jr., "Caius Plinius Secundus," *Catalogus Translationum et Commentariorum* 4 (1980): 300.

90. Erotian, *Vocum Hippocraticarum*, p. 51.

91. Meyer, *Geschichte*, 2:134–136; Cohn, "Erotianos," *P.W.* 6, pt. 1 (1907): 544–549; Sarton, *Introduction*, 1:264; P. M. Fraser, *Ptolemaic Alexandria*, 1:365–366, 2:540–541 refs.

92. Pliny, *Natural History*, XXVI. 4. 5 (hereafter referred to as *N.H.*); Tacitus, *Annals*, XV. 33; Max Wellmann, "Bassus," *P.W.* 10 (1918): 180–181.

93. Magie, *Roman Rule*, 2:1582 refs., on inscriptionary evidence. Dioscorides refers to L. Bassus with the title of address *κρατίστια*, or "his excellency." The Greek term is used as an equivalent for both *clarissimus* (the Latin address for senatorial rank) and *egregius* (equestrian rank). Because of the imprecision in meaning we cannot discover Bassus' rank and, therefore, the stage of his career when Dioscorides referred to him—assuming that the two identities belong to the same person. On Bassus, see Scarborough and Nutton, "Preface," p. 217.

94. Wellmann, "Sextius Niger," pp. 530–569. The first to propose that similarities between Pliny's and Dioscorides' works could be explained best by postulating a mutual source was Claude de Saumaise, or Salmasius (1588–1653), *Plinianae exercitationes in Caii Julii Soilini Polyhistoria*.

95. Galen calls it a small book: Βιβλίδιον τὶ σμικρόν (*De comp. med. secundum locos*, IX. 4, 13:271).

96. Pliny, *N.H.*, XXV. 38. 78.

97. *De materia medica*, III. 82.

98. John Scarborough, "Nicander's Toxicology I: Snakes," *Pharmacy in History* 19 (1977): 3–23, esp. 4, and "Nicander's Toxicology II: Spiders, Scorpions, Insects and Myriapods," ibid., 21 (1979): 3–34, 73–92. Nicander, *Nicander: The Poems and Poetical Fragments*.

99. Susemihl, *Geschichte der griechischen Litteratur*, 1:784. Evidence for Diocles' material is presented by Wellmann, "Sextius Niger," pp. 557–560, and for Apollodorus, pp. 560–563. *De materia medica*, III. 74, from Theophrastus; Theophrastus, *Enquiry*, IX. 11. 11; *De materia medica*, V. 108, from *Enquiry*, IX. 18. 3.

100. Meyer, *Geschichte*, 2:114–115; Wellmann, "Sextius Niger," pp. 24, 549–557; Allbutt, *Greek Medicine in Rome*, pp. 377–378; more recently John Scarborough has studied Theophrastus and connected many passages with those in Dioscorides, but he judiciously avoids venturing an opinion about whether Dioscorides directly used Theophrastus ("Theophrastus on Herbals and Herbal Remedies," *Journal of the History of Biology* 11 [1978]: 353–385).

101. Wellmann, "Sextius Niger," pp. 549–557.

102. Ibid., pp. 530–569.

103. Ibid., pp. 536–548.

104. Ibid., p. 541.

105. Caesar, *Gallic Wars*, VI. 36; Galen, *De simplicium medicamentorum*, VIII. 29, 12:127; cf. Theophrastus, *Enquiry*, III. 10. 2, and Vergil, *Eclogues*, IX. 30, who spoke of its toxicity. Nicander's alleged mention of it (*Alexipharmaca*, 611) is supposed to be an interpolation.

106. Pliny the Younger, *Letters*, III. 5.

107. *De materia medica*, III. 52; cf. Pliny, *N.H.*, XX. 15. 31–32. Wellmann, "Sextius Niger," pp. 559–560; Susemihl, *Geschichte der griechischen Litteratur*, 1:879n; Hans Diller, "Philistion," *P.W.* 19, pt. 2 (1938): 2405–2408; Max Wellmann, *Die Fragmente der sikelischen Ärzte Akron, Philistion und des Diokles von Karystos*.

108. *De materia medica*, II. 125; cf. Pliny, *N.H.*, XX. 43. 111. Wellmann, "Sextius Niger," p. 560; idem, "Chrysippos," *P.W.* 3, pt. 2 (1899): 2509–2510.

109. *De materia medica*, II. 66; cf. Pliny, *N.H.*, XXVIII. 30. 119–120, although Sextius Niger may be this direct source, he at least being the only author cited by Pliny. Wellmann ("Sextius Niger," pp. 538–540) believes Sostratus to be a source for Dioscorides. Nicander also relied on Sostratus and was consequently an indirect source for Dioscorides. See Scarborough, "Nicander's Toxicology I," pp. 4, 19n, and "Nicander's Toxicology II," pp. 6, 13–14; also Gossen, "Sostratus," *P.W.* 3A suppl. (1927): 1203–1204.

110. *De materia medica*, III. 39; cf. Athenaeus, *Deipnosophistae*, XV. 681b, and Pliny, *N.H.*, XXI. 35. 61. *De materia medica*, IV. 162; cf. Erotian, *Vocum Hippocraticum*, 72. 72, 119. 50 (41, 5; 81, 16 Nachmanson ed.), Pliny, *N.H.*, XXV. 47. *De materia medica*, II. 110; cf. Pliny, *N.H.*, XXV. 6. 18–19. Wellmann, "Sextius Niger," pp. 557–559, and *Fragmente*; Scarborough, "Nicander's Toxicology II," p. 6. I do not find the evidence persuasive that Dioscorides used Diocles directly.

111. *De materia medica*, IV. 16; Wellmann, "Diagoras," p. 311.

112. Bernert, "Philonides," pp. 73–74.

113. Wellmann, *Krateuas*, and fragments of Crateuas published by Wellmann in *Pedanii Dioscuridis*, 3:139–146.

114. Pliny, *N.H.*, XXV. 4. 48.

115. Dioscorides cites Crateuas by name in I. 29, II. 127, III. 125, and IV. 35 (IV. 119 is an interpolation).

116. Wellmann, "Sextius Niger," p. 548.

117. Pauly-Wissowa-Kroll, *Realencyclopaedie der classischen Altertumswissenschaft*, 3:1131–1142.

118. The essay is dated October 6, 1905, at Potsdam, but it did not appear until volume 2 of the text edition, *Pedanii Dioscoridis*.

119. It is interesting to speculate about the size of his predecessors' works. Juba wrote a small book called Περὶ λιβύης, which Galen called Βιβλίδιον τὶ σμικρόν (*De comp. med. secundum locos*, IX. 4; 13:271, on one plant. Chrysippus devoted a special volume (*privatem volumen*) to the cabbage plant (Pliny, *N.H.*, XX. 33. 78). At the other extreme, Philonides' work on drugs extended to at least eighteen books since Galen quoted from the eighteenth book (*De differentia pulsuum*, IV. 10, 8:748). Despite Dioscorides' criticism that Crateuas left out some important root herbs, Crateuas included some that Dioscorides did not have in his own work.

120. "Iollas," *P.W.* 9, pt. 2 (1916): 1855; Wellmann, "Zur Geschichte der Medicin," p. 561; "Herakleides," *P.W.* 8, pt. 1 (1912): 493–496; Scarborough and Nutton, "Preface," p. 203.

121. *De materia medica*, Pref., 2–3.

122. The Greek word δύναμις is generally translated as "power," "strength," "elementary force," or "function." The Latin equivalent is *virtus*, but, when both the Greek and Latin are applied to drugs, I am following Scarborough and Nutton's translation of "property" ("Preface," p. 200).

123. Pref., 3, Scarborough and Nutton trans.

124. *De materia medica*, III. 126–127.

125. The σαξίφραγον (Latin: *saxifraga* = *saxum fraga*, lit., "rock breaking") was variously identified throughout antiquity and the Middle Ages. The plant was interpolated in some of Dioscorides' manuscripts (incl. Vienna MS. gr. 1, s. VI, and Naples MS. gr. 28, s. VII), but it was not listed by Dioscorides (2:182 Wellmann ed.). Galen said that the Celts refer to *betonikē* as *saxifragon* (*De sanitate tuenda*, V. 5, 6, 339). The plant identification of *saxifragon*(*a*) varied from time to time, writer to writer (e.g., Jacques André, *Lexique des termes de botanique en latin*, p. 283; A. Carnoy, *Dictionnaire étymologique des noms grecs de plantes*, p. 235; Herman Fischer, *Mittelalterliche Pflanzerkunde*, pp. 269, 273, 287, and passim).

126. Jerry Stannard writes: "This is the so-called 'Doctrine of Signatures' which, in both the primitive and sophisticated forms, played an enormously important role in the history of therapeutics. Logically, the belief in the signature(s) of a plant substance (or animal substance) depends upon the acceptance of two premises, though seldom are both made explicit. First is the admission of a recognition of a similarity, fanciful or real, between the morphological appearance of a plant (color, habit, armature, etc.) or some portion thereof (seed, capsule, root, leaf, etc.) and a symptom or abnormal condition of the human body. Then, once that similarity is asserted, it is further assumed that, *because* of that similarity, the plant (or specified portion thereof) is specifically and therapeutically effective for that symptom or abnormal condition. The second of these two premises of *Signaturenlehre* is thus one of several variants of the well-known axiom *similia similibus curantur* that is found to underlie many 'sympathetic' cures and remedies" ("Medicinal Plants and Folk Remedies in Pliny, *Historia Naturalis*," *History and Philosophy of the Life Sciences* 4, no. 1 (1982): 14.

127. See articles in *P.W.*

128. L. W. Daly, *Contributions to a History of Alphabetization in Antiquity and the Middle Ages*, p. 35.

129. Wellmann, *Krateuas*, p. 21. Daly (*Alphabetization*, p. 36) expresses doubt about whether Niger's work was alphabetized but accepts the order for Crateuas.

130. Pref., 5, Scarborough and Nutton trans.

131. Galen, *De simpl. med.*, VI. pref., 11:795.

132. P. H. Davies and V. H. Heywood, *Principles of Angiosperm Taxonomy*, p. 13.

133. John Sibthorp and James E. Smith, *Flora Graeca*; William T. Stearn,

"From Theophrastus and Dioscorides to Sibthorp and Smith: The Background and Origin of the *Flora Graeca*," *Biological Journal of the Linnean Society* 8 (1976): 285–318.

134. The great historian of botany, Edward Lee Greene, was intrigued by Dioscorides' taxonomical ability when he wrote: "The whole subject of Dioscorides as a taxonomist merits a fuller development. A thorough study of his text might show that classification had progressed somewhat during those three centuries that had then elapsed since Theophrastus" (*Landmarks of Botanical History*, 1:223).

2. *One Plant, One Chapter*

1. Charles Schmidt, "Theophrastus," *Catalogus Translationum et Commentariorum* 2 (1971): 239–322.
2. Pliny, *N.H.*, XXV. 27. 63.
3. Carnoy, *Dictionnaire étymologique*, p. 265.
4. Oleg Polunin, *Flowers of Europe*, no. 1098.
5. Ibid., no. 1103.
6. M. Grieve, *A Modern Herbal*, 1:353.
7. Polunin, *Flowers of Europe*, no. 1099.
8. John Riddle, "Pseudo-Dioscorides' *Ex herbis femininis* and Early Medieval Medical Botany," *Journal of the History of Biology* 14 (1981): 47–50.
9. Laura Georgi, "Pollination Ecology of the Date Palm and Fig Tree: Herodotus 1. 193. 4–5." *Classical Philology* 77 (1982): 224–228.
10. Bailey, *Manual of Cultivated Plants*, p. 421.
11. *De materia medica*, Pref., 7, Scarborough-Nutton trans.
12. Georg Harig, "Verhältnis zwischen den Primär- und Sekundärqualitaten in der theoretischen Pharmakologie Galens," *N.T.M. Schriftenreihe für Geschichte der Naturwissenschaften, Technik, und Medizin* 10 (1973): 64–81; and G. E. R. Lloyd, "The Hot and the Cold, the Dry and the Wet in Greek Philosophy," *Journal of Hellenic Studies* 84 (1964): 92–106.
13. Pliny, *N.H.*, XXIV. 22. 35.
14. Compare I. 42, which has warming and binding qualities but not the same medicinal usages as oil of myrtle (I. 39).
15. Soranus, *Gynecology*, III. 4. 26–30. Also described by Celsus, *De medicina*, IV. 27; Aretaeus, *De causis et signis acutorum morborum libri II*, 11; Aetios, *The Gynaecology and Obstetrics of the VIth Century, A.D.*, 68.
16. Paulus Aegineta, *Seven Books*, III. 71, 1:633.
17. Soranus, *Gynecology*, III. 4. 29. Hippocrates (*Aphorismi*, V. 34) said: "When a women suffers from hysteria or difficult labor an attack of sneezing is beneficial."
18. Wolfgang Schneider, *Lexikon zur Arzneimittelgeschichte*, 5: pt. 2, 214–219.
19. George Edward Trease, *A Text-book of Pharmacognosy*, p. 180.
20. Ibid., pp. 257–260; Friedrich A. Flückiger and Daniel Hanbury, *Pharmacographia*, pp. 595–598; *Merck Index*, pp. 480, 1012.
21. Schneider, *Lexikon*, 5: pt. 2, 339–343; Trease, *Pharmacognosy*, pp. 298–299; Flückiger and Hanbury, *Pharmacographia*, pp. 508–509; *Merck Index*, p. 709.

22. John Edmund Driver and George Edward Trease, *The Chemistry of Crude Drugs*, p. 59; Henry Kramer, *A Textbook of Botany and Pharmacognosy*, pp. 476–477.

23. Flückiger and Hanbury, *Pharmacographia*, p. 498.

24. Harig, "Primär-," p. 68.

25. Dioscorides' words: στυπτικός, στυφελός, στῦψις; Galen, στῦφον and στρυφνόν (see Harig, "Primär-," p. 71).

26. For a discussion of the relation between chemicals and organoleptic perception, see R. W. Moncrieff, *The Chemical Senses*.

27. Carl Pfaffmann, "Smell and Taste," *Encyclopaedia Britannica*, 20:685.

28. Flückiger and Hanbury, *Pharmacographia*, p. 396.

29. Paulus Aegineta, *Seven Books*, 3:181.

30. See H. Flück, "The Influence of the Soil on the Content of Active Principles in Medicinal Plants," *Journal of Pharmacy and Pharmacology* 6 (1954): 153–163, and "The Influence of Climate on the Active Principles in Medicinal Plants," ibid. 7 (1955): 361–383; W. H. Lewis and Memory P. F. Elvin-Lewis, "Systematic Botany and Medicine," in *Systematic Botany, Plant Utilization and Biosphere Conservation*, ed. Inga Hedberg, p. 27.

31. See "General Principles Regarding Plant Environment," below.

32. E. F. Steinmetz, "Crude Vegetable Drugs and Their Galenical Preparations versus Active Principles Derived Therefrom," *Quarterly Journal of Crude Drug Research* 1 (1961): 3–5; Scarpa, "Pre-Scientific Medicines," p. 319.

33. Korolkovas and Burchhater, *Essentials of Medicinal Chemistry*, pp. 7–8, name thirteen individual patient variable factors affecting drug metabolism, ten variable factors with drug administration, and thirteen variable factors with external environmental factors.

34. J. W. Fairbairn, "Perspectives in Research on the Active Principles of Traditional Herbal Medicine," *Journal of Ethnopharmacology* 2 (1980): 101.

35. Foster and Anderson, *Medical Anthropology*, pp. 156–157 and passim.

36. *De materia medica*, I. 7; cf. Harald Nielsen, *Ancient Ophthalmological Agents*, p. 49.

37. Scarborough and Nutton, "Preface," p. 192.

38. Adam Patrick, "Disease in Antiquity: Ancient Greece and Rome," in *Diseases in Antiquity*, ed. Don Brothwell and A. T. Sandison, p. 245; Celsus, *De medicina*, 1:342–343n.

39. Pliny, *N.H.*, 6:viii.

40. Julius Preuss, *Biblical and Talmudic Medicine*, p. 340.

41. Ibid., p. 340; Paulus Aegineta, *Seven Books*, 2:1–14; Vivian Nutton wrote to me (London, November 22, 1983) that the discovery that Pliny's lepra and elephantiasis were not the same is perhaps owed to Niccolo Leoniceno, *De morbo Gallico* (Venice, 1497). He also reports that the problem of *lepra* is reported by M. D. Grmek, *Les maladies a l'aube de l'histoire* (Paris, 1983), which I have not seen.

42. Letter, Vivian Nutton to Riddle, November 22, 1983.

43. Albert F. Hill, *Economic Botany*, pp. 319–321, 488–489; Robert James Forbes, *Studies in Ancient Technology*, 3:63–70. Professor Gerald Elkin pointed out to me the possibility of microorganisms in nonaerated brewing.

44. Hippocrates, *Hippocrates*, 1:lvi.

45. Pliny, *N.H.*, 6:xi; W. G. Spencer (Celsus, *De medicina*, 1:463–465) believes that the form of gout described by Pliny and Galen as being new was chronic lead poisoning. New, collaborative evidence is presented by Jerome O. Nriagu, "Saturnine Gout among Roman Aristocrats," *New England Journal of Medicine* 308 (1983): 660–663. Spencer said (p. 464) that the first definite indication of true gout is found in a Nubian cemetery of the 5th c. A.D., but Philip Salib ("Trauma and Disease of the Post-Cranial Skeleton in Ancient Egypt," in *Diseases in Antiquity*, ed. Don Brothwell and A. T. Sandison, p. 601) points to ancient Egyptian (i.e., pre-Roman) skeletons with concretions of uric acid crystals at their joints.

46. Andres Goth, *Medical Pharmacology*, pp. 533–534; Walter H. Lewis and Memory P. F. Elvin-Lewis, *Medical Botany*, pp. 199, 219.

47. Lewis and Elvin-Lewis, *Medical Botany*, pp. 150–151; Lucius E. Sayre, *A Manual of Organic Materia Medica and Pharmacognosy*, p. 137.

48. Dixon M. Woodburn and Edward Fingl, "Analgesic-Antipyretics, Anti-inflammatory Agents, and Drugs Employed in the Therapy of Gout," in *The Pharmacological Basis of Therapeutics*, ed. Louis S. Goodman and Alfred Gilman, pp. 338–339; Lewis and Elvin-Lewis, *Medical Botany*, p. 151.

49. James A. Duke, "Phytotoxin Tables," *C.R.C. Critical Reviews in Toxicology* 5 (November 1977): 224.

50. *Merck Index*, p. 781, but Paul Greengard ("The Vitamins," in *The Pharmacological Basis of Therapeutics*, ed. Louis S. Goodman and Alfred Gilman, p. 1559) gives some symptoms of the deficiency.

51. Duke, "Phytotoxin Tables," p. 215.

52. Ibn Māsawaih Yūhannā, *Mesue qui Graecorum*, 61.4 G.14.

53. George E. Trease and William C. Evans, *Pharmacognosy*, p. 119.

54. V. E. Tyler et al., *Pharmacognosy*, p. 255.

55. Nielsen, *Ophthalmological Agents*, pp. 58 ff.

56. Ibid., p. 10.

57. William Emmott, "Ophthalmology in Classical Medicine," *Ophthalmic Optician* 5 (January 1965): 14, 19–22, 81–82.

58. E.g., I. 12, 15, 68, 74, 109, 112; II. 99, 107, 129, 131, 134, 135.

59. E.g., I. 64, 76, 105.

60. E.g., II. 78, 136, 151. Argema occurred on the circle of the iris but extended over a surrounded area so that the part on the external side of the iris was red and on the internal side, white (Emmott, "Ophthalmology," p. 20).

61. Conversation with Sid L. Gulledge, M.D., Raleigh, N.C.

62. Celsus, *De medicina*, VII. 7.

63. Burton Chance, *Ophthalmology*, p. 15; cf. Liddell and Scott, *Greek English Lexicon*.

64. Trease, *Pharmacology*, pp. 404–407; *Dispensatory of the United States of America*, pp. 875–876.

65. *Dispensatory*, p. 877.

66. Nielsen, *Ophthalmological Agents*, p. 44.

67. *Dispensatory*, pp. 1184–1185.

68. Driver and Trease, *Chemistry of Crude Drugs*, pp. 125–127.

69. Liddell and Scott, *Greek English Lexicon*, p. 1171. Pliny's *nubecula*, the Latin equivalent, possibly is a cataract (Pliny, *N.H.*, 8:581). Chance (*Ophthalmology*, p. 17) says that the ancients had no treatment for cataract, but apparently they did.

70. Nielsen, *Ophthalmological Agents*, pp. 83–86.

71. Ibid., p. 84.

72. Pliny, *N.H.*, XXXI. 47. 125.

73. Nielsen, *Ophthalmological Agents*, p. 86.

74. Vivian Nutton wrote to me (November 11, 1983) and suggested that the warm bread in a bag might have been intended for external use as a "hot water bottle."

75. Dennis P. Van Gerven, "Nubia's Last Christians: The Cemeteries of Kulubnarti," *Archaeology* 34 (1981): 30.

76. Lewis and Elvin-Lewis, *Medical Botany*, p. 359.

77. Lester A. Mitscher, "Plant-Derived Antibiotics," in *Antibiotics, Isolation, Separation, and Purification*, ed. Marvin J. Weinstein and Gerald H. Wagman, p. 464.

78. Berendes, *Dioskurides*, pp. 117–118; Gunther, *Greek Herbal*, p. 238; cf. Carnoy, *Dictionnaire étymologique*, p. 37.

79. Mitscher, "Plant-Derived Antibiotics," pp. 467–469.

80. Lewis and Elvin-Lewis, *Medical Botany*, p. 360.

81. Mitscher, "Plant-Derived Antibiotics," p. 464.

82. Celsus, *De medicina*, V. 9; Paulus Aegineta, *Seven Books*, IV. 25; cf. definition in Galen, *In Hippocratis aphorismos commentarii*, V. 26, 17B:636. Inexplicably in the tract, *On abnormal swellings*, or *De tumoribus praeter naturam* (7: 705–732), Galen does not use the term *phuma*. In this work, *anthrakes* are described as a type of abnormal swelling (*onkos*); cf. D. G. Lytton and L. M. Resuhr, "Galen on Abnormal Swellings," *Journal of the History of Medicine and Allied Sciences* 33 (1978): 531– 549.

83. Celsus, *De medicina*, III. 10. 2. Rudolf Virchow's claim that Galen added a fifth sign, "disturbed function," is disproven; see Guido Majno, *The Healing Hand: Man and Wound in the Ancient World*, pp. 372–373, 412–413, and L. J. Rather, *The Genesis of Cancer*, p. 11.

84. Galen, *Ad Glauconem*, II. 1, 11:77.

85. Paulus Aegineta, *Seven Books*, IV. 25, 2:76.

86. For a definition and discussion of *nomas*, see Galen, *De compositione medicamentorum per genera*, IV. 10, 13:731–733, and *De methodo medendi*, V. 4, 10:326. The Old Latin translation of Dioscorides translated the Greek νόμας as *pascentia vulnera*, or "growing wound/sore" (*Dioscoride Latino Materia Medica Libro Primo*, ed. H. Mihaescu, p. 46).

87. The Latin translation of this verb was *curo*.

88. Lewis and Elvin-Lewis, *Medical Botany*, p. 360.

89. Trease and Evans, *Pharmacognosy*, p. 425.

90. Tyler et al., *Pharmacognosy*, p. 149.

91. Lewis and Elvin-Lewis, *Medical Botany*, p. 341.

92. John M. Kingsbury, *Poisonous Plants of the United States and Canada*, p. 485.

93. Grieve, *Modern Herbal*, 2:640.

94. Tyler et al., *Pharmacognosy*, pp. 50–51.

95. Lewis and Elvin-Lewis, *Medical Botany*, p. 127, citing A. P. Dustin, "Nouvelles applications des poisons caryoclassique à la cancerologic," *Sang* 12 (1938): 677–697. Goth, *Medical Pharmacology*, p. 654, places the beginning of antineoplastic chemotherapy, however, during World War II with the research on nitrogen mustards. Also see Paul Calabresi and Robert E. Parks, Jr., "Alkylating Agents, Antimetabolics, Hormones and Other Antiproliferative Agents," in *The Pharmacological Basis of Therapeutics*, ed. Louis S. Goodman and Alfred Gilman, p. 1254.

96. Dioscorides' ἐφημέρον is identified by Thiselton-Dyer in Theophrastus (*Enquiry*, IX. 16. 6, 2:301) as meadow saffron and by Liddell and Scott (*Greek English Lexicon*, p. 744) as *Colchicum autumnale*. Gunther (Dioscorides, *Greek Herbal*, p. 482) identified it as *Colchicum parnassicum*, which he mistakenly said was meadow saffron. The chapter preceding is κολχίκον (IV. 83), which I identified as autumn crocus (saffron = crocus or *Colchicum autumnale*) on the basis of almost all authorities, the manuscript pictures, and Dioscorides' description. Sprengel thought ἐφημέρον might be *Convallaria verticillata* L., but all evidence, including pharmacological, points to it as being a *Colchicum* as all except Sprengel have indicated. Since there are sixty or more species of *Colchicum* (Bailey, *Manual of Cultivated Plants*, p. 235), there is a range of possibilities as to the exact species, one or more, that Dioscorides intended, but all species would have the active component of the chemical colchicine. For the purposes here the unresolved question is superfluous. For the use of colchicine as an antitumor drug in China, see Bin Hsu, "The Use of Herbs as Anticancer Agents," *American Journal of Chinese Medicine* 8 (1980): 302–304.

97. See above.

98. Don Brothwell, "The Evidence for Neoplasms," in *Diseases in Antiquity*, ed. Don Brothwell and A. T. Sandison, pp. 320–345, using paleopathological evidence.

99. Galen, *Hippocratic de acutorum morborum victu liber*, 15: 770; 17A:801.

100. Galen, *De usu partim*, III. 9, 1:174 (cf. *On the Usefulness of the Parts of the Body*, p. 193).

101. Berendes (*Dioskurides*, p. 212) identified the plant as *Vicia ervilia* L., while W. Schneider (*Lexikon*, 5: pt. 3, 397–399) says that it could be either *V. ervilia* or *V. faba* L.

102. Some ancient descriptions of "gangrene" clearly indicate our gangrene but others point to a "running ulcer." Certainly where Dioscorides indicated that it favorably responded to therapy (e.g., II. 100, 108, 112), something like an ulcer was meant. See also Jeremiah Reedy, "Galen on Cancer and Related Diseases," *Clio Medica* 10 (1975): 234.

103. Dioscorides (II. 135) said that it could be cured; cf. Galen, *De tumoribus praeter naturam*, 7:728, whose context suggests the same. W. G. Spencer (Celsus, *De medicina*, 2:158) translated Celsus' use of the Latin term as follicular abscess, but Celsus (*De medicina*, V. 28, 13) said that there are two kinds. Pliny (*N.H.*, XX. 4. 11) said that they were "hard," which is not descriptive of follicular abscesses.

104. Jonathan L. Hartwell, "Plants Used against Cancer: A Survey," *Llloydia* 33 (1970): 120–122.

105. R. J. McIlroy, *The Plant Glycosides*, pp. 22–23; Duke, "Phytotoxin Tables," p. 236; *Merck Index*, p. 1107.

106. Kingsbury, *Poisonous Plants*, pp. 362–363.

107. Lewis and Elvin-Lewis, *Medical Botany*, pp. 125–126.

108. McIlroy, *Plant Glycosides*, p. 20.

109. Hartwell, "Plants Used against Cancer," 30 (1967): 379–436; 31 (1968): 71–170; 32 (1969): 79–107, 153–205, 247–296; 33 (1970): 97–194, 288–392; 34 (1971): 103–160, 204–255, 310–360, 386–425.

110. W. S. Stone, "A Review of the History of Chemical Theory in Cancer," *Medical Record* 90 (1916): 628.

111. A call was made by Jonathan L. Hartwell, "Plant Remedies for Cancer," *Cancer Chemotherapy Reports*, July 1960, pp. 19–24.

112. Keith Hopkins, "Contraception in the Roman Empire," *Comparative Studies in Society and History* 8 (1965): 143.

113. Richard Harrow Feen, "Abortion and Exposure in Ancient Greece: Assessing the Status of the Fetus and 'Newborn' from Classical Sources," in *Abortion and the Status of the Fetus*, ed. William B. Bondeson et al., pp. 283–300.

114. Ludwig Edelstein, "The Hippocratic Oath," in *Ancient Medicine*, ed. Oswei and C. Lilian Temkin, pp. 4–63, esp. 13–20; D. Nickel, "Ärztliche Ethik und Schwangerschaftsunterbrechung bei den Hippokratikern," *N.T.M.* 9 (1972): 73–80; Georg Harig and Jutta Kollesch, "Der hippokratische Eid, Zur Entstehung der antiken medizinischen Deontologie," *Philologus* 122 (1978): 157–176.

115. Donald Engles, "The Problem of Female Infanticide in the Graeco-Roman World," *Classical Philology* 75 (1980): 112–120; William V. Harris, "The Theoretical Possibility of Extensive Infanticide in the Graeco-Roman World," *Classical Philology* 32 (1982): 114–116.

116. Jérôme Carcopino, *Daily Life in Ancient Rome*, pp. 42, 77.

117. Richard Duncan-Jones, *The Economy of the Roman Empire: Quantitative Studies*, pp. 291–310.

118. Jerome, *Letters*, XXXVIII. 3; XXII. 13, 17, in *Patrologiae cursus completus*. Series latina, 22:401–402, 464.

119. The intellectual history of contraception has been brilliantly written by John T. Noonan (*Contraception: A History of Its Treatment by the Catholic Theologians and Canonists*), but Professor Noonan expressed only a faith that, since there was so much attention to contraception in the sources, there must have been some technical basis for it (pp. 158–159). Still useful is Norman E. Himes, *Medical History of Contraception*.

120. Pliny, *N.H.*, XXV. 7. 25.

121. Hopkins, "Contraception," p. 125; Sheila K. Dickinson, "Abortion in Antiquity," *Arethusa* 6 (1973): 159–166; John Scarborough, "On the Understanding of Medicine among the Romans, *Historian* 39 (1977): 217. Even today there is some general confusion between contraception and abortion. On a physiological basis, a contraceptive agent prevents ovulation and/or fertilization; any agent that interferes with implantation is an interceptive; and an

agent that terminates the pregnancy after implantation is an abortifacient. Since Dioscorides could not have distinguished between contraceptive and interceptive, I am using contraception the way he used it, that is, to include any prevention of fertilization or pregnancy within the short period after intercourse.

122. Soranus, *Gynaeciorum*, I. 60, 45.

123. Trease, *Pharmacognosy*, p. 180; on uterine stimulants, see Lewis and Elvin-Lewis, *Medical Botany*, pp. 321–322.

124. Luigi Palma, *Le piante medicinali d'Italia*, pp. 67–69.

125. Norman R. Farnsworth et al., "Potential Value of Plants as Sources of New Antifertility Agents I," *Journal of Pharmaceutical Sciences* 64 (1975): 562.

126. J. W. C. Gunn, "The Action of the 'Emmenagogue Oils' on the Human Uterus," *Journal of Pharmacology and Experimental Therapeutics* 15 (1920): 485–489.

127. Based on survey of plants evaluated in animals or humans for antifertility effects by N. R. Farnsworth et al. ("Sources of New Antifertility Agents," pp. 547–554), but one plant, *Thuja occidentalis*, a Cupressaceae, the same family as juniper, has been shown to have an anovulatory effect (p. 549). Juniper berries appear in one antifertility pill for human use (see E. Schifferli, "Abtreibungen und Abtreibungsversuche mit pflanzlichen Materialien," *Deutsches Zeitschrift für gesamte gerichtliche Medizin* 31 [1939]: 244).

128. M. L. Gujral et al., "Preliminary Observations on the Antifertility Effect of Some Indigenous Drugs," *Indian Journal of Medical Research* 48 (1960): 46–51.

129. Henry de Laszlo and Paul S. Henshaw, "Plant Materials Used by Primitive Peoples to Affect Fertility," *Science* 10 (1954): 630.

130. George Usher, *Dictionary of Plants Used by Man*, p. 602; cf. Grieve, *Modern Herbal*, 1:188.

131. Hopkins, "Contraception," p. 131n.

132. Murand and Gilman, "Estrogens and Progestins," pp. 1423–1434.

133. Lewis and Elvin-Lewis, *Medical Botany*, p. 318.

134. Boleslaw Skarzynski, "An Oestrogenic Substitute from Plant Material," *Nature* 131 (1933): 766.

135. *Zeitschrift für Physiologische Chemie* 218 (1933): 104–112, as reported by J. B. Harborne, *Introduction to Ecological Biochemistry*, p. 85.

136. Harborne, *Ecological Biochemistry*, p. 86.

137. Ibid., pp. 83–89.

138. R. R. Chaudhury, "Plants with Possible Antifertility Activity," *Indian Council for Medical Research, Special Reports Series* 55 (1966): 12, 15.

139. Harborne, *Ecological Biochemistry*, p. 85.

140. Farnsworth et al. ("Sources of New Antifertility Agents," p. 545) report two references in science journals (*Science* 119 [1954]: 629, and *Planta Medica* 23 [1973]: 169) to folk usage of white poplar (*Populus alba*), but the source for both references is Dioscorides through J. Berendes.

141. Laszlo and Henshaw, "Plant Materials," pp. 626–631; B. E. Finch and Hugh Green, *Contraception through the Ages*, for a general survey.

142. *Dispensatory*, p. 1710; R. Ullsperger, "Die Entwicklung der Crataegusforschung," *Planta Medica* 1 (1953): 43–50.

143. Mieczaslaw Mazure et al., "Pharmacology of Lupanine and 13-Hydroxylupanine," *Acta Physiologiae Polononica* 17, no. 2, pp. 299–309, as reported in *Chemical Abstracts* 65 (1966): 11163q.

144. P. I. Sizov, "Experimental Parturifacient Action of Pachycarpine Brevicolline and Thalictrimine," *Zdravookhranenie Belorusii* 15 (1969): 44–46 as reported in *Chemical Abstracts* 72 (1970): 119957u. See also *Chemical Abstracts* 78 (1973): 66914t. N. R. Farnsworth et al., "Sources of New Antifertility Agents," p. 566.

145. Pinaeus, *Historia plantarum*, no. 187.

146. Farnsworth et al., "Sources of New Antifertility Agents," pp. 32, 554–577.

147. Finch and Green (*Contraception*, p. 47) believe that the Romans limited condoms to the prevention of disease; however, there is some evidence suggesting wider uses and purposes: see John Scarborough, *Roman Medicine*, p. 209n. 50; Himes, *Contraception*, p. 188.

148. Hopkins, "Contraception," p. 131.

149. Pliny (*N.H.*, XXV. 37. 75) apparently misread or translated incorrectly his Greek source because he thought in another section (*N.H.*, XXVI. 61. 94) that a single dose suppressed sexual desire for forty days (see note, W. H. S. Jones, Pliny, *N.H.*, 7:190).

150. Plants can stimulate sexual activity; for instance, a species of vole has a substance that increases fertility and triggers sexual activity in animals who eat it (Edward H. Sanders et al., "6-Methoxybenzoxazolinone: A Plant Derivative That Stimulates Reproduction in *Microtus montanus*," *Science* 214, [1981]: 67–69).

151. Jay M. Arena, *Poisoning: Toxicology—Symptoms—Treatments*, pp. 210–212 and passim.

152. Κοιλία, as it is generally spelled, and στομάχος pose difficult translation problems. *Koilia* has a broad meaning of the entire body cavity (thorax and abdomen), but it can have specialized meanings of stomach, intestines, bowels, or, in fact, any body cavity, even heart chamber or womb. *Stomachos* ranges in meaning from throat to gullet, neck of the bladder, orifice of the stomach, and the stomach itself. Clearly, when Dioscorides has something good for one and bad for the other, he is making a distinction. In the majority of his usages the meaning "lower digestive tract" and "upper digestive tract" seems about as precise as he intended. If some Greeks employed the words interchangeably, did Dioscorides edit their works before recording their usages? Since Dioscorides was consistent, it seems likely that he was a careful editor.

153. Arena (*Poisoning*, p. 442) reports that the principal symptom of the volatile oil from juniper berries is vomiting and circulatory collapse.

154. McIlroy, *Plant Glycosides*, pp. 79–82; *Dispensatory*, p. 1708.

155. Berendes, *Dioskurides*, p. 446; cf. W. Schneider, *Lexikon*, 5:pt. 2, p. 26.

156. Arbutus is discussed also by Theophrastus, *Enquiry*, III. 16. 4; Pliny,

N.H., XV. 28. 98–99; and Galen, *De simpl. med.*, VII. 39, 12:34, who most likely abridged Dioscorides' account.

157. Arena, *Poisoning*, p. 319.

158. H. Kramer, *Botany and Pharmacognosy*, p. 357; Duke, "Phytotoxin Tables," p. 214. I acknowledge John Scarborough's assistance in relating this information.

159. Pinaeus, *Historia plantarum*, no. 304.

160. Another entry without any beneficial use is II. 122.

161. Berendes, *Dioskurides*, p. 59; Adams, Paulus, *Seven Books*, 3:102.

162. Arena, *Poisoning*, p. 592.

163. Sayre, *Organic Materia Medica*, p. 376.

164. *Dispensatory*, p. 1426.

165. *De materia medica*, Pref., 3, 7.

166. About the same plant, Theophrastus wrote (*Enquiry*, IX. 11. 6): ". . . three-twentieths of an ounce in weight is given, if the patient is to become merely sportive and to think himself a fine fellow; twice this dose if he is to have delusions; thrice the dose if he is to be permanently insane; . . . four times the dose is given if the man is to be killed." See comments on this passage by Scarborough, "Theophrastus on Herbals and Herbal Remedies," pp. 367–368.

167. Directly or indirectly, Dioscorides apparently employed Theophrastus (*Enquiry*, IX. 11. 6), who had the same dosages for similar effects. Lloyd (*Science, Folklore and Ideology*, p. 128) observed an apparent incongruity in comparison with the Hippocratic work *On Internal Affairs* (27, L VII 238, 3 ff.), which prescribed half a cotyle (.226 liters) of jimsonweed juice be taken daily as a painkiller together with a quarter of a cotyle of *melikrēton* (milk-honey mixture) and the yolk of a boiled chicken egg. The toxic effects of the jimsonweed would be reduced by the absorptive and demulcent countereffects of the *melikrēton* and egg.

168. V. E. Tyler et al., *Pharmacognosy*, p. 37; E. N. Croom, Jr., "Ethnobotanical Documentation in the Evaluation of the Safety and Efficacy of Herbal Medicine by Pharmacological Testing," *Journal of Ethnopharmacology* (forthcoming).

169. Tyler et al., *Pharmacognosy*, pp. 9, 100.

170. Croom, "Ethnobotanical Documentation."

171. Scarpa, "Pre Scientific Medicines," p. 318.

172. In a personal conversation, Dr. David Timothy (Crop Science Department, North Carolina State University), an expert in northern South American grasses, speculates that the gaucho is tasting varying concentrations of salt. In past geological eras the pampa was dotted with salt lakes, now dried. Dr. Timothy does not, however, verify the authenticity of this legend.

173. Polunin, *Flowers of Europe*, nos. 1176–1177; Trease, *Pharmacognosy*, pp. 534–536; William A. R. Thomson, *Medicines from the Earth*, no. 126, p. 74, and passim.

174. Croom, "Ethnobotanical Documentation," p. 9.

175. Tyler et al., *Pharmacognosy*, p. 10.

176. Scarborough and Nutton, "Preface," p. 227, identify the tree as *Tilia*

rubra D. C. or *T. platyphyllos* Scop. Theophrastus (*Enquiry*, V. 3. 3) discussed the character of the wood. Usher (*Plants Used by Man*, p. 577) reports that today the wood of *T. japonica* Simk is used in Japan to manufacture boxes.

177. Tyler et al., *Pharmacognosy*, p. 150.

178. Pliny, *N.H.*, XI. 14 (3:13, John Bostock ed., London, 1855–1857), as cited by Ernst W. Stieb, "Drug Adulteration and Its Detection in the Writings of Theophrastus, Dioscorides and Pliny," *Journal Mondial de Pharmacie* 2 (1958): 117.

179. Tyler et al., *Pharmacognosy*, pp. 30–31.

180. Stieb, "Drug Adulteration," p. 121.

181. Ibid.

182. Professor John Scarborough writes me: "This one is a puzzle: it could be one of two things as μετώπιον; either this is 'oil of almonds' as in Dioscorides I. 33. 1 . . . ἀμυγδάλινον ἔλαιον, ὅ τινες μετώπιον καλοῦσι, and would be from *Amygdalus communis* L.; or it is the name of a fancy Egyptian ointment into which χαλβάνη is mixed (Diosc. I. 59. 1). I would lean toward 'almond-oil,' since adulterating balsam with an ointment already containing balsam might not make much practical sense."

183. For this last sentence, clearly both Dioscorides and Pliny were using the same source. Pliny (*N.H.*, XII. 54. 119) wrote: "Of the wood the sort resembling boxwood is the best, and also has the strongest scent; the best seed is that which is largest in size and heaviest in weight, which has a biting taste and is hot in the mouth. Balsam is adulterated with the ground-pine [*hyperico*] of Petra, which can be detected by its size, hollowness and long shape and by its weak scent and its taste like pepper" (H. Rackham trans., 4:85).

184. Pliny, *N.H.*, XII. 54. 111.

185. Ibid., XII. 54. 123.

186. For references, see Stieb, "Drug Adulteration," pp. 118–120.

187. Scarborough, *Roman Medicine*, p. 171; Emmanuel Leclainche, *Histoire de la médecine vetérinaire*, pp. 40–63; R. E. Walker, "Roman Veterinary Medicine," in *Animals in Roman Life and Art*, ed. J. M. C. Toynbee, pp. 303–343, 404–414.

188. Varro, *Rerum rusticarum*, II. 5. 11, and Pliny, *N.H.*, VIII. 41. 97, as cited by Scarborough, *Roman Medicine*, pp. 171–173.

189. For a discussion of ancient views on ectoparasites and the identification of lice, see John Scarborough, "Roman Medicine and Public Health," in *Public Health*, ed. Teizo Ogawa, pp. 37–38.

190. D. C. Blood and J. A. Henderson, *Veterinary Medicine*, pp. 675–681.

191. *Merck Veterinary Manual*, p. 1504.

192. Ibid., p. 910; Blood and Henderson, *Veterinary Medicine*, p. 678.

193. *Dispensatory*, pp. 364–365.

194. Sextus Empiricus, *Against the Mathematicians*, XI. 50 (2:387 Mutschmann ed.); cf. translation and discussion, P. M. Fraser, *Ptolemaic Alexandria*, 2:524.

195. E.g., Sarton, *History of Science*, 1:19: "The historian of science cannot devote much attention to the study of superstition and magic, that is of unreason . . ."

196. Perhaps beginning in the 1890s with J. G. Frazer's *The Golden Bough* and Bronislaw Malinowski, *Magic, Science, and Religion and Other Essays* (1925). Among the newer works: Claude Lévi-Strauss' *The Savage Mind* and E. E. Evans-Pritchard's *Witchcraft, Oracles and Magic among the Azande*. Perhaps the first historian to see the importance of magic in developing empirical science was Lynn Thorndike (*The Place of Magic in the Intellectual History of Europe* and *A History of Magic and Experimental Science*).

197. G. E. R. Lloyd, *Magic, Reason and Experience: Studies in the Origins and Development of Greek Science*, p. 2.

198. John Riddle, "Quid pro Quo: Pharmacy in the Middle Ages," *Medical Heritage* 5 (1985–1986); Ludwig Edelstein, "Greek Medicine in Its Relation to Religion and Magic," *Bulletin of the Institute of the History of Medicine* 5 (1937): 230–234.

199. Lynn White, Jr., *Machina ex Deo: Essays in the Dynamism of Western Culture*, p. 54.

200. Henry E. Sigerist, *A History of Medicine*, vol. 1; for a modern separation, see Charles Singer, *From Magic to Science*.

201. Lloyd, *Magic*, p. 231.

202. Hippocrates, *On the Sacred Disease*, XVIII. 1 (trans. adapted from Jones, *Hippocrates*, vol. 2).

203. See especially E. R. Dodds, *The Greeks and the Irrational*.

204. Lloyd, *Magic*, p. 6.

205. Vergil, *Aeneid*, VI. 60–68; cf. much the same sentiments in Aeschylus, *Prometheus*, 484–499, where the benefits given to man include medicine, navigation, and divination.

206. E.g., *Papyri Graecae Magicae*.

207. E.g., *Hermetica: The Ancient Greek and Latin Writings*.

208. Galen, *De comp med. secundum locos*, VI. 8, 12:966.

209. Theophrastus, *Enquiry*, IX, is notable for folk traditions.

210. Soranus, *Gynecology*, II. 2, 4, p. 7.

211. Pliny, *N.H.*, XXVII. 13. 30, has the same statement.

212. Lewis and Elvin-Lewis, *Medical Herbal*, pp. 183–184; *Dispensatory*, p. 1305; Grieve, *Modern Herbal*, 2:766–769.

213. Jerry Stannard, "Squill in the Ancient and Medieval Materia Medica with Special Reference to Its Employment for Dropsy," *Bulletin of the New York Academy of Medicine* 50, 2d ser. (1974): 684–713, esp. 686–687; cf. Theophrastus, *Enquiry*, IX. 18. 3.

214. Stannard, "Squill," esp. p. 696.

215. Pliny, *N.H.*, XX. 39. 101.

216. Stannard, "Squill," p. 689.

217. Rufos of Ephesos, *Oeuvres*, frag. 90; cf. Theophrastus, *Enquiry*, IX. 19. 2–3, and Lloyd, *Magic*, p. 42.

218. Liddell and Scott, *Greek English Lexicon*.

219. Lewis and Elvin-Lewis, *Medical Botany*, p. 347; Grieve, *Modern Herbal*, 1:258–260.

220. Lewis and Elvin-Lewis, *Medical Botany*, p. 135.

221. Pliny, *N.H.*, XXV. 21. 50; cf. Theophrastus, *Enquiry*, IX. 10. 4.

222. E. A. Wallis Budge, *The Divine Origin of the Craft of the Herbalist*; cf. ritual in *Papyri Graecae Magicae*, IV. 2967–3006 (English translation forthcoming, ed. H.-D. Betz [University of Chicago Press]; manuscript made available to me by John Scarborough, who translated this particular section, along with most of the medical and pharmaceutical sections of the *Papyri Graecae Magicae*).

223. Josephus, *Wars of the Jews*, VII. 6. *Baaras* is the name in Hebrew for *mangragora*. For other ancient sources but without references, see C. J. S. Thompson, *The Mystic Mandrake*.

224. Galen, *De comp. med. secundum locos*, VI. 8, 12:966; cf. Edelstein, "Greek Medicine," p. 231.

225. Galen, *De libris propriis*, 2.19.19.

226. Fridolf Kudlien, "Galen's Religious Belief," in *Galen: Problems and Prospects*, ed. Vivian Nutton, p. 126.

227. Exceptions are various Hippocratic pharmaceutical works that also excluded magical elements and, according to Lloyd (*Science, Folklore and Ideology*, p. 129), never mentioned the use of amulets—in contrast with Theophrastus, who freely related folk beliefs and practices. Nevertheless, Lloyd cogently notes that these same authors did not acknowledge that most (all?) of the medicinal uses were derived from folk discoveries and that the authors, while taking a "hard-headed rationalist stance" (p. 132), adopted the vocabulary of drugs and spells.

228. Harborne, *Ecological Biochemistry*, pp. 107 ff.; Scarborough, "Roman Medicine and Public Health," pp. 37–38.

229. Kudlien, *Der griechische Arzt*, pp. 104–111; Forbes, *Ancient Technology*, 3:1–49; Alfred Schmidt, *Drogen und Drogenhandel im Altertum*, pp. 25–38.

230. Kudlien, *Der griechische Ärzt*, pp. 104–111.

231. Berendes, *Dioskurides*, pp. 52–53.

232. Translated with the assistance of John Scarborough, whose translation of this text will appear shortly in *Papyri Graecae Magicae in English*, ed. H.-D. Betz, translated from the Greek and Coptic texts, ed. Karl Preisendanz (University of Chicago Press, forthcoming). I am grateful to Professor Scarborough for making this translation available to me.

233. Compared by Berendes, *Dioskurides*, p. 52; cf. *Papyrus Ebers*, no. 98, p. 114.

234. Pliny, *N.H.*, XIII. 32–59, in direct reference to frankincense.

235. Ibid., XIII. 4. 20.

236. Ibid., XIII. 4. 23.

237. Forbes, *Ancient Technology*, 3:32.

238. In his work on perfumes, *Concerning Odors*, Theophrastus (14–15) mentioned almond oil as a base; cf. Forbes, *Ancient Technology*, 3:29. Dioscorides (I. 31) gave the recipe for almond oil, but he did not use it in the perfume formula.

239. But see *De materia medica*, V. 6.

240. For further details on Egyptian manufacture, see Forbes, *Ancient Technology*, 3:9–10.

241. Athenaeus, *Deipnosophists*, XII. 553 D.

3. *Drug Affinities*

1. Through the sixteenth century, there was much confusion over Dioscorides' *akoron* (I. 2) and the *acorus* of the related arum family. I presume that the confusion is reflected in the English common names: yellow flag for *Iris pseudacorus* L. and sweet flag for *Acorus calamus* L. Later writers often thought Dioscorides' *akoron* to be *Acorus calamus* L. This later plant was, according to the best modern thinking, Dioscorides' *kalamos arōmatikos* (I. 18 and also in the *kupi* recipe). To Dioscorides, *akoron* was *Iris pseudoacorus* of the iris family. For the unravelling of the confusion, see Kurt Ruegg, *Beiträge zur Geschichte der offizinellen Drogen: Crocus, Acorus Calamus und Colchicum*, pp. 141–207, esp. 150–153, 203–205.

2. Schneider, *Lexikon*, 2:70.

3. Sayre, *Manual*, p. 120.

4. Tyler et al., *Pharmacognosy*, p. 35.

5. See Flückiger and Hanbury, *Pharmacographia*, pp. 519–534; Hill, *Economic Botany*, pp. 467–470; *Dispensatory*, pp. 328–333; I. H. Burkill, *A Dictionary of the Economic Products of the Malay Peninsula*, 1:549–566.

6. Theophrastus, *Enquiry*, IX. 5. 1–3; Pliny, *N.H.*, XII. 42. 85–94, 43. 95–98.

7. J. Innes Miller, *The Spice Trade of the Roman Empire, 29 B.C. to A.D. 641*, p. 43.

8. Pliny, *N.H.*, XII. 42. 85–91.

9. *Periplus of the Erythraean Sea*, 8, 10, 12, 13, and pp. 127–128, 134. The various translators of the *Periplus* have consistently said that the *casia* is the *Cinnamomum* genus. The *Periplus* said there were three grades: 1, *gizir* and *douaka*; 2, *moto* and *magla*; 3, *asuphe*. See discussion in Berendes, *Die Pharmazie*, 2:183.

10. John Mitchell Watt and Maria Gerdina Breyer-Brandwijk, *The Medicinal and Poisonous Plants of Southern and Eastern Africa*, pp. 566–574; Flückiger and Hanbury, *Pharmacographia*, pp. 216–224; Schneider, *Lexikon*, 5: pt. 1, 246–252.

11. *Periplus*, pp. 99–100; Miller, *Spice Trade*, pp. 153–172 and passim.

12. Wilhelm Dittenberger, *Orientis Graeci Inscriptiones Selectae*, 1:328.

13. The list is found in the *Corpus Juris Civilis*, Civil Law sec., 9.39.4.16 (7) (Scott ed.) and reprinted in Miller, *Spice Trade*, pp. 279–280. On cinnamon leaf, see "Manuscript Illuminations and Dioscorides' Original Version," Chap. 5, below.

14. *Dispensatory*, pp. 1226–1231.

15. Literature reviewed by Schneider, *Lexikon*, 5: pt. 1, 248–251.

16. Dioscorides' chapter μαλάβαθρον (I. 12) has been interpreted to mean cinnamon leaves and the word was listed in the list of taxed imports at Alexandria (see Berendes, *Dioskurides*, pp. 34–35; Paulus Aegineta, *Seven Books*, 3:238; and Pliny, *N.H.*, XII. 46. 129). Since there is this uncertainty, I have omitted this chapter from our discussion.

17. Σῦριγξ (also in Paulus Aegineta, *Seven Books*, 7. 22. 5; συριγγίς in Andromachus, a medical poet, quoted by Galen, *De antidotis*, XIV. 73). The fine bark was stripped from the branches and tender tips, dried, and rolled into

tubes that resembled, to the Greeks, "shepherd's pipes," thereby giving a synonym for *cassia*. The Greek σῦριγξ went into Latin as *fistula*. This should not necessarily mean a confusion with *Cassia fistula*, which is a modern species of cassia.

18. Hebrew לגת, or *āhū*.

19. Mentioned also by Galen (*De antidotis*, XIV. 72). There is in Arabic and medieval Latin an "Alexandrian senna," which is the twigs of cassia and used as a substitute for senna, a purgative drug made from the fruit of the modern cassia plant.

20. The *Periplus* names *gizir* as a grade or kind of cassia/cinnamon (see n. 9, above). Galen (*De antidotis*, XIV. 72–73) gives varieties or grades as *moto*, *arebo*, *daphnitis*, and *gizi*, the last being best, better even than cinnamon. The Greek is related to the Hebrew *geziʿah* in Psalms 45:8: "All thy garments *smell* of myrrh, and aloes, *and* cassia, out of the ivory palaces, whereby they have made thee glad"; also in Job 42:14 as a personal name.

21. Seemingly named for the place name in Greek Cape Guardafiu, the northern tip of Somalia, sometimes referred to in antiquity as Arōmatōn, and south of it as Cinnamon country. See *Periplus*, 12, 30, under Arōmatōn.

22. *Periplus*, 12.

23. *Dispensatory*, p. 1226; Schneider, *Lexikon*, 5: pt. 1, 248–251, who lists other species as well.

24. A. Hermann and H. Grapow, *Wörterbuch der ägyptische Sprache*; V. Loret, *Le flore pharaonique d'après les documents hiéroglyphiques et les spécimens decouverts dans les tombes*, p. 51; Miller, *Spice Trade*, p. 144.

25. Miller, *Spice Trade*, pp. 144, 154, citing James Breasted, *History of Egypt*, but I am unable to find the citation in Breasted's work.

26. Miller, *Spice Trade*, p. 47.

27. Strabo, *Geography*, II. 5. 12; Ptolemy, Map. 1, cited by Miller, *Spice Trade*, p. 45.

28. *Dispensatory*, p. 1227; Usher, *Plants Used by Man*, p. 128, Burkill, *Economic Products of the Malay Peninsula*, 1:480.

29. Moses Maimonides, a twelfth-century Jewish writer in Arabic, gave cassia the term *dār čīnī*, which he said meant "wood from China" (*Glossary of Drug Names*, p. 74). Meyerhof says that the Arabic form is from the Persian *dār čīnī*, meaning "wood from China." Burkill (*Economic Products of the Malay Peninsula*, 1:550–551) says of the suggested connection between *dār sīnī* and "wood from China" that "the argument is not as forcible as it once seemed to be."

30. Tyler et al., *Pharmacognosy*, p. 34.

31. Watt and Breyer-Brandwijk, *Plants of Southern and Eastern Africa*, p. 566. Lewis and Elvin-Lewis (*Medical Botany*, pp. 42, 282–283, 325, 333, 342, 345–346, 351, 353, 362, 387) give a number of usages for cassia and the list reveals that Dioscorides' usages appear worldwide in folk and medical practice.

32. McIlroy, *Plant Glycosides*, p. 95; Lewis and Elvin-Lewis, *Medical Botany*, p. 363; Watt and Breyer-Brandwijk, *Plants of Southern and Eastern Africa*, p. 567.

33. Watt and Breyer-Brandwijk, *Plants of Southern and Eastern Africa*, p. 566.

34. Lewis and Elvin-Lewis, *Medical Botany*, p. 346.

35. Galen, *De simpl. med.*, 10. 11, 12:13.
36. Watt and Breyer-Brandwijk, *Plants of Southern and Eastern Africa*, pp. 530–531.
37. *Dispensatory*, p. 330.
38. Grieve, *Modern Herbal*, 1:169.
39. *Dispensatory*, pp. 605–606, 1799–1780.
40. Ibid., pp. 1799–1780; Schneider, *Lexikon*, 5: pt. 3, 79–82.
41. Lewis and Elvin-Lewis, *Medical Botany*, pp. 250–346; Watt and Breyer-Brandwijk, *Plants of Southern and Eastern Africa*, pp. 846–847.
42. *Dispensatory*, p. 606.
43. P. C. Das, *British Pat.*: 1, 025, 372 (CL. A Glk), April 6, 1956; *Indian Appl.*, July 25, 1963, 2 pp.; through *Chem. Abstr.*, 64:19328h (1966). See also, Farnsworth et al., "Sources of New Antifertility Agents," p. 552.
44. Farnsworth et al., "Sources of New Antifertility Agents," pp. 545, 571.
45. Trease and Evans, *Pharmacognosy*, pp. 449–454, 559–560.
46. S. van Straten, Flora de Vrijer, and J. C. de Beauveser, eds., *Lists of Volatile Compounds in Foods*, pp. 34.1–2–38.1–2; J. S. Govindarajan, "Pepper—Chemistry, Technology, and Quality Evaluation," *CRC Critical Reviews in Food Science and Nutrition* 9 (1977): 115–225.
47. Maxime McKendry, *The Seven Centuries Cookbook*, pp. 56–57.
48. Driver and Trease, *Chemistry of Crude Drugs*, p. 75.
49. Arena, *Poisoning*, p. 345.
50. Kingsbury, *Poisonous Plants*, pp. 275–294; Arena, *Poisoning*, pp. 499–500.
51. *Dispensatory*, pp. 1070–1071; not listed as a poisonous plant by Arena or Kingsbury.
52. *Dispensatory*, p. 1071; cf. Grieve, *Modern Herbal*, 2:644.
53. Ibid.
54. Lewis and Elvin-Lewis, *Medical Botany*, p. 331.
55. Arena, *Poisoning*, pp. 345–346.
56. Fisher, *Mittelalterliche Pflanzenkunde*, p. 279; Schneider, *Lexikon*, 5: pt. 3, 88–90.
57. Driver and Trease, *Chemistry of Crude Drugs*, p. 81.
58. Korolkovas and Burchhater, *Essentials of Medicinal Chemistry*, p. 225.
59. Ibid., pp. 225–231; Goth, *Medical Pharmacology*, pp. 115–151; Lewis and Elvin-Lewis, *Medical Botany*, p. 164.
60. I am comparing here papaverine from one species of the opium family with its chemical analogues in the Solanaceae family. Judging, however, by the toxic symptoms shown by grazing animals when ingesting a variety of poppy species, there is justification for Dioscorides including the poppy plants together; see Kingsbury, *Poisonous Plants*, pp. 148–153.
61. Schneider, *Lexikon*, 5: pt. 2, 35; Behrendes, *Dioskurides*, p. 412.
62. Aconitine is $C_{34}H_{47}O_{11}N$, although there are other proposals, $C_{34}H_{45}O_{11}N$ (Driver and Trease, *Chemistry of Crude Drugs*, p. 89; *Merck Index*, p. 15); hyoscamine is $C_{17}H_{23}O_3N$.
63. Arena, *Poisoning*, p. 319.
64. Driver and Trease, *Chemistry of Crude Drugs*, pp. 71–72.
65. These two Greek MSS, I observed, place the two hellebores side by side

as Sprengel's reading: Paris MS gr. 2183, vol. 113v and Salamanca MS 2659, vols. 130v–131.

66. Lewis and Elvin-Lewis, *Medical Botany*, pp. 187–189.

67. *Physician's Desk Reference*, 20th ed., pp. 566, 806, 808, 865, 949; *Merck Index*, pp. 881, 1104; Trease, *Pharmacognosy*, pp. 198–200.

68. Bernet, "Philonides," pp. 73–74.

69. Wellmann's numbering for large and small *sesamoides* is 149 and 163, but I believe that there is sufficient manuscript and pharmaceutical evidence to postulate that Dioscorides put these two species of the same plant genera together.

70. Lewis and Elvin-Lewis, *Medical Botany*, p. 187.

71. Friedrich Ludwig Meissner, *Encyclopëdia der medizinischen Wissenschaften*, cited by Schneider, *Lexikon*, 2:63.

72. Arena, *Poisoning*, pp. 505–506.

73. *Merck Index*, p. 18.

74. Alexander Tschirch, *Handbuch der Pharmakognosie*, 1:566: "Dioscorides' 'system,' if one can speak of a system, is a mixture, having as a controlling force both a morphological and a physical basis, as—if one may say so—a chemical and therapeutic theme on a systematic botanical starting point. One knows clearly to take by itself the effort, but one sees the inability to find a correct principle on which to operate."

75. Allbutt, *Greek Medicine in Rome*, p. 377.

76. Driver and Trease, *Chemistry of Crude Drugs*, p. 125.

77. Kingsbury, *Poisonous Plants*, pp. 363–364.

78. Duke, "Phytotoxin Tables," p. 216.

79. *Merck Index*, pp. 4, 771–772; hydrocyanic acid (p. 544) is toxic and its antidote is sodium nitrite, which raises a question whether the sodium in Dioscorides' prescription was to counter the hydrocyanic acid.

80. Tschirch's apt phrase is: "ein echter Naturforscher," a genuine investigator of Nature (*Handbuch*, 1:552).

4. Animals, Wines, and Minerals

1. Korolkovas and Burchhater, *Essentials of Medicinal Chemistry*, p. 12.

2. As based on 101 chapters for animal drugs and 102 for mineral drugs, as determined by Hermolaus Barbarus, Venice, 1516 ed.

3. Gossen, "Sostratos." For a survey, see Loren C. MacKinney, "Animal Substances in Materia Medica: A Study in the Persistence of the Primitive," *Journal of the History of Medicine and Allied Sciences* 1 (1946): 149–170.

4. For references to dung as a medicine, see Scarborough, "Nicander's Toxicology II," p. 82.

5. Sayre, *Manual*, pp. 437–451.

6. The most recent and systematic attempt is by Zoltán Kádár, *Survivals of Greek Zoological Illuminations in Byzantine Manuscripts*, pp. 56–58 and passim; also see Ed. Bonnet, "Etude sur les figures de plantes et d'animaux peintes dans une version arabe, manuscrite, de la matière médicale de Dioscoride," *Janus* 14 (1909): 294–303.

7. *Dispensatory*, pp. 223–224, 755–756; *Physicians' Desk Reference*, 20th ed., p. 737.

8. Forbes, *Ancient Technology*, 3:180–181.

9. *Merck Index*, p. 194.

10. A symptom of fox mange is progressive balding. Dioscorides said that this quicklime drug "fills up the hair" of those with alopecia, which we believe to be fox mange. Quicklime today is used commercially to remove hair from animal skins in preparation for tanning (*Merck Index*, p. 194), but in two other chapters (II. 7, 9) Dioscorides said it stops hair from coming out.

11. In his treatise *On Stones* (62), Theophrastus used the word *γύψος* (from which English derives *gypsum*) to mean quicklime. See discussion by Earle R. Caley and John C. Richards, Theophrastus, *On Stones*, 240:215–216, 220–221.

12. *Dispensatory*, pp. 757–758.

13. Ibid., p. 223.

14. Achille Morricone, "I medicamenti di origine animale ricavati dal mare nell' opera di Dioscoride," *Pagine di Storia della medicina* 7, no. 5 (1963): 25–26.

15. Léon Moulé, "La zoothérapie au temps de Dioscoride et de Pline," *International Congress for the History of Medicine* 1 (1920): 457.

16. On cockroaches in medicine, cf. Sayre, *Manual*, p. 440.

17. On the viper, see Scarborough, "Nicander's Toxicology I," pp. 8–9; Moulé, "La zoothérapie," pp. 456–457.

18. The Greek term, *θηρίον*, *θηριακή*, first was applied to venomous beasts but came to mean also an antidote against animal bites and, more broadly, an antidote against all poisons.

19. Pliny, *N.H.*, XXIX. 21. 70.

20. Ibid., XXIX. 21. 121.

21. For instance in *N.H.*, XXX. 1. 1–3, Pliny denounced magic, but shortly thereafter in his narrative he wrote (XXX. 11. 51): "I find that a heavy cold [*gravedinem*] clears up if the sufferer kisses a mule's muzzle."

22. See Scarborough, "Nicander's Toxicology I," pp. 3–23, and "Nicander's Toxicology II," pp. 3–34, 73–92.

23. Scarborough, "Nicander's Toxicology I," p. 16.

24. Moulé, "La zoothérapie," p. 459.

25. On asps, see Scarborough, "Nicander's Toxicology I," pp. 7–8.

26. Ibid., p. 8.

27. Arena, *Poisoning*, p. 543.

28. He used the words together regarding the walnut (II. 125): *θανασίμων θαρμάκων ἀντιθάρμακον*, taken internally with rue and figs, *before and after* the poisoning.

29. Arena, *Poisoning*, pp. 40, 73.

30. Kenneth G. V. Smith, "Coleoptera and Other Insects: Beetles, Mayflies and Caddisflies," in *Insects and Other Arthropods of Medical Importance*, ed. K. Smith, pp. 413–415; Schneider, *Lexikon*, 1:26; Sayre, *Manual*, pp. 437–438; for a thorough study of the ancients' knowledge, see Scarborough, "Nicander's Toxicology II," pp. 20–21, 74–79.

31. Scarborough, "Nicander's Toxicology II," p. 21.

32. *Dispensatory*, pp. 236–239; *Merck Index*, p. 201.

33. Bin Hsu, "Herbs as Anticancer Agents," p. 304.
34. Paulus Aegineta, *Seven Books,* 3:162–163; cf. Scarborough, "Nicander's Toxicology I," p. 13.
35. Sayre, *Manual,* 451; Schneider, *Lexicon,* 1:27.
36. Trease and Evans, *Pharmacognosy,* pp. 628–637, esp. 637.
37. Moulé, "La zoothérapie," p. 460.
38. Ibid., p. 461.
39. John Riddle, "Amber in Ancient Pharmacy," *Pharmacy in History* 15 (1973): 3–17.
40. Pliny, *N.H.,* XXIX. 8. 17.
41. Forbes, *Ancient Technology,* 3:120.
42. Ibid., 3:114.
43. Ibid., 3:110–111.
44. E.g., Pliny, *N.H.,* XIV. 11. 80. For other references, see Nriagu, *Lead and Lead Poisoning,* pp. 333–352.
45. E.g., Pliny, *N.H.,* XIV. 27. 136: "leaden and not copper jars should be used [for boiling]."
46. Nriagu, *Lead and Lead Poisoning,* p. 350. See also Josef Eisinger, "Lead and Wine: Eberhard Gockel and the *Colica Pictonum,*" *Medical History* 26 (1982): 279–302. For other references to lead poisoning, see "Minerals," below.
47. Pliny, *N.H.,* XXII. 53. 114.
48. Cf. ibid., XIV. 20. 113–115; XXII. 52. 112.
49. Stannard, "Squill," pp. 693–695.
50. Lewis and Elvin-Lewis, *Medical Botany,* pp. 132–133, 183–186, 323.
51. Forbes, *Ancient Technology,* 3:118.
52. Ibid., 3:226–228.
53. Ibid., 3:220.
54. Ibid., 3:215, but Dietlinde Goltz, *Studien zur Geschichte der Mineralnamen in Pharmazie, Chemie und Medizin von den Anfängen bis Paracelsus,* p. 147, does not identify *kuanos.*
55. Goltz, *Mineralnamen,* p. 147.
56. Theophrastus, *On Stones.*
57. Forbes, *Ancient Technology,* 8:260–278; Goltz, *Mineralnamen,* pp. 130–134; André Rosenfeld, *The Inorganic Raw Materials of Antiquity,* pp. 141–142, 151–152; N. F. Moore, *Ancient Mineralogy,* pp. 66–68 (old but still valuable).
58. J. F. Healy, *Mining and Metalurgy in the Greek and Roman World,* pp. 65–66; Forbes, *Ancient Technology,* 8:261–263; Rosenfeld, *Inorganic Raw Materials,* pp. 141–142, 151–152.
59. Cornelius S. Herlbut, Jr., and Cornelis Klein, *Manual of Mineralogy after James D. Dana,* pp. 302–303.
60. *Dispensatory,* p. 1517.
61. Cf. explanation for pharmacologic action by Stewart C. Harvey, "Antiseptics and Disinfectants; Fungicides; Ectoparasiticides," in *Pharmacological Basis of Therapeutics,* p. 1001. For a historical survey of its use, see Schneider, *Lexikon,* 6:207–211.
62. Forbes, *Ancient Technology,* 8:266.
63. Goltz, *Mineralnamen,* pp. 132–134.

64. Helmut Wilsdorf, "Die architektonische Rekonstruktion antiker Produktionsanlagen für Bergbau und Hüttenwesen," *Klio. Beiträge zur alten Geschichte* 59 (1977): 17.

65. In making this translation, I was guided in places by the partial translation by Wyndham Hume (cited by Forbes, *Ancient Technology*, 8:203–204) and the German translation by Wilsdorf, "Die architektonische Rekonstruktion," pp. 16, 18–20.

66. Forbes, *Ancient Technology*, 8:204.

67. Ibid.

68. *Dispensatory*, p. 264.

69. Ibid.

70. Victor Herbert, "Drugs Effective in Iron Deficiency and Other Hypochromic Activity," in *Pharmacological Basis of Therapeutics*, p. 1320.

71. Stewart C. Harvey, "Heavy Metals," in *Pharmacological Basis of Therapeutics*, pp. 938–942; *Dispensatory*, p. 746; Schneider, *Lexikon*, 6:171–175.

72. More-recent assertions are made by S. C. Gilfillan, "Lead Poisoning and the Fall of Rome," *Journal of Occupational Medicine* 7 (1965): 53–60.

73. Vitruvius (*De architectura*, VIII. 6. 10) said that "water is much more wholesome from earthenware than from lead pipes. For it seems to be made injurious by lead, because white lead is produced by it; and this is said to be harmful to the human body."

74. Tony Waldron and Calvin Wells, "Exposure to Lead in Ancient Populations," *Transactions and Studies. College of Physicians of Philadelphia* ser. 5, 1 (1979): 102–115; less conclusively, R. Ted Steinbock, "Lead Ingestion in Ancient Times," *Paleopathology Newsletter*, no. 27 (1979): 9–11.

75. Eisinger, "Lead and Wine," pp. 279–302, esp. 284–288; cf. H. A. Waldron, "Lead Poisoning in the Ancient World," *Medical History* 17 (1973): 391–399.

76. L. Ahlgren, J. O. Christoffersson, and S. Mattsson, "Lead and Barium in Archaeological Roman Skeletons Measured by Nondestructive X-Ray Fluorescence Analysis," *Advances in X-Ray Analysis* 24 (1980): 377–382. Roman skeletons from various grave sites were examined in comparison with prehistoric and twelfth-century medieval skeletons from Sweden as control groups as well as an *in vivo* group. The prehistoric and medieval skeletons revealed a low level of lead concentration in comparison with the Roman artifacts.

77. *Dispensatory*, p. 745.

78. Goltz, *Mineralnamen*, p. 138; Nielsen, *Ancient Ophthalmological Agents*, p. 56.

79. Forbes, *Ancient Technology*, 8:200–205; Goltz (*Mineralnamen*, pp. 139–143) adds other lead compounds as being included in the terms.

80. Harvey, "Heavy Metals," pp. 928–930.

81. Leonard J. Goldwater, *Mercury: A History of Quicksilver*.

82. Pliny, *N.H.*, XXXIII. 38. 115: "milton vocant Graeci miniumque cinnabarim."

83. Theophrastus, *On Stones*, 58, pp. 193–194.

84. Pliny, *N.H.*, XXXIII. 38. 115.

85. Pliny, *N.H.*, 9:86; Grieve, *Modern Herbal*, 1:262.
86. Pliny, *N.H.*, XXXIII. 38. 116.
87. Theophrastus, *On Stones*, 58.
88. Goldwater, *Mercury*, p. 254.
89. Ibid.; Harvey, "Heavy Metals," pp. 935–938.
90. Goldwater, *Mercury*, p. 178.
91. Ibid., p. 78.
92. Goldwater (*Mercury*) does not see Dioscorides' errors regarding confusion of terms; cf. Schneider, *Lexikon*, 6:115–116.
93. Goldwater, *Mercury*, p. 299; Theophrastus, *On Stones*, pp. 178–180; Forbes, *Ancient Technology*, 3:206–207.
94. Moore, *Ancient Mineralogy*, pp. 128–130; Liddell and Scott, *Greek English Lexicon*, p. 1972; cf. more-complex analysis by Goltz, *Mineralnamen*, pp. 152–153, and Schneider, *Lexikon*, 6:86–87.
95. Goltz, *Mineralnamen*, p. 156.
96. Ibid., p. 157; Schneider, *Lexikon*, 3:41.
97. Forbes, *Ancient Technology*, 3:215; Goltz, *Mineralnamen*, pp. 158–160; Schneider, *Lexikon*, 6:52–53.
98. Goltz, *Mineralnamen*, p. 160; Schneider, *Lexikon*, 6:53–55.
99. Harvey, "Heavy Metals," p. 924.
100. Rosenfeld (*Inorganic Raw Materials*, p. 86) identifies it as a glass froth, but E. R. Caley and J. C. Richards (Theophrastus, *On Stones*, p. 92) decline to identify it except to say that it is associated with volcanoes; Goltz (*Mineralnamen*, p. 162) identifies Dioscorides' word as *Bimstein*, or pumice.
101. Gerald L. Geison, "Louis Pasteur," *Dictionary of Scientific Biography*, 10:357; *Dispensatory*, p. 1387.
102. Uno Boklund, "Carl Wihelm Scheele," *Dictionary of Scientific Biography*, 12:146; *Dispensatory*, p. 1387.
103. Pliny, *N.H.*, XXII. 27. 86; Paulus Aegineta, *Seven Books*, 3:33.
104. Paulus Aegina (*Seven Books*, 7. 3, 3:22) describes it as "a sort of froth of salt water, collecting about rubbish and weeds."
105. Riddle, *Marbode of Rennes' De Lapidibus*, pp. 35–43.
106. Cf. John M. Riddle, "Lithotherapy in the Middle Ages . . . Lapideries Considered as Medical Texts," *Pharmacy in History* 12 (1970): 39–50.
107. John M. Riddle and James A. Mulholland, "Albert on Stones and Minerals," in *Albertus Magnus and the Sciences*, ed. J. A. Weisheipl, p. 213; cf. Schneider, *Lexikon*, 6:72–73.
108. *Dispensatory*, p. 773.
109. Cf. for copper, V. 76–90, 89–90, 99–103; for iron, 80, 96–97.
110. Pliny, *N.H.*, XXXVI. 11. 57.
111. In 1688 Nicolas Lemery proposed that the Memphis stone was an ordinary stone that was near where poppy juice had impregnated it because of its proximity. Another theory proposed that limestone near Memphis was acted on by vinegar causing CO_2 which had an anesthetic effect. E. S. Ellis (*Ancient Anodynes: Primitive Anaesthesia, and Allied Conditions*, p. 118) called this suggestion "absurd," and Lemery's idea as "not very satisfactory." Adams (Paulus Aegineta, *Seven Books*, 3:228) says that the Memphis stone contains bitumen

and ethereal oil and may be retinasphatum or retinite; Eichholz (Pliny, 10:45) suggests it might be dolomite.

112. Rackham, Pliny, 9:283; Forbes, *Ancient Technology*, 3:227; *Dispensatory*, pp. 772–773, 778.

113. Theophrastus, *On Stones*, pp. 62–64.

114. Scarborough, "Nicander's Toxicology II," p. 77; Rackham, Pliny, 9:282.

115. Cf. Eichholz, Pliny, 10:121.

116. *Dispensatory*, pp. 734–736.

117. Cf. Pliny, *N.H.*, XXXVI. 40. 152.

118. Forbes, *Ancient Technology*, 3:220.

119. Scarborough and Nutton, "Preface."

120. Ibid.

121. Ibid.

122. Lloyd, *Magic*, p. 125.

123. Lévi-Strauss, *The Savage Mind*, pp. 9–10.

5. *Done and Undone*

1. André Bernand, *Alexandrie la Grand*, p. 116; cf. Majno, *The Healing Hand*, pp. 337–338. The box was not necessarily the depository for Dioscorides of Anazarbus but likely belonged to him. There are other authors bearing the same name, but only one of them is known to have written a multibook work and that was Dioscorides Phacas of Alexandria.

2. Erotian, *Vocum Hippocraticarnum*, 31. 7–9 (85).

3. Galen, *De simpl. med.*, VI. pref., 11:794–795.

4. E.g., ibid., IX. 2, 12:171, and *De Antidotis*, II, 14:191; for other refs, see Kühn's Index to *Opera Omnia*, vol. 20.

5. Galen, *De comp. med. per genera*, V. 15, 13:857.

6. For 473 count, see Max Neuburger, *Geschichte der Medizin*, 1:396, and L. Garcia Ballester, *Galeno*, p. 238; for ca. 434 count, see Jerry Stannard, "Byzantine Botanical Lexicography," *Episteme* 5 (1971): 171 refs.

7. Galenic pharmaceutical theory and its basis in comprehensive Galenic thought are found scattered throughout various works ascribed to Galen, and the details must rest on a determination of the authorship of each treatise. To avoid some of these problems, I am following the suggestion of John Scarborough ("The Galenic Question," *Sudhoffs Archiv* 65 [1981]: 1–31) and use the adjectival form of his name just as we do with "Hippocratic" theory. No single work has studied comprehensively Galenic pharmaceutical theory, but works by Michael McVaugh and Georg Harig provide a good genesis. See esp. Michael McVaugh, "The Mediaeval Theory of Compound Medicines," dissertation, Princeton, 1965, and *Arnaldi de Villanova . . . II. Aphorisimi de gradibus*. For Georg Harig's works, see nn. 9–10 and 16, below. One whose reading is in English will gain insight into Galenic theory *as it evolved* through the explanation by Avicenna in *The Canon of Medicine*. The explanation of Galenic theory here comes from attempts to understand and summarize it with indebtedness and apologies to McVaugh, Harig, and Avicenna.

8. The charts are adapted and expanded versions based on those done by

Hans Biedermann, *Medicina Magica: Metaphysische Heilmethoden in spätantiken und mittelalterlichen Handschriften*, pp. 16–17.

9. Georg Harig, *Bestimmung der Intensität im medizinischen System Galens: Ein Beiträg zur theoretische Pharmakologie, Nosologie und Therapie in der Galenischen Medizin*, p. 74.

10. Harig, "Primär-," pp. 64–81, esp. 68.

11. Galen, *De simpl. med.*, I. 7, 392–393; cf. discussion by McVaugh, "Theory of Compound Medicines," pp. 8–9.

12. Galen, *De simpl. med.*, I. 11, 11:398–399.

13. Lloyd, "The Hot and the Cold," pp. 102–104.

14. When discussing the qualities, Galen used ποιότης ("quality") and δύναμις ("property") almost interchangeably, and so shall I.

15. Galen, *De simpl. med.*, VIII. 20, 12:148.

16. Ibid., III. 10, 11:561, and III. 13, 11:571; cf. discussion by Georg Harig, "Der Begriff der lauen Wärme in der theoretischen Pharmakologie Galens," *NTM* 13 (1976): 70–76, esp. 72.

17. Galen, *De simpl. med.*, VI. 73, 11:843; cf. Harig, "Der Begriff," p. 72.

18. ("Der Begriff," p. 74) discounts a mathematical concept for Galen's intent although it was an effect from interpreting his ideas.

19. Galen, *De simpl. med.*, VII. 43, 12:36–40.

20. Pliny, *N.H.*, 6:x–xi.

21. Galen, *De simpl. med.*, VII. 43, 12, 36.

22. Paulus Aegineta, *Seven Books*, 3:189 for ibn Māsawaih and Sarābiyūn; also see Matthaeus Platearius, *Circa instans*, p. 42, who has coriander warm in the 2°; Al-Kindi (*Medical Formulary*, 21:48, 326–327) used it for a cooling remedy; ibn Sīnā (*Canon*, II. 2. 144, pp. 104–105, Venice, 1507 ed.) repeats the controversy, as does Rufinus (*Herbal*, fol. 45ra&b, pp. 102–103). Of interest is that the action of coriander is still a matter of interpretation. Gathercoal and Wirth (*Pharmacognosy*, p. 525) says that it is a stimulant, which would make it warming in ancient terminology, but Grieve (*Herbal*, 1:222) says that its seeds used too freely have a narcotic effect, which would be cooling.

23. Lloyd, "The Hot and the Cold," p. 94.

24. Kurt Weitzmann, *Illustrations in Roll and Codex*, pp. 69–70; Leighton Durham Reynolds and N. G. Wilson, *Scribes and Scholars*, pp. 29–31, date the codex in the second century despite references to a form of it by Martial in the first century.

25. Weitzmann, *Roll and Codex*, p. 47.

26. Pliny, *N.H.*, XXV. 4. 8.

27. Wellmann, *Krateuas*, pp. 24–25.

28. Tebtunis II, no. 679, published and discussed by J. de M. Johnson, "A Botanical Papyrus with Illustrations, "*Archiv für die Geschichte de Naturwissenschaften und der Technik* 4 (1913): 403–408; cf. Kurt Weitzmann, *Ancient Book Illumination*, pp. 11–12.

29. Johnson, "Botanical Papyrus," p. 404.

30. Campbell Bonner, "A Papyrus of Dioscorides in the University of Michigan Collection," *Transactions and Proceedings of the American Philological Association* 53 (1922): 142–168.

31. Ibid., pp. 142–145.

32. E. O. Winstedt, "Some Greek and Latin Papyri in Aberdeen Museum," *Classical Quarterly* 1 (1907): 263–264; and Wellmann, "Preface," p. xx.

33. C. Leemans, ed., *Papyri Graeci Musei Antiquarii Publici Lugduni-Batavi*, 2:242–249. The fragment is fairly large and begins, "Διοσκορίδου ἐκ τοῦ περὶ ὕλης." It contains sizable and accurate text from the following chapters in order: *arsenikon* (V. 104), *sandarakē* (105), *misu* (100), *kadmia* (74), *chrusokolla* (89), *militos sunopikē* (96), *stuptēria* (106), *nitrōn* (113), *kinnabarei* (94), and *udrarguros* (95).

34. Text and discussion by Singer, "The Herbal in Antiquity," pp. 31–33.

35. J. W. B. Barns and H. Zilliacus, *The Antinoopolis Papyri*, vol. III, no. 123, pp. 31–39; cf. review by U. Fleischer in *Gnomon* 41 (1969): 640–646, esp. 642.

36. So unoriginal did Oribasius' first modern editors think these books to be that they omitted them in their edition: Charles Daremberg and C. Bussemaker, *Oeuvres*. A new edition, however, includes Books XI–XIII: Johannes Raeder, *Oribasii collectionum medicarum reliquiae* (Corpus Medicorum Graecorum, vol. 6), 2 vols in 4 pts, XI–XIII in 1, pt. 2.

37. Max Wellmann, "Die Pflanzennamen des Dioskurides," *Hermes* 33 (1898): 373–375, and repeated in his article on Dioscorides for *P.W.* 5 (1903): 114. Earlier in the *Hermes* article (p. 369), Wellmann suggested that the Alphabetical Dioscorides could date back to the second half of the first century. Galen's tract *On simple medicines* partially uses the alphabet to organize material but one can assume that Galen did not use an Alphabetical Dioscorides because he referred to *De materia medica* as being in five books (see quotation in "Published and Misread," above). The extant early MSS of the Alphabetical Dioscorides dropped Dioscorides' Preface (where he said the work was in five books) and did not divide the work into books. Later extant MS copies (see below), however, which retain Dioscorides' Preface, are divided into five books.

38. Oribasius, *Collectionum medicarum*, V. 22–46, 1: pt. 1, pp. 140–143.

39. There are two facsimile printings: *De codicis Dioscuridei Aniciae Iulianae nunc Vindobonensis Med. Gr. 1*, ed., Joseph de Karabacek, and *Dioscurides Codex Vindobonesis Med. Gr. 1*.

40. Folios 2–12 are various frontispieces, including 4r, 5r, and 7r, interspersed with an index by Johannes Chortasmenos (ca. A.D. 1406); fols. 12v–387, text of Dioscorides in alphabetical order, fragments of Crateuas and Galen, 383 illustrations, 391 plant descriptions; fols. 388–392, an anonymous poem, "Carmen de viribus herbarum"; fols. 393–437v, Euteknios' paraphrase of Nicander's *Theriaka*; fols. 438v–459v, paraphrase of Nicander's *Alexipharmaka*; fols. 460–473, anonymous paraphrase of Oppianos' *Halieutika*; fols. 474–485v, anonymous paraphrase of Dionysios of Philadelphia's *Ornithiaka*; fols. 486–491v, various short fragments described by Herbert Hunger, *Katalog der griechischen Handschriften der oesterreichischen Nationalbibliothek*, 2: pt. 1, 37–41.

41. For a partial listing, see, Riddle, "Dioscorides," 4:14–15; and Ioannis Spatharakis, *Corpus of Dated Illuminated Greek Manuscripts to the Year 1453*,

1:5–6; Otto Mazal, *Pflanzen, Wurzeln, Säfte, Samen: Antike Heilkunst in Miniaturen des Wiener Dioskurides.*

42. Singer, "The Herbal in Antiquity," p. 6.

43. The case is presented by Wellmann, *Krateuas*, with additional comments by Hermann Stadler, "Neues zur alten Botanik," *Bayerische Blaetter für das Gymnasialschulwesen* 34 (1898): 609–614. Max Wellmann published Crateuas' fragments, including those in the Anicia MS in *Pedanii Dioscuridis Anazarbei De materia medica libri quinque*, 3:139–146.

44. Singer ("The Herbal in Antiquity," pp. 8–17) traced and published the suspected Crateuas' drawings from the Anicia manuscript. Wilfrid Blunt and Sandra Raphael, *The Illustrated Herbal*, pp. 18–19, reproduced two illustrations in color. The plant illustrations are, according to Singer's identifications: greater aristolochia (*Aristolochia sempervirens*), fol. 17v, Anicia MS, III. 4, Wellmann; round aristolochia (*A. pallida*), fol. 18v, IV. 4 W.; achilleios (*Salvia multifida*), fol. 24v, IV. 36 W.; purple anemone (*Papaver dubium*), fol. 25v, II. 176 W.; asphodel (*Asphodelus* sp.), fol. 26v, II. 169 W.; argemone (*Adonis aestivalis*), fol. 28v, II. 177 W.; arnoglosson (*Plantago* sp.), fol. 29v, II. 126 W.; asaron (*Asarum europaeum*), fol. 30v, I. 9 W.; asterion (*Silene linifolia*), fol. 32v, IV. 119 W.; and the two anagallides (*Anagallis arvensis* and *A. foemina*), fols. 39v, 40v, II. 178. W.

45. Wellmann, *Krateuas*, pp. 30–32; Antony de Premerstein, in *De codicis Dioscuridei Aniciae Iulianae nunc Vindobonensis Med. Gr. 1*, pp. 88–92; Singer, "The Herbal in Antiquity," p. 7; Blunt and Raphael, *Illustrated Herbal*, p. 17; Weitzmann, *Roll and Codex*, p. 135.

46. Wellmann, *Krateuas*, p. 21; Premerstein, *De codicis Dioscuridei*, pp. 90–91. Wellmann's evidence is somewhat teleological since it is based on the alphabetical order produced by the Crateuas fragments in the Anicia MS.

47. Pliny, *N.H.*, XXV. 4. 8.

48. Wellmann, *Krateuas*, pp. 26–27; Premerstein, *De codicis Dioscuridei*, p. 78.

49. Daubeny (*Roman Husbandry*) compared the pictures in the Anicia MS with Dioscorides' text as identified "by Sibthorp, Lindley, and others." Of the 345 plants, he thought 93 as being a good likeness, 36 as fictitious, 17 as bad, 16 with some resemblance, 127 as "pretty good," 9 as "tolerably like," and 44 as "indifferent." He explained, "When the term *fictitious* is attached, the meaning is, that the artist, in ignorance of the plant named, has given a representation of some other, totally unconnected with the real ones, if indeed he has not in this instance drawn from his own fancy alone." In fairness to the artists, however, Dioscorides sometimes included two or more plant species in one chapter. A judgment would have to be made. One must assume that there might have been one person, the author of an archetype to the Anicia, who had before him copies of Dioscorides', Crateuas', and others' illustrations and he had to fit the pictures to Dioscorides' text, especially, we suppose, when he judged Dioscorides' illustrations to be inferior. Daubney's catalogue is reprinted in the Appendix to *Greek Herbal*, ed. Gunther, pp. 661–679. Gunther has sketches from the Anicia tradition throughout the Goodyer translation and has attempted to update the fitting of picture with plant.

50. A. von Salis, "Images Illustrium," in *Eumusia Festgabe für Ernst Howald*, pp. 11–29.

51. Premerstein, in *De codicis Dioscuridei*, pp. 93–94.

52. Salis, "Images Illustrium," p. 15; cf. Pliny, *N.H.*, XXXV. 2. 11.

53. Wellmann, "Dioskurides," pp. 1139–1140.

54. Paul Buberl, "Die antiken Grundlager der Miniaturen des Wiener Dioskurideskodex," *Jahrbuch des deutschen archäologischen Instituts* 51 (1936): 129–133. The similarity of Dioscorides' portraits in folios 3v and 5v is also observed by Kurt Weitzmann, *Late Antique and Early Christian Book Illumination*, p. 65.

55. Premerstein, in *De codicis Dioscuridei*, pp. 113–114. See also Pietro Capparoni, "Intorno ad una copia delle scene raffiguranti l'estrazione della mandragora . . . ," in *Atti del V congresso internazionale di studi bizantini*, 2: sec. 4, pp. 63–69.

56. Paul Buberl, *Die byzantinischen Handschriften*, 8: pt. 4, p. 23, as cited by Kurt Weitzmann, *Studies in Classical and Byzantine Manuscript Illumination*, p. 136n.

57. Weitzmann, *Manuscript Illumination*, p. 136.

58. Weitzmann, *Roll and Codex*, pp. 81–83.

59. R. Bianchi Bandinelli, "Il Dioscoride di Napoli," in *Accademia Nazionale dei Lincei, Roma, classe di scienze morale, storiche, e filologiche*, ser. 8a, 11:78 (77–104); for a history and description of the MS, see G. Pierleoni, *Catalogus codicum graecorum bibliothecae*, 1:v–xxii, 1–7. Singer, "The Herbal in Antiquity," 24, says incorrectly that the MS is in St. Mark's Library at Venice.

60. Weitzmann, *Manuscript Illumination*, p. 136.

61. Bandinelli, "Il Dioscoride di Napoli," 11:85–94. Bandinelli provides a suggested reconstruction of the order of the leaves because they are misbound.

62. Weitzmann, *Roll and Codex*, pp. 71–72.

63. Ed. Bonnet, "Essai d'identification des plantes médicinales mentionnées par Dioscoride, d'après les peintures d'un manuscrit de la Bibliothèque Nationale de Paris Ms. grec. No. 2179," *Janus* 8 (1903): 167–177, 225–232, 280–285, proposed identifications of 200 of the 415 figures in the MS. The Egyptian original was first proposed by B. de Montfaucon, *Palaegraphica Graeca*, pp. 265 ff.; cf. Weitzmann, *Manuscript Illumination*, p. 28n.

64. Wellmann, *Krateuas*, p. 23.

65. Weitzmann, *Roll and Codex*, pp. 71–72.

66. Singer, "The Herbal in Antiquity," pp. 27–29; Blunt and Raphael, *Illustrated Herbal*, pp. 24–26; Weitzmann, *Manuscript Illumination*, pp. 29–30; see also Plate 6, from fol. 124 in *Bibliothèque Nationale, Departement des manuscrits: Facsimilés de manuscrits Grecs, Latins et Français du Ve au XIVe siècle exposés dans la Galerie Mazarine*.

67. Photographs of the flyleafs of the Yerevan MS (s. XIV) were obtained in 1888 by F. C. Conybeare and deposited in the Oxford Bodleian Library, where they have a shelf mark of Bodl. MS gr. class. e. 19 (31, 538); see Falconer Madan and H. E. Craster, *A Summary Catalogue of Western Manuscripts in the Bodleian Library at Oxford*, 5:62. Notice of the Dioscorides leaves was made by Ernest Bihain, "Les manuscrits grecs du maténadaran d'Erévan," *Byzantion*

42 (1972): 256n. Professor John Scarborough obtained photographs of the Yerevan manuscript from Yerevan and they are the same as those obtained by Conybeare. (I am grateful to Scarborough for supplying me with copies.)

68. This manuscript was known to Wellmann as Matritensis palat. Reg. 44 (2: p. xiii), and now it is in the Biblioteca de Universidad in Salamanca.

69. Berendes, *Dioskurides*, p. 258, suggested *Parietaria cretica* L., and others think it may be *Asperugo procumbens* L. or *Myosotis palustris* L. or *Lithosperum purpureo-coruleum*; cf. Carnoy, *Dictionnaire étymologique*, p. 261; Gunther, *Herbal*, p. 228.

70. Weitzmann, *Manuscript Illumination*, p. 30.

71. On *thapsia*, cf. Theophrastus, *Enquiry*, IX. 11. 2.

72. Also in the same MS in Book II, PNB *Dracontea*, there is a nude man with genitals drawn who, standing beside the plant, looks toward the plant while pointing to a snake. Other human figures appear throughout.

73. For a description and references, see Riddle, "Dioscorides," 4:20–22.

74. Daubeny, *Roman Husbandry*, reprinted in Gunther, *Herbal*, p. 668.

75. Hermann Stadler, "Der lateinische Dioscorides der Münchener Hof- und Staatsbibliothek und die Bedeutung dîeser Uebersetzung für einem Teil der mittelalterlichen Medizin," *Janus* 4 (1899): 548–549.

76. Weitzmann, *Manuscript Illumination*, p. 43.

77. Leiden, Bibliotheek der Rijksuniversiteit, MS or. 289. Ernst J. Grube, "Materialien zum Dioskurides Arabicus," *Aus der Welt der islamischen Kunst. Festschrift für Ernst Kühnel*, p. 169 refs (163–194). The folio on *malabathrum* is reproduced and described by Weitzmann, *Manuscript Illumination*, pp. 28–29.

78. On *malabathron*, see Berthold Laufer, "Malabathron," *Journal Asiatique* 193 (1918): 5–49.

79. Weitzmann, *Manuscript Illumination*, p. 29.

80. Padua, Seminario di Padova, MS 193, described by Elpidio Mioni, "Un novo erbario greco di Dioscoride," *Rassegna Medica Convivum Sanitatis* 36, no. 3 (1959): 169–184.

81. Actually, there are pictures of animals in the Anicia Codex, but most of them illustrate the works of other authors included in the codex, e.g., Euteknios' paraphrase of Nicander's *Theriaka* with 66 pictures of plants and animals (fols. 393–437v) and an anonymous paraphrase of Dionysius of Philadelphia's *Ornithiaka* with pictures of 24 birds. Also there is the picture of the dead dog in the frontispiece (fol. 4v) where the mandrake is drawn. For a discussion of the depictions of this dog, see Kádár, *Greek Zoological Illuminations*, pp. 52–53.

82. But Paris MS gr. 2179, fols. 159v–163v, has animal pictures illustrating the pseudo-Dioscorides' treatise(s) *On poisons*. For a reproduction of these pictures, see Kádár, *Greek Zoological Illuminations*, plates 101–112, p. 71.

83. Singer, "The Herbal in Antiquity," p. 25; cf. Wellmann, *Dioskurides*, 2:xvii–xx.

84. There is a published facsimile edition: *Pedanii Dioscorides Anazarbei De Materia Medica accedunt Nicandri et Eutecni Opuscula Medica*. Before New York became its home, Max Wellmann employed the text for his critical edition, citing it as Phillippicus 21975 and dating it in the eleventh century. Although there are many published notices of the codex, the most comprehensive is the

unpublished notes (46 pp.) made by Samuel A. Ives, August 1953, and kept in the Pierpont Morgan Library. Ives discusses the reasons for the ca. 890 date.

85. Little notice is made of this codex. For a brief description, see Iohannes Mercati and Pius Franchi de' Cavalieri, *Bibliothecae Apostolicae Vaticanae. Codices Vaticani graeci*, 1:393; and Kurt Weitzmann, *Die byzantinische Buchmalerei des 9. und 10. Jahrunderts*, p. 34. Identification of the animals is made by Zoltán Kádár, "Etude comparée des miniatures zoologiques dans trois manuscrits byzantins . . . ," *Acta Biologica Debrecina* 7–8 (1969–1970): 257–263.

86. Spyridon and Sophronios Eustratiades, *Catalogue of the Greek Manuscripts in the Library of the Laura on Mount Athos with Notices from Other Libraries*, 12:343. Wellmann used the text for his edition. Plates of its pictures are published by Weitzmann, *Manuscript Illumination*, pp. 31, 146–148; Weitzmann, *Roll and Codex*, pp. 86–87, pl. 24, no. 68 (I have not seen this MS).

87. J. Théodoridès, "Remarques sur l'iconographie zoologique dans certains manuscrits médicaux byzantins et étude des miniatures zoologique du Codex Vaticanus Graecus," in *Jahrbuch der oesterreiches byzantinische Gesellschaft*, pp. 24–27, esp. 26.

88. Pius F. de' Cavalieri, *Codices Graeci Christiani et Borigiani*, pp. 104–106.

89. A. Olivieri, catalogue of Bologna MSS as printed in Christa Samberger, *Catalogi Codicem Graecorum qui in monoribus Bibliothecis Italicis Asservantur*, 1:60–74. Also see Capparoni, "Intorno ad una copia," pp. 62–69.

90. Otto Penzig, *Contribuzioni alla Storia della Botanica*, pp. 246–247 (pp. 241–279, plus plates for full discussion of the Chigi MS).

91. Weitzmann, *Manuscript Illumination*, p. 148.

92. New York, Pierpont Morgan MS 652, fol. 214v; Vatican Chigi MS 53 (F. VII. 159), fol. 209. For photographs of these pictures, Kádár, *Greek Zoological Illuminations* pp. 58–59.

93. J. Théodoridès, "Intérêt scientifique des miniatures zoologiques d'un manuscrit de Matiere médicale de Dioscuride," *Acta Biologica Debrecina* 7–8 (1969–1970): 268.

94. Kádár, *Greek Zoological Illuminations*, p. 62.

95. Théodoridès, "Intérêt scientifique," p. 267; Kádár, *Greek Zoological Illuminations*, pp. 58–59.

96. Kádár, *Greek Zoological Illuminations*, pp. 58–59

97. Ibid.

98. Premerstein, *De codicis Dioscuridei*, pp. 101–110; Charles Diehl, *Manuel de l'art byzantin*, 1:237–239; H. Gerstinger, *Die griechische Buchmalerei*, pp. 19–21; Weitzmann, *Roll and Codex*, p. 136; Singer, "The Herbal in Antiquity," pp. 20–29; P. Burberl, "Wiener Dioskurideskodex," pp. 114–136; Kádár, *Greek Zoological Illuminations*, pp. 13, 69.

99. Wellmann, *Dioscurides*, 2:vi.

100. Eugen Oder, "Revue of *Pedanii Dioscuridis*," *Berliner philologische Wochenschrift*, no. 17 (April 28, 1906), col. 520; Premerstein, *De codicis Dioscuridei*, p. 118, also rejected Wellmann's Joannine recension.

101. Bonner, "A Papyrus of Dioscurides," pp. 167–168.

102. Described by P. A. Revilla, *Catálogo de los códices griegos de la Biblioteca de el Escorial*, pp. 268–271; cf. Wellmann, *Dioscurides*, 2:xi–xii.

103. Kádár, *Greek Zoological Illuminations*, p. 65.

104. Weitzmann, *Manuscript Illumination*, p. 148.

105. Kádár, *Greek Zoological Illuminations*, p. 68.

106. Ibid., p. 61.

107. Ibid., p. 46.

108. Wilhelmina F. Jashemski, *The Gardens of Pompeii, Herculaneum and the Villas Destroyed by Vesuvius*, pp. 55–87; idem, "The Campanian Peristyle Garden," in *Ancient Roman Gardens*, ed. Elizabeth B. MacDougall and Wilhelmina F. Jashemski, pp. 47–48.

109. Max Wellmann, "Dorion," no. 4, *P.W.* 5 (1905): 1563; cf. Kádár, *Greek Zoological Illuminations*, p. 63 refs.

110. Kádár, *Greek Zoological Illuminations*, p. 117.

111. Weitzmann, *Christian Book Illumination*, pp. 70–71; cf. his *Ancient Book Illumination*, pp. 16–17.

WORKS CITED

ANCIENT AUTHORS AND WORKS

Aeschylus. *Prometheus*. In *Aeschylus*. 2 vols. Chicago: University of Chicago Press, 1953–1956.

Aetios of Amida. *The Gynaecology and Obstetrics of the VI*[th] *Century, A.D.: Translated from the Latin Edition of Cornarius, 1542*. Trans. James V. Ricci. Philadelphia: Blakiston, 1950.

Aretaeus. *De causis et signis acutorum morborum libri II*. In *Aretaeus*, ed. Karl Hüde. 2 vols. Corpus medicorum Graecorum. Leipzig and Berlin: Teubner, 1923; repr. Berlin: Academiae Scientiarum, 1958.

———. *The Extant Works of Aretaeus, the Cappadocian*. Ed. and trans. Francis Adams. London: Sydenham Society, 1856; repr. Boston: Longwood, 1977.

Aristotle. *Physics*. Trans. Philip H. Wicksteed and Francis M. Cornford. 2 vols. Cambridge, Mass.: Harvard University Press; London: Heinemann, [1934?]–1935.

Athenaeus. *Deipnosophists*. Ed. and trans. Charles Burton Gulick. 7 vols. Cambridge, Mass.: Harvard University Press; London: Heinemann, 1927–1941.

Caelius Aurelianus. *On Acute Diseases and on Chronic Diseases*. Ed. and trans. I. E. Drabkin. Chicago: University of Chicago Press, 1950.

Caesar, Julius. *Gallic Wars*. Rev. ed. Arthur T. Walker. Chicago: Scott, Foresman, 1926.

Celsus, *De medicina*. Ed. and trans. W. G. Spencer. 3 vols. Cambridge, Mass.: Harvard University Press; London: Heinemann, 1935–1938.

Crateuas. [Fragments]. In Max Wellmann, *Pedanii Dioscoridis Anazarbei De materia medica libri quinque*. 3 vols. Berlin: Weidmann, 1906–1914 [vol. 1, 1907]; repr. Berlin: Weidmann, 1958.

Diodorus. *Library*. Ed. and trans. C. H. Oldfather. 12 vols. Cambridge, Mass: Harvard University Press; London: Heinemann, 1939–1967.

Dioscorides. *De materia medica.*

Modern Editions

Dioscoride Latino Materia Medica Libro Primo. Ed. H. Mihaescu. Iaşi: A. A. Terek, 1938.
Sprengel, Curtius. *Pedanii Dioscoridis Anazarbei De materia medica libri quinque.* Medicorum graecorum opera quae exstant, vols. 25–26. Leipzig: Cnoblochii, 1829–1830.
Wellmann, Max. *Pedanii Dioscoridis Anazarbei De materia medica libri quinque.* 3 vols. Berlin: Weidmann, 1906–1914 [vol. 1, 1907]; repr. Berlin: Weidmann, 1958.

Modern Translations

Berendes, Julius. *Des Pedanios Dioskurides aus Anazarbos Arzneimittellehre in fünf Buchern.* Stuttgart: F. Enke, 1902.
Gunther, Robert T. *The Greek Herbal of Dioscorides: Illustrated by a Byzantine A.D. 512. Englished by John Goodyer A.D. 1655. Edited and First Printed by Robert T. Gunther.* New York: Hafner, 1934; repr. 1959, 1968.
Scarborough, John, and Vivian Nutton. "The Preface of Dioscorides' *De materia medica*: Introduction, Translation, Commentary." *Transactions and Studies of the College of Physicians of Philadelphia* 4, no. 3 (1982): 187–227.

Manuscripts Cited

Bologna. Biblioteca Universitaria. MS gr. 3632. s. xii.
Cambridge. University Library. MS Ee 15, s. xvi.
El Escorial. Real Biblioteca. MS 37 (R III 3), s. xi.
Leiden, Bibliotheek der Rijksuniversiteit. MS gr. 289, anno 1083.
Mount Athos. Library of the Laura. MS Omega 75, s. xii.
Munich. Bayrische Staatsbibliothek. MS lat. 337, s. x.
Naples. Biblioteca Nazionale. MS gr. 1, s. vii.
New York. Pierpont Morgan Library. MS 652, s. x.
———. Facsimile: *Pedanii Dioscorides Anazarbei De Materia Medica accedunt Nicandri et Eutechi Opuscula Medica.* Paris, 1935.
Oxford. Bodleian Library. MS gr. class. e. 19 (31528), photographs and transcription made in 1888 of Yrevan fragment.
Padua. Biblioteca del Seminario. MS 194, s. xiv.
Paris. Bibliothèque Nationale. MS gr. 2179, s. ix; MS gr. 2182, anno 1481; MS gr. 2183, s. xv.
Salamanca. Biblioteca Universitaria. MS 2659, s. xv.
Vatican. Biblioteca Apostolica. MS Chigi F. VII. 159 (53), s. xv, illustrations only; MS gr. 284, s. x, with illustrations added in s. xv.
Vienna. Nationalbibliothek. MS med. gr. 1, s. vi.
———. Facsimile: *De codicis Dioscuridei Aniciae Iulianae nunc Vindobonensis Med. Gr. 1.* Ed. Joseph de Karabacek; comm. Anthony de Premerstein, Carol Wessely, and Josephus Mantuani. 4 vols. Leiden: A. W. Sijthoff, 1906.

———. Facsimile: *Dioscurides Codex Vindobonensis Med. Gr. 1.* Comm. J. Gerstinger. 5 vols. Graz: Akademische Druck- u. Verlagsanstalt, 1965–1970.

Erotian. *Erotiani vocum Hippocraticarum collectio cum fragmentis.* Ed. Ernst Nachmanson. Uppsala: Appelbergs, 1918.

Galen. *Claudii Galeni Opera Omnia.* Ed. Claude G. Kühn. 20 vols. in 22 pts. Leipzig: Car. Cnoblochii, 1821–1833; repr. Hildesheim: G. Olms, 1964–1965:

Ad Glauconem de medendi methodo. 11:1–146.

De antidotis. 14:1–209.

De compositione medicamentorum per genera libri VII. 13:362–1058.

De compositione medicamentorum secundum locos libri X. 12:378–13:361.

De differentia pulsum. 8:493–765[?].

De fasciis liber 1. 18a:768–838.

De libris propriis. 19:8–48.

De methodo medendi. 10:1–1021.

De sanitate tuenda. 6:1–452.

De tumoribus praeter naturam. 7:705–732.

De venae sectione adversus Erasistratum. 11:147–378.

Hippocratis de acutorum morborum victu liber et Galeni Commentarius IV. 15: 732–919.

In Hippocratis aphorismos commentarii, VII. 17b:345–18a:195.

———. "Galen on Abnormal Swellings." Trans. and comm. D. G. Lytton and L. M. Resuhr. *Journal of the History of Medicine and Allied Sciences* 33 (1978): 531–549.

———. "On Medical Sects: For Beginners." In *Greek Medicine,* ed. and trans. A. J. Brock, pp. 130–151. London: Dent, 1929.

———. *On the Usefulness of the Parts of the Body.* Trans. with introd. and comm. Margaret Talmadge May. 2 vols. Ithaca: Cornell University Press, 1968.

Hermetica: The Ancient Greek and Latin Writings Which Contain Religious or Philosophic Teachings Ascribed to Hermes Trismegistus. Ed. and trans. Walter Scott. 4 vols. Oxford: Clarendon Press, 1924.

Hippocrates, *Aphorismi.* In *Hippocrates,* ed. and trans. W. H. Jones, 4:98–221. 4 vols. Cambridge, Mass.: Harvard University Press; London: Heinemann, 1923–1931.

———. *The Art.* In *Hippocrates,* ed. and trans. W. H. Jones, 2:185–217. 4 vols. Cambridge, Mass.: Harvard University Press; London: Heinemann, 1923–1931.

———. *The Canon.* In *Hippocratic Writings,* ed. G. E. R. Lloyd; trans. J. Chadwick and W. N. Mann, pp. 68–69. New York: Penguin, 1978.

———. *On the Sacred Disease.* In *Hippocrates,* ed. and trans. W. H. Jones, 2:138–183. 4 vols. Cambridge, Mass.: Harvard University Press; London: Heinemann, 1923–1931.

Jerome. *Letters.* In *Patrologiae cursus completus. Series latina,* ed. J. P. Migne, 22:235–1182. 221 vols. Paris, 1845.

Josephus. *Wars of the Jews.* In *Josephus,* ed. and trans. H. St. Thackeray. 9 vols. Cambridge, Mass.: Harvard University Press; London: Heinemann, 1926–1965.

Lucianus. *How to Write History*. In *Dialogues*, ed. and trans. A. M. Harmon, 6:1–73. 8 vols. Cambridge, Mass.: Harvard University Press; London: Heinemann, [1913]–1967.

Nicander. *Nicander: The Poems and Poetical Fragments*. Ed. and trans. A. S. F. Gow and A. F. Scholfield. Cambridge: Cambridge University Press, 1953.

Oribasius. *Oeuvres*. Ed. Charles Daremberg and C. Bussemaker. 6 vols. Paris: J. B. Bailliere, 1851–1876.

———. *Oribasii collectionum medicarum reliquiae*. Ed. Johannes Raeder. 2 vols. in 4 pts. Corpus medicorum Graecorum. Leipzig and Berlin: Teubner, 1928; repr. Amsterdam: Hakkart, 1964.

Papyri Graeca Magicae. Die griechischen Zauberpapyri. 2d ed. Ed. Karl Preisendanz. 2 vols. Stuttgart: Teubner, 1973–1974.

Papyrus Ebers: The Greatest Egyptian Medical Document. Trans. B. Ebbell. Copenhagen: Levin and Munksgaard; London: Oxford University Press, 1937.

Paulus Aegineta. *Seven Books of Paulus Aegineta*. Trans. Francis Adams. 3 vols. London: Syndenham Society, 1844.

Periplus of the Erythraean Sea. Ed. and trans. G. W. B. Huntingford. London: Hakluyt Society, 1980.

Philo Judaeus. *On Husbandry*. Ed. and trans. F. H. Colson and G. H. Whitaker. 10 vols. Cambridge, Mass.: Harvard University Press; London: Heinemann, 1929–1962.

Pliny. *Natural History*. Ed. W. H. Jones, H. Rackham, and D. E. Eichholz. 10 vols. Cambridge, Mass.: Harvard University Press; London: Heinemann, 1938–1963.

Pliny the Younger. *Letters*. Ed. and trans. Betty Radice. 2 vols. Cambridge, Mass.: Harvard University Press; London: Heinemann, 1969.

Rufos of Ephesus. *Oeuvres*. Ed. C. Daremberg and Emile Ruelle. Paris: Imprimerie Nationale, 1879; repr. Amsterdam: Hakkart, 1963.

Scribonius Largus. *Conpositiones*. Ed. George Helmreich. Leipzig: Teubner, 1887.

Sextus Empiricus. *Against the Mathematicians*. In *Opera*, ed. H. Mutschmann. 4 vols. Leipzig: Teubner, 1912–1964.

———. *Sextus Empiricus*. Ed. and trans. R. G. Bury. 4 vols. Cambridge, Mass.: Harvard University Press; London: Heinemann, 1961.

Soranus. *Gynecology*. Trans. Owsei Temkin. Baltimore: Johns Hopkins University Press, 1956.

———. *Soranii Gynaeciorum libri IV. De signis fracturarum. De fascii. Vita Hippocratis secundum Soranum*. Ed. Johannes Ilberg. Leipzig and Berlin: Teubner, 1927.

Strabo. *Geography*. Ed. and trans. Horace Leonard Jones. 8 vols. Cambridge, Mass.: Harvard University Press; London, Heinemann: 1917–1935.

Tacitus. *Annals*. Ed. and trans. John Jackson. 3 vols. Cambridge, Mass.: Harvard University Press; London: Heinemann, 1951.

Theophrastus. *Enquiry into Plants*. Ed. and trans. Arthur Hort. 2 vols. Cambridge, Mass.: Harvard University Press; London: Heinemann, 1948.

———. *On Stones*. Ed. and trans. Earle R. Caley and John C. Richards. Columbus: Ohio State University Press, 1956.

Varro. *Rerum rusticarum.* In *Cato and Varro,* ed. William Davis Hooper; rev. Harrison Boyd Ash. Cambridge, Mass.: Harvard University Press; London: Heinemann, 1934.

Vergil. *Aeneid.* Ed. and trans. H. Rushton Fairclough. 2 vols. Cambridge, Mass.: Harvard University Press; London: Heinemann, 1946.

———. *Eclogues.* Ed. Robert Coleman. Cambridge: Cambridge University Press, 1977.

Vitruvius. *De architectura.* Ed. and trans. Frank Granger. 2 vols. Cambridge, Mass.: Harvard University Press; London: Heinemann, 1931–1934.

MEDIEVAL AND MODERN AUTHORS AND WORKS

Acta Phytotherapeutica. 1– (1954–).

Adams, Francis. See Paulus Aegineta.

Ahlgren, L., J. O. Christofferson, and S. Mattsson. "Lead and Barium in Archaeological Roman Skeletons Measured by Nondestructive X-Ray Fluorescence Analysis." *Advances in X-Ray Analysis* 24 (1980): 377–382.

Al-Kindi. *Medical Formulary.* Ed. and trans. Martin Levey. Madison: University of Wisconsin Press, 1966.

Allbutt, T. Clifford. *Greek Medicine in Rome.* New York: Thomas, 1921.

André, Jacques. *Lexique des termes de botanique en latin.* Paris: C. Klincksieck, 1956.

Archila, Richardo. "Pedacio Dioscoridas." *Sociedad Mexicana de Historia y Filosofía de la Medicina Boletín* suppl. (1980): 2–20.

Arena, Jay M. *Poisoning: Toxicology—Symptoms—Treatments.* 3d ed. Springfield: Thomas, 1974.

Avicenna. *Liber Canonis.* Venice: Paganinum de paganinis Burieniem, 1507; repr. in fasc. Hildesheim: Georg Olms, 1964.

———. *A Treatise of the Canon of Medicine of Avicenna Incorporating a Translation of the First Book.* Trans. O. Cameron Gruner. New York: Augustus M. Kelley, 1970.

Baader, Gerhard. "Ärzte auf pannonischen Inschriften." *Klio. Beiträge zur alten Geschichte* 55 (1973): 273–279.

———. "Der Ärztliche Stand in der Antike." In *Jahrbuch der Universität Düsseldorf 1977/8,* pp. 301–315. Düsseldorf, 1978.

Bailey, L. H. *Manual of Cultivated Plants Most Commonly Grown in the Continental United States and Canada.* Rev. ed. New York: Macmillan, 1949.

Ballester, L. Garcia. *Galeno en la sociedad y en la ciencia de su tiempo (c. 130 c. 200 d. de C.).* Madrid: Ediciones Guadarrma, 1972.

Bandinelli, R. Bianchi. "Il Dioscoride di Napoli." *Accademia Nazionale dei Lincei, Roma classe di scienza morale, storiche, e filologiche* ser. 8a. 11 (fasc., 3–4, 1956): 77–104.

Barns, J. W. B., and H. Zilliacus. *The Antinoopolis Papyri,* vol. III. London: Egypt Exploration Society, 1967.

Benson, Herbert, and David P. McCallie, Jr. "Angina Pectoris and the Placebo Effect." *New England Journal of Medicine* 300, no. 25 (1979): 1423–1429. 1891; repr. Hildesheim: Georg Olms, 1965.

Berendes, Julius. *Die Pharmazie bei den alten Kulturvolkern, Historische-Kritsche.* 2 vols. Halle: Tausch and Grosse, 1891; repr. Hildesheim: George Olms, 1965.

———. See Dioscorides.

Bernand, André. *Alexandrie la Grand.* Paris: Arthaud, 1966.

Bernert, Ernst. "Philonides." No. 6 *P. W.* 20 (1941): 73–74.

Bibliothèque Nationale, Departement des manuscrits. Facsimilés de Manuscrits Grecs, Latins et Francais du Ve au XIVe siècle exposés dans la Galerie Mazarine. Paris, [1900].

Biedermann, Hans. *Medicina Magica: Metaphysische Heilmethoden in spätantiken und mittelalterlichen Handschriften.* Graz: Akademische Druck, 1972.

Bihain, Ernest. "Les manuscrits grecs du maténadaran d'Erévan." *Byzantion* 42 (1972): 254–256.

Bin Hou. "The Use of Herbs as Anticancer Agents." *American Journal of Chinese Medicine* 8 (1980): 301–306.

Blood, D. C., and J. A. Henderson. *Veterinary Medicine.* 4th ed. Baltimore: Williams and Wilkins, 1974.

Blunt, Wilfrid, and Sandra Raphael. *The Illustrated Herbal.* New York: Thames and Hudson, 1979.

Boklund, Uno. "Carl Wilhelm Scheele." In *Dictionary of Scientific Biography,* 12:143–150. 1975.

Bonner, Campbell. "A Papyrus of Dioscorides in the University of Michigan Collection." *Transactions and Proceeding of the American Philogical Association* 53 (1922): 142–168.

Bonnet, Ed. "Essai d'identification des plantes médicinales mentionnées par Dioscoride, d'après les peintures d'un manuscrit de la Bibliothèque Nationale de Paris Ms. grec. No. 2179." *Janus* 8 (1903): 167–177, 225–232.

———. "Etude sur les figures de plantes et d'animaux peintes dans un version arabe, manuscrite, de la matière médicale de Dioscoride." *Janus* 14 (1909): 294–303.

Bourne, Henry R. "Rational Use of Placebo." In *Clinical Pharmacology,* ed. Kenneth L. Melmon and Howard F. Morelli, pp. 1052–1062. 2d. ed. New York: Macmillan, 1978.

Brock, A. J., trans. and ed. *Greek Medicine.* London, 1929.

Brothwell, Don. "The Evidence for Neoplasms." In *Diseases in Antiquity: A Survey of the Diseases, Injuries, and Surgery of Early Populations,* ed. Don Brothwell and A. T. Sandison, pp. 320–346. Springfield: Thomas, 1967.

Buberl, Paul. "Die antiken Grundlager der Miniaturen des Wiener Dioskurideskodex." *Jahrbuch des deutschen archäologischen Instituts* 51 (1936): 114–136.

———. *Die byzantinischen Handschriften.* Beschreibendes Verzeichnis der illuminierten Handschriften in Östereich, 8, pt 4. Leipzig: K. Hiersemann, 1937.

Budge, E. A. Wallis. *The Divine Origin of the Craft of the Herbalist.* London: Society of Herbalists, 1928.

Burkill, I. H. *A Dictionary of the Economic Products of the Malay Peninsula.* 2 vols. Kuala Lumpur: Ministry of Agriculture and Cooperatives, 1966.

Calabresi, Paul, and Robert E. Parks, Jr. "Alkylating Agents, Antimetabolics, Hormones and Other Antiproliferative Agents." In *The Pharmacological Basis of Therapeutics*, ed. Louis S. Goodman and Alfred Gilman, pp. 1254–1308. 5th ed. New York: Macmillan, 1975.

———, ———. "Chemotherapy of Neoplastic Diseases." In *The Pharmacological Basis of Therapeutics*, ed. Louis S. Goodman and Alfred Gilman, pp. 1248–1253. 5th ed. New York: Macmillan, 1975.

Caley, Earle R., and John C. Richards. See Theophrastus.

Capparoni, Pietro. "Intorno ad una copia delle scene raffiguranti l'estrazione della mandragora, che ornavano il Codice così detto 'Dioscoride di Giuliana Ancia', da lungo tempo scomparse." *Atti del V Congresso internazionale di studi bizantini, Roma 20–26 settembre 1936*. Vol. 2: *Archeologia*, sec. IV, pp. 63–69. Rome, 1936.

Carcopino, Jérôme. *Daily Life in Ancient Rome*. Trans. E. O. Lorimer; ed. Henry T. Rowell. New Haven: Yale University Press, 1940.

Carnoy, A. *Dictionnaire étymologique des noms grecs de plantes*. Bibliothèque de Muséon, vol. 46. Louvain, 1959.

Cavalieri, Pius F. de. *Codices Graeci Christiani et Borigiani*. Rome: Typis Polyglottis Vaticanis, 1927.

Chance, Burton. *Ophthalmology*. New York: P. B. Hoeber, 1939.

Chaudhury, R. R. "Plants with Possible Antifertility Activity." *Indian Council for Medical Research, Special Reports Series* 55 (1966): 3–19.

Chemical Abstracts. 1907–.

Cohn. "Erotianos." *P.W.* 6, pt. 1 (1907): 544–549.

Cohn-Haft, Louis. *The Public Physicians of Ancient Greece*. Northampton, Mass.: Department of History of Smith College, 1956.

Comaroff, Jean. "A Bitter Pill to Swallow: Placebo Therapy in General Practice." *Sociological Review* n.s. 24 (1976): 79–96.

Croom, E. N., Jr., "Ethnobotanical Documentation in the Evaluation of the Safety and Efficacy of Herbal Medicine by Pharmacological Testing." *Journal of Ethnopharmacology* (forthcoming).

Daly, L. W. *Contributions to a History of Alphabetization in Antiquity and the Middle Ages*. Brussels: Latomus, 1967.

Daubeny, Charles. *Lectures on Roman Husbandry*. Oxford: J. Wright, 1857.

Davies, P. H., and V. H. Heywood. *Principles of Angiosperm Taxonomy*. Huntington, N.Y.: R. E. Krieger, 1973.

Davies, R. W. "The Medici of the Roman Armed Forces." *Epigraphische Studien* 8 [1969]: 83–99.

———. "Some More Military Medici." *Epigraphische Studien* 9 (1972): 1–11.

Dickinson, Sheila K. "Abortion in Antiquity." *Arethusa* 6 (1973): 159–166.

Diechgräber, Karl. *Die griechische Empirikerschule: Sammlung der Fragmente und Darstellung der Lehre*. Berlin: Weidmann, 1930.

———. "Petronius." No. 1. *P.W.* 19 (1937): 1193–1194.

———. *Professio medici-Zum Vorwort des Scribonius Largus*. Abhandunger Akademic der Wissenschaften und der Literatur, Mainz, no. 9. Wiesbaden: F. Steiner, 1950.

———. "Sextius Niger." No. 33A, *P.W.* 5 suppl. (1931): 971–972.

Diehl, Charles. *Manuel de l'art byzantin.* 2 vols. Paris: A. Pickard, 1925–1926.
Dierbach, Johann Heinrich. *Die Arzneimittel des Hippokrates.* Heidelberg, 1824; repr. Hildesheim, 1969.
Diller, Hans. "Philistion." No. 4. *P.W.* (1938): 2405–2408.
———. "Thessalos." *P.W.* (1936): 168–182.
Dispensatory of the United States of America. 28th ed. Philadelphia: Lippincott, 1955.
Dittenberger, Wilhelm. *Orientis Graeci Inscriptiones Selectae.* 2 vols. Leipzig: S. Hirzel, 1903.
Dodds, E. R. *The Greeks and the Irrational.* Berkeley: University of California Press, 1951.
———. *Pagan and Christian in an Age of Anxiety.* New York: Norton, 1970.
Dowling, Henry F. *Medicines for Man.* New York: Knopf, 1973.
Drabkin, I. E. See Caelius Aurelianus.
Driver, John Edmund, and George Edward Trease. *The Chemistry of Crude Drugs.* London: Longman, Green & Co., 1928.
Duke, James A. "Phytotoxin Tables." *C.R.C. Critical Reviews in Toxicology* 5 (November 1977): 189–237.
Duncan-Jones, Richard. *The Economy of the Roman Empire: Quantitative Studies.* Cambridge: Cambridge University Press, 1974.
DuPinet, Antoine. See Pinaeus, Antonius.
Dustin, A. P. "Nouvelles applications des poisons caryoclassique à la cancerologic." *Sang* 12 (1938): 677–697.
Edelstein, Emma Jeannette, and Ludwig Edelstein. *Asclepius: A Collection and Interpretation of the Testimonies.* 2 vols. Baltimore: Johns Hopkins University Press, 1945.
Edelstein, Ludwig. "Empiricism and Skepticism in the Teaching of the Greek Empiricist School." In *Ancient Medicine,* ed. Oswei and C. Lilian Temkins, pp. 195–203. Baltimore: Johns Hopkins University Press, 1967.
———. "Greek medicine in Its Relation to Religion and Magic." *Bulletin of the Institute of the History of Medicine* 5 (1937): 201–246; repr. in *Ancient Medicine,* ed. Oswei and C. Lilian Temkin, pp. 205–246. Baltimore: Johns Hopkins University Press, 1967.
———. "The Hippocratic Oath." In *Ancient Medicine,* ed. Oswei and C. Lilian Temkins, pp. 3–63. Baltimore: Johns Hopkins University Press, 1967.
———. "The Methodists." In *Ancient Medicine,* ed. Oswei and C. Lilian Temkin, pp. 173–191. Baltimore: Johns Hopkins University Press, 1967.
Eisinger, Josef. "Lead and Wine: Eberhard Gockel and the *Colica Pictonum.*" *Medical History* 26 (1982): 279–302.
Ellis, E. S. *Ancient Anodynes: Primitive Anaesthesia and Allied Conditions.* London: Heinemann, 1946.
Emmott, William. "Ophthalmology in Classical Medicine." *Ophthalmic Optician* 5 (1965): 14, 19–22, 81–82.
Engles, Donald. "The Problem of Female Infanticide in the Graeco-Roman World." *Classical Philology* 75 (1980): 112–120.
Erman, Adolf, and H. Grapow. *Wörterbuch der ägyptische Sprache.* 5 vols. Leipzig: Heinrichs, 1926–1950.

Estes, J. Worth. "Making Therapeutic Decisions with Protopharmacologic Evidence." *Transactions and Studies of the College of Physicians of Philadelphia* 1, no. 2 (1979): 116–137.

Eustratiades, Spyridon and Sophronios. *Catalogue of the Greek Manuscripts in the Library of the Laura on Mount Athos with Notices from Other Libraries.* Cambridge, Mass.: Harvard University Press, 1925.

Evans-Pritchard, E. E. *Witchcraft, Oracles and Magic among the Azande.* Oxford: Clarendon Press, 1937.

Fabricius, Ioannes. *Bibliotheca Graeca.* Ed. G. C. Harles. 12 vols. Hamburg: Christian Liebezeit, 1790–1809.

Fairbairn, J. W. "Perspectives in Research on the Active Principles of Traditional Herbal Medicine." *Journal of Ethnopharmacology* 2 (1980): 99–104.

Farnsworth, Norman R. "The Phytochemistry of Vinca Species." In *The Vinca Alkaloids,* ed. William I. Taylor and Norman Farnsworth. New York: M. Dekker, 1973.

———, Audrey S. Bingel, Geoffrey A. Cordell, Frank A. Crane, and Harry H. S. Fong. "Potential Value of Plants as Sources of New Antifertility Agents I." *Journal of Pharmaceutical Sciences* 64 (1975): 535–598.

Feen, Richard Harrow. "Abortion and Exposure in Ancient Greece: Assessing the Status of the Fetus and 'Newborn' from Classical Sources." In *Abortion and the Status of the Fetus,* ed. William B. Bondeson et al., pp. 283–300. Dordrecht: Reidel, 1983.

Finch, B. E., and Hugh Green. *Contraception through the Ages.* Springfield: Thomas, 1963.

Fingl, Edward. "Laxative and Cathartics." In *The Pharmacological Basis of Therapeutics,* ed. Louis S. Goodman and Alfred Gilman, pp. 976–986. 5th ed. New York: Macmillan, 1975.

Fischer, Hermann. *Mittelalterliche Pflanzenkunde.* Munich: Münchner Drucke, 1929.

Fleischer, U. "Review of *Antinoopolis Papyri.*" *Gnomon* 41 (1969): 640–646.

Flück, H. "The Influence of Climate on the Active Principles in Medicinal Plants." *Journal of Pharmacy and Pharmacology* 7 (1955): 361–383.

———. "The Influence of the Soil on the Content of Active Principles in Medicinal Plants." *Journal of Pharmacy and Pharmacology* 6 (1954): 153–163.

Flückiger, Friedrich A., and Daniel Hanbury. *Pharmacographia: A History of the Principal Drugs of Vegetable Origin Met with in Great Britain and British India.* 2d ed. London: Macmillan, 1879.

Forbes, Robert James. *Studies in Ancient Technology.* 9 vols. Leiden: Brill, 1955–1964.

Foster, George M., and Barbara Gallatin Anderson. *Medical Anthropology.* New York: Knopf, 1978.

Fraser, Peter Marshal. *Ptolemaic Alexandria.* 3 vols. Oxford: Clarendon Press, 1972.

Frazer, J. G. *The Golden Bough.* 3d ed. 12 vols. London: Macmillan, 1911–1915.

Gathercoal, Edmund N., and Elmer H. Wirth. *Pharmacognosy.* Philadelphia, 1936.

Geison, Gerald L. "Louis Pasteur." In *Dictionary of Scientific Biography*, 10: 351–416. 1974.

Georgi, Laura. "Pollination Ecology of the Date Palm and Fig Tree: Herodotus 1. 193. 4–5." *Classical Philology* 77 (1982): 224–228.

Gerstinger, H. *Die griechische Buchmalerei.* Vienna: Verlag der Öesterreichischen Staatsdruckesei, 1926.

Gilfillan, S. C. "Lead Poisoning and the Fall of Rome." *Journal of Occupational Medicine* 7 (1965): 53–60.

Goldwater, Leonard J. *Mercury: A History of Quicksilver.* Baltimore: York Press, 1972.

Goltz, Dietlinde. *Studien zur Geschichte der Mineralnamen in Pharmazie, Chemie und Medizin von den Anfängen bis Paracelsus.* Sudhoffs Archiv, Beiheft 14. Wiesbaden: F. Steiner, 1972.

Goodman, Louis S., and Alfred Gilman, eds. *The Pharmacological Basis of Therapeutics.* 5th ed. New York: Macmillan, 1975.

Goodyer, John. See Dioscorides.

Gossen, "Sostratos." No. 13, *P.W.* 3A suppl. (1927): 1203–1204.

Goth, Andres. *Medical Pharmacology.* 9th ed. St. Louis: Mosby, 1978.

Govindarajan, J. S. "Pepper—Chemistry, Technology, and Quality Evaluation." *CRC Critical Reviews in Food Science and Nutrition* 9 (1977): 115–225.

Gow, A. S. F., and A. F. Scholfield. See Nicander.

Greene, Edward Lee. *Landmarks of Botanical History.* Ed. Frank N. Egerton. 2 vols. Stanford: Stanford University Press, 1983.

Greengard, Paul. "The Vitamins." In *Pharmacological Basis of Therapeutics*, ed. Louis S. Goodman and Alfred Gilman, pp. 1544–1548. 5th ed. New York: Macmillan, 1975.

Grieve, M. *A Modern Herbal.* 2 pts. New York: Harcourt Brace, 1931; rep. New York: Dover, 1971.

Grube, Ernst J. "Materialien zum Dioskurides Arabicus." In *Aus der Welt der islamischen Kunst. Festschrift für Ernst Kühnel*, pp. 163–194. Berlin: Gebr. Mann, 1959.

Gujral, M. L., D. R. Varma, K. N. Sareen, and A. K. Roy. "Preliminary Observations on the Antifertility Effect of Some Indigenous Drugs." *Indian Journal of Medicinal Research* 48 (1960): 46–51.

Gunn, J. W. C. "The Action of the 'Emmenagogue Oils' on the Human Uterus." *Journal of Pharmacology and Experimental Therapeutics* 15 (1920): 485–489.

Gunther, Robert T. See Dioscorides.

Harborne, J. B. *Introduction to Ecological Biochemistry.* London: Academic Press, 1977.

Harig, Georg. *Bestimmung der Intensität im medizinischen System Galens: Ein Beiträg zur theoretische Parmakologie, Nosologie und Therapie in der Galenischen Medizin.* Berlin: Akademie-Verlag, 1974.

———. "Der Begriff der lauen Wärme in der theoretischen Pharmakologie Galens." *NTM: Schriftenreihe für Geschichte der Naturwissenschaften, Technik, und Medizin* 13 (1976): 70–76.

———. "Verhältnis zwischen den Primär- und Sekundärqualitaten in der theoretischen Pharmakologie Galens." *NTM: Schriftenreihe für Geschichte der Naturwissenschaften, Technik, und Medizin* 10 (1973): 64–81.

———, and Jutta Kollesch. "Der hippokratische Eid, Zur Entstehung der antiken medizinischen Deontologie." *Philologus* 122 (1978): 157–176.

Harris, William V. "The Theoretical Possibility of Extensive Infanticide in the Graeco-Roman World." *Classical Philology* 32 (1982): 114–116.

Hartwell, Jonathan L. "Plant Remedies for Cancer." *Cancer Chemotherapy Reports*, July 1960, pp. 19–24.

———. "Plants Used against Cancer: A Survey." *Lloydia* 30 (1967): 379–436; 31 (1968): 71–170; 32 (1969): 79–107, 153–205, 247–296; 33 (1970): 97–194, 288–392; 34 (1971): 103–160, 204–255, 310–360, 386–425.

Harvey, Stewart C. "Antiseptics and Disinfectants; Fungicides; Ectoparasiticides." In *The Pharmacological Basis of Therapeutics*, ed. Louis S. Goodman and Alfred Gilman, pp. 987–1017. 5th ed. New York: Macmillan, 1975.

———. "Heavy Metals." In *The Pharmacological Basis of Therapeutics*, ed. Louis S. Goodman and Alfred Gilman, pp. 924–945. 5th ed. New York: Macmillan, 1975.

Hava, Milos. "The Pharmacology of Vinca Species and Their Alkaloids." In *The Vinca Alkaloids*, ed. W. I. Taylor and N. Farnsworth, pp. 305–338. New York: M. Dekker, 1973.

Healy, J. F. *Mining and Metalurgy in the Greek and Roman World*. London: Thames and Hudson, 1978.

"Herakleides." No. 54, *P.W.* 8, pt. 1 (1912): 493–496.

Herbert, Victor. "Drugs Effective in Iron Deficiency and Other Hypochromic Activity." In *The Pharmacological Basis of Therapeutics*, ed. Louis S. Goodman and Alfred Gilman, pp. 1309–1323. 5th ed. New York: Macmillan, 1975.

Hill, Albert F. *Economic Botany*. New York: McGraw-Hill, 1937.

Himes, Norman E. *Medical History of Contraception*. Baltimore: Williams and Wilkins, 1936.

Hopkins, Keith. "Contraception in the Roman Empire." *Comparative Studies in Society and History* 8 (1965): 124–151.

Hort, Arthur. See Theophrastus.

Hunger, Herbert. *Katalog der griechischen Handschriften der oesterreichischen Nationalbibliothek*. 2 vols. Vienna: G. Prachner, 1969.

Hurlbut, Cornelius S., Jr., and Cornelius Klein. *Manual of Mineralogy after James D. Dana*. 19th ed. New York: Wiley, 1977.

Hurlbut, Cornelius S., Sr. *Dana's Manual of Minerals*. 16th ed. New York: Wiley, 1952.

ibn Másawayh, Yūhannā. *Mesue qui Graecorum ac Arabum postremus medicinam practicam illustravit*. Venice: Junta, 1558.

ibn Sīnā. See Avicenna.

"Iollas." *P.W.* 9 (1916): 1855.

Jashemski, Wilhelmina. "The Campanian Peristyle Garden." In *Ancient Roman Gardens*, ed. Elizabeth B. MacDougall and Wilhelmina Jashemski, pp. 31–48. Dumbarton Oaks Colloquium, no. 8. Washington: Dumbarton Oaks, 1981.

———. *The Gardens of Pompeii, Herculaneum and the Villas Destroyed by Vesuvius.* New Rochelle, N.Y.: Caratzas, 1979.

Johnson, J. de M. "A Botanical Papyrus with Illustrations." *Archiv für die Geschichte der Naturwissenschaften und der Technik* 4 (1913): 403–408.

Jones, A. H. M. *The Cities of the Eastern Roman Provinces.* 2d ed. Oxford: Clarendon Press, 1971.

Jones, W. H. S. See Pliny.

Journal of Animal Sciences, July 25, 1963.

Kádár, Zoltán. "Etude comparée des miniatures zoologiques dans trois manuscrits byzantins de la matière médicale de Dioscoride (manuscrit de New York et ceux de Rome) et leur intérêt scientifique." *Acta Biologica Debrecina* 7–8 (1969–1970): 257–263.

———. *Survivals of Greek Zoological Illuminations in Byzantine Manuscripts.* Trans. T. Wilkinson. Budapest: Akadémiai Kiadó, 1978.

Kingsbury, John M. *Poisonous Plants of the United States and Canada.* Englewood Cliffs, N.J.: Prentice-Hall, 1964.

Korolkovas, Andrejus, and Joseph P. Burchhater. *Essentials of Medicinal Chemistry.* New York: Wiley, 1976.

Kraemer, Henry. *A Textbook of Botany and Pharmacognosy.* 4th rev. ed. Philadelphia: Lippincott, 1910.

Kremers, Edward, and George Urdang. *A History of Pharmacy.* Ed. Glenn Sonnendecker. 4th ed. Philadelphia: Lippincott, 1979.

Kudlien, Fridolf. *Der griechische Ärtz im Zeitalter des Hellenismus: Seine Stellung in Staat und Gesellschaft.* Abh. d. Geistes- und Sozialwissen, Kl. Jahrgang, no. 6. Wiesbaden: F. Steiner, 1979.

———. "Diodors Zwitter-exkurs als Testimonium hellenistischer Medizin." *Clio Medica* 1 (1960): 319–324.

———. "Galen's Religious Belief." In *Galen: Problems and Prospects*, ed. Vivian Nutton. London: Wellcome Institute, 1981.

———. "Medical Education in Classical Antiquity." In *The History of Medical Education*, ed. C. D. O'Malley, pp. 3–37. Berkeley: University of California Press, 1970.

Lambecius, Petrus. *Commentarorium de augustissima Bibliotheca Caesarea Vindobonensi.* 8 vols. Vienna: M. Cosmorovii, 1665–1679.

Langkavel, Bernhard. *Botanik der spaeteren Griechen.* Berlin: F. Berggold, 1866; repr. Amsterdam: Hakkart, 1964.

Laszlo, Henry de, and Paul S. Henshaw. "Plant Materials Used by Primitive Peoples to Affect Fertility." *Science* 10 (1954): 626–631.

Laufer, Berthold. "Malabathron." *Journal Asiatique* 193 (1918): 5–49.

Lavie, David, and Shlomo Szinai. "The Constituents of *Ecballium elaterium* L. II: a-Elaterin[1,2]." *Journal of the American Chemical Society* 80 (1958): 707–710.

———. "The Constituents of *Ecballium elaterium* L. III: Elatericin A and B[1,2]." *Journal of the American Chemical Society* 80 (1958): 710–714.

Leake, Chauncey D. *An Historical Account of Pharmacology to the 20th Century.* Springfield: Thomas, 1975.

Leclainche, Emmanuel. *Histoire de la médecine vetérinaire.* Toulouse: Office du livre, 1936.

Leemans, C., ed. *Papyri Graeci Musei Antiquarii Publici Lugduni-Bataui.* 2 vols. Leiden: H. W. Hazenberg, 1885.

Lévi-Strauss, Claude. *The Savage Mind.* Chicago: University of Chicago Press, 1973.

Lewis, Naphtali. *Life in Egypt under Roman Rule.* Oxford: Clarendon Press, 1983.

Lewis, Walter H., and Memory P. F. Elvin-Lewis. *Medical Botany.* New York: Wiley, 1977.

———, ———. "Systematic Botany and Medicine." In *Systematic Botany, Plant Utilization and Biosphere Conservation,* ed. Inga Hedberg. Uppsala, 1979.

Liddell, Henry G., and Robert Scott. *A Greek English Lexicon with Supplement.* Rev. Henry Stuart Jones. 9th ed. Oxford: Clarendon Press, 1968.

Lloyd, G. E. R. "The Hot and the Cold, the Dry and the Wet in Greek Philosophy." *Journal of Hellenic Studies* 84 (1964): 92–106.

———. *Magic, Reason and Experience: Studies in the Origins and Development of Greek Science.* Cambridge: Cambridge University Press, 1979.

———. *Science, Folklore and Ideology.* Cambridge: Cambridge University Press, 1983.

Loew, Elias A. *The Beneventan Script: A History of the South Italian Minuscule.* Oxford: Clarendon Press, 1914.

Loret, V. *Le flore pharaonique d'après les documents hiéroglyphiques et les spécimens découverts dans les tombes.* Paris: Ernest Leroux, 1892; repr. Hildesheim: G. Ohms, 1975.

Lytton, D. G., and L. M. Resuhr. See "Galen on Abnormal Swellings."

McIlroy, R. J. *The Plant Glycosides.* London: Arnold, 1951.

McKendry, Maxime. *The Seven Centuries Cookbook.* Ed. Arabelle Boxer. New York: McGraw-Hill, 1973.

MacKinney, Loren C. "Animal Substances in Materia Medica: A Study in the Persistence of the Primitive." *Journal of the History of Medicine and Allied Sciences* 1 (1946): 149–170.

McVaugh, Michael. *Arnaldi de Villanova. Opera medica Omnia, II. Aphorisimi de gradibus.* Granada-Barcelona: Seminarium Historiae Medicae Granatensis, 1975.

———. "The Mediaeval Theory of Compound Medicines." Dissertation, Princeton, 1975

Madan, Falconer, and H. E. Craster. *A Summary Catalogue of Western Manuscripts in the Bodleian Library at Oxford.* 7 vols. Oxford: Clarendon Press, 1895–1953.

Magie, David. *Roman Rule in Asia Minor.* 2 vols. Princeton: Princeton University Press, 1950.

Maimonides, Moses. *Glossary of Drug Names.* Trans. Max Meyerhof; ed. Fred Rosner. Philadelphia: American Philosophical Society, 1979.

Majno, Guido. *The Healing Hand: Man and Wound in the Ancient World.* Cambridge, Mass.: Harvard University Press, 1975.

Malinowski, Bronislaw. *Magic, Science and Religion and Other Essays.* Garden City, N.Y.: Doubleday, 1954.

Mazal, Otto. *Pflanzen, Wurzeln, Säfte, Samen: Antike Heilkunst in Miniaturen des Wiener Dioskurides*. Graz: Akademische Druck, 1981.

Mazure, Mieczaslaw, Przedzislw Polakowski, and Anna Szdowske. "Pharmacology of Lupanine and 13-Hydroxylupanine." *Acta Physiol. Polon.* 17:299–309, as reported in *Chemical Abstracts* 65 (1966): 11163q.

Meissner, Friedrich Ludwig. *Encyclopëdia der medizinischen Wissenschaften*. 14 vols. Leipzig, 1830–1835.

Mercati, Iohannes, and Pius Franchi de' Cavalieri. *Bibliotheca Apostolica Vaticana. Codices Vaticani graeca*. 3 vols. Rome: Typis Polyglottis Vaticanis, 1923.

Merck Index: An Encyclopedia of Chemicals and Drugs. 9th ed. Rahway, N.J.: Merck, 1978.

Merck Veterinary Manual. 4th ed. Rahway, N.J.: Merck, 1973.

Meyer, Ernst H. F. *Geschichte der Botanik*. 4 vols. Konigsberg: G. Bornträger, 1854–1857.

Miller, J. Innes. *The Spice Trade of the Roman Empire, 29 B.C. to A.D. 641*. Oxford: Clarendon Press, 1969.

Mioni, Elpidio. "Un novo erbario greco di Dioscride." *Rassegna Medica Convivum Sanitatis* (Milan) 36, no. 3 (1959): 169–184.

Mitscher, Lester A. "Plant-Derived Antibiotics." In *Antibiotics, Isolation, Separation, and Purification*, ed. Marvin J. Weinstein and Gerald H. Wagman. Amsterdam: Elsevier, 1978.

Moe, Gordon K., and J. A. Abildskou. "Antiarrhythmic Drugs." In *The Pharmacological Basis of Therapeutics*, ed. Louis S. Goodman and Alfred Gilman, pp. 683–704. 5th ed. New York: Macmillan, 1975.

Moncrieff, R. W. *The Chemical Senses*. 3rd ed. London: L. Hill, 1967.

Montfaucon, B. de. *Palaegraphia Graeca*. Paris: L. Guerin, 1708.

Moore, N. F. *Ancient Mineralogy*. New York: Harper & Brothers, 1859.

Morel, W. "Pharmakopoles." *P.W.* 19, pt. 2 (1938): 1840–1841.

Morricone, Achille. "I medicamenti di origine animale ricavati dal mare nell' opera di Dioscoride." *Pagine di Storia della medicina* 7 (1963): 24–28.

Morton, Julia F. *Major Medicinal Plants*. Springfield: Thomas, 1977.

Moulé, Léon. "La zoothérapie au temps de Dioscoride et de Pline." *International Congress for the History of Medicine* (Antwerp) 1 (1920): 451–461.

Murad, Ferid, and Alfred G. Gilman. "Estrogens and Progestins." In *The Pharmacological Basis of Therapeutics*, ed. Louis S. Goodman and Alfred Gilman, pp. 1423–1450. 5th ed. New York: Macmillan, 1975.

Nauert, Charles G., Jr. "Caius Plinius Secundus." *Catalogus Translationum et Commentariorum* 4 (1980): 297–422.

Neuburger, Max. *Geschichte der Medizin*. 2 vols. Stuttgart: F. Enke, 1906–1911.

Nickel, D. "Ärztliche Ethik und Schwangerschaftsunterbrechung bei den Hippokratikern." *N.T.M. Schriftenreihe für Geschichte der Naturwissenschaften, Technik, und Medizin* 9 (1972): 73–80.

Nielson, Harald. "Ancient Ophthalmological Agents." Trans. Lars McBridge. In *Acta Historica Scientarium Naturalium et Medicinalium*. Ed. Bibl. Univ. Havensis, vol. 31. Odense: Odense University Press, 1974.

Nissen, C. *Die botanische Buchillustration*. Stuttgart: Hiersemann, 1951.

Noonan, John T. *Contraception: A History of Its Treatment by the Catholic Theologians and Canonists.* Cambridge, Mass.: Harvard University Press, 1966.

Nriagu, Jerome O. *Lead and Lead Poisoning in Antiquity.* New York: Wiley, 1983.

———. "Saturnine Gout among Roman Aristocrats." *New England Journal of Medicine* 308 (1983): 660–663.

Nutton, Vivian. "The Chronology of Galen's Early Career." *Classical Quarterly* 23 (1973): 158–171.

———. "Medicine and the Roman Army." *Medical History* 13 (1969): 260–270.

———. See Dioscorides.

Oder, Eugen. "Revue of *Pedanii Dioscurides.*" Ed. M. Wellmann. *Berliner Philologische Wochenschrift*, no. 17 (April 28, 1906), col. 520.

Oliver-Bever, B. "Vegetable Drugs for Cancer Therapy." *Quarterly Journal of Crude Drug Research* 11 (1971): 1668–1677.

P.W. See Pauly-Wissowa-Kroll.

Palma, Luigi. *Le piante medicinali d'Italia. Botanica. Chimica. Farmacodinamica. Terapia.* [Torino]: Società Editorice Internazionale, 1964.

Panova, D., and S. Nilolov. "Steriodal sapogenins and sterois of Ruscus aculeatus var ponticus (woronov)." *Farmtsiya* 29 (1979): 25–29.

Patrick, Adam. "Disease in Antiquity: Ancient Greece and Rome." In *Disease in Antiquity*, ed. Don Brothwell and A. T. Sandison, pp. 238–246. Springfield: Thomas, 1967.

Pauly-Wissowa-Kroll. *Realencyclopaedie der classischen Altertumswissenschaft.* Stuttgart: Metzlerscher, 1894–.

Penzig, Otto. *Contribuzioni alla Storia della Botanica.* Milan: V. Hoepli, 1905.

Pfaffmann, Carl. "Smell and Taste." *Encyclopaedia Britannica*, 20: 684–687. 1971.

Physicians' Desk Reference. 20th ed. Oradell, N.J.: Medical Economics, 1966.

———. 37th ed. Oradell, N.J.: Medical Economics, 1983.

Pierleoni, G. *Catalogus codicum graecorum Bibliothecae.* New series, 8. Rome: Instituto poligrafico dello Stato, 1962.

Pinaeus, Antonius. *Historia plantarum.* Lyons: Gabriel Coterius, 1561.

Platearius, Matthaeus. *Circa instans.* In *Das Arzneidrogenbuch Circa Instans.* Berlin, 1939. [Photocopy available from A. Preilipper, Hamburg.]

Polunin, Oleg. *Flowers of Europe.* London: Oxford University Press, 1969.

———. *Flowers of Greece and the Balkans.* Oxford: Oxford University Press, 1980.

Power, Frederick B., and Charles W. Moore. "Chemical Examination of Elaterium and Elaterin." *Pharmaceutical Journal and Pharmacist*, October 23, 1909, pp. 501–504.

Premerstein, Antony de. See Dioscorides.

Preuss, Julius. *Biblical and Talmudic Medicine.* Trans. and ed. Fred Rosner. New York and London: Sanhedrin Press, 1978.

Quarterly Journal of Crude Drug Research 1– (1961–).

Raeder, Johannes. See Oribasius.

Ramsay, W. M. *Cities of St. Paul.* London: Hodder and Stoughton, 1907.

Rather, L. J. *The Genesis of Cancer: A Study in the History of Ideas.* Baltimore: Johns Hopkins University Press, 1978.

Rawson, Elizabeth. "The Life and Death of Asclepiades of Bithynia." *Classical Quarterly* 32 (1982): 358–370.

Reedy, Jeremiah. "Galen on Cancer and Related Diseases." *Clio Medica* 10 (1975): 227–238.

Revilla, P. A. *Catálogo de los códices griegos de la Biblioteca de el Escorial.* Madrid: Imprenta Helénica, 1936.

Reynolds, Leighton Durham, and N. G. Wilson. *Scribes and Scholars.* London: Oxford University Press, 1968.

Riddle, John. "Amber in Ancient Pharmacy." *Pharmacy in History* 15 (1973): 3–17.

———. "Dioscorides." In *Catalogus Translationum et Commentariorum,* ed. Paul O. Kristeller, 4:1–143. Washington: Catholic University Press, 1980.

———. "Lithotherapy in the Middle Ages. Lapidaries Considered as Medical Texts." *Pharmacy in History* 12 (1970): 39–50.

———. *Marbode of Rennes' De lapidibus.* Sudhoffs Archiv, Beiheft 20. Wiesbaden: F. Steiner, 1977.

———. "Pseudo-Dioscorides' *Ex herbis femininis* and Early Medieval Medical Botany." *Journal of the History of Biology* 14 (1981): 43–81.

———. "Quid pro Quo: Pharmacy in the Middle Ages." *Medical Heritage* (forthcoming).

———, and James A. Mulholland. "Albert on Stones and Minerals." In *Albertus Magnus and the Sciences,* ed. J. A. Weisheipl, pp. 203–234. Toronto: Pontifical Institute, 1980.

Rosenberg, Charles E. "The Therapeutic Revolution: Medicine, Meaning, and Social Change in Nineteenth-Century America." *Perspectives in Biology and Medicine* 20 (1977): 485–506.

Rosenfeld, André. *The Inorganic Raw Materials of Antiquity.* Washington, 1965.

Ruegg, Kurt. *Beiträge zur Geschichte der offizinellen Drogen: Crocus, Acorus Calamus und Colchicum.* Dissertation. Stetten and Basel: Karl Schahl, 1936.

Rufinus. *The Herbal of Rufinus.* Ed. Lynn Thordike and Francis Benjamin. Chicago: University of Chicago Press, 1946.

Salib, Philip. "Trauma and Disease of the Post-Cranial Skeleton in Ancient Egypt." In *Diseases in Antiquity,* ed. Don Brothwell and A. T. Sandison, pp. 599–605. Springfield: Thomas, 1967.

Salis, A. von. "Images Illustrium." In *Eumusia Festgabe für Ernst Howald.* Zurich: E. Rentsch, 1947.

Samberger, Christa. *Catalogi Codicem Graecorum qui in monoribus Bibliothecis Italicis Asservantur.* 2 vols. Leipzig: Zentral-Antiquariat, 1965.

Sanders, Edward H., Pete D. Gardner, Patricia J. Berger, and Norman C. Negus. "6-Methoxybenzoxazolinone: A Plant Derivative That Stimulates Reproduction in *Microtus montanus.*" *Science* 214 (1981): 67–69.

Saracenus, Janus Antonius. *Τὰ σωζόμενα ἅπαντα . . .: Opera quae extant omnia.* Frankfurt a/m, 1598.

Sarton, George. *Introduction to the History of Science.* 3 vols in 5 parts. Baltimore: Williams and Wilkins, 1927–1947.

Saumaise, Claude de. *Plinianae exercitationes in Caii Julii Soilini Polyhistoria.* Paris, 1689.

Sayre, Lucius E. *A Manual of Organic Materia Medica and Pharmacognosy.* 4th ed. Philadelphia: P. Blakiston, 1917.

Scarborough, John. "The Drug Lore of Asclepiades of Bithynia." *Pharmacy in History* 17 (1975): 43–57.

———. "The Galenic Question." *Sudhoffs Archiv* 65 (1981): 1–31.

———. "Nicander's Toxicology I: Snakes." *Pharmacy in History* 19 (1977): 3–23.

———. "Nicander's Toxicology II: Spiders, Scorpions, Insects and Myriapods." *Pharmacy in History* 21 (1979): 3–34, 73–92.

———. "On the Understanding of Medicine among the Romans." *Historian* 39 (1977): 213–227.

———. *Roman Medicine.* Ithaca: Cornell University Press, 1969.

———. "Roman Medicine and Public Health." In *Public Health: Proceedings of the 5th International Symposium on the Comparative History of Medicine—East and West, Suosono, Japan, October 26–November 1, 1980,* ed. Teizo Ogawa, pp. 33–74. Tokyo, c. 1981.

———. "Roman Medicine and the Legions." *Medical History* 12 (1968): 296–306.

———. "Theophrastus on Herbals and Herbal Remedies." *Journal of the History of Biology* 11 (1978): 353–385.

———, and Vivian Nutton. See Dioscorides.

Scarpa, Antonio. "Pre-Scientific Medicines: Their Extent and Value." *Social Science and Medicine* A, 15A (1981): 317–326.

Schauenberg, Paul, and Ferdinand Paris. *Guide des plantes médicinales.* Nauchâtel, 1977. English trans. by Maurice Pugh-Jones, Guildford, Conn.: Lutterworth, 1977.

Schifferli, E. "Abtreibungen und Abtreibungsversuche mit pflanzlichen Materialien." *Deutsches Zeitschrift für gesamte gerichtliche Medizin* 31 (1939): 238–245.

Schmidt, Alfred. *Drogen und Drogenhandel im Altertum.* Leipzig: J. A. Barth, 1924; repr. New York: Arno, 1979.

Schmidt, Charles. "Theophrastus." Ed. Paul O. Kristeller. *Catalogus Translationum et Commentariorum* 2 (1971): 239–322.

Schneider, Wolfgang. *Lexikon zur Arzneimittelgeschichte.* 7 vols. Frankfurt: Govi-Verlag, 1968–1975.

Sesse, Hubert, Jean Ray, and Jean Pierre Tarye. "Pharmaceutical Composition with Antiinflammatory and Vasculotropic Activity." *France Demande.* [Patent] 2, 377, 201 Cl. A61K37/48, 11 Aug. 1978, as reported by *Chemical Abstracts* 91 (1979): 91: 9494a.

Shapiro, Arthur K. "The Placebo Effect in the History of Medical Treatment: Implications for Psychiatry." *American Journal of Psychiatry* 116 (1959): 298–304.

Sibthorp, John, and James E. Smith. *Flora Graeca.* 10 vols. London: Richard Taylor, 1806–1840.

Sigerist, Henry E. *A History of Medicine.* 2 vols. New York and London: Oxford University Press, 1951–1961.

Singer, Charles. *From Magic to Science.* London: E. Benn, 1928.

———. "Greek Biology and Its Relation to the Rise of Modern Biology." In *Studies in the History and Method of Science,* 2:1–101. Oxford: Clarendon Press, 1921.

———. "The Herbal in Antiquity." *Journal of Hellenic Studies* 47 (1927): 1–52.

Sizov, P. I. "Experimental Parturifacient Action of Pachycarpine Brevicolline and Thalictrimine." *Zdravookhranenie Belorussii* 15 (1969): 44–46, as reported in *Chemical Abstracts* 72 (1970): 119957u.

Skarzynski, Boleslaw. "An Oestrogenic Substitute from Plant Materials." *Nature* 131 (1933): 766.

Smith, Kenneth G. V. "Coleoptera and Other Insects: Beetles, Mayflies and Caddisflies." In *Insects and Other Arthropods of Medical Importance,* ed. K. Smith. London: Trustees of the British Museum, 1973.

Smith, Wesley. "Galen on Coans versus Cnidians." *Bulletin of the History of Medicine* 47 (1973): 569–585.

———. *The Hippocratic Tradition.* Ithaca: Cornell University Press, 1979.

Spatharakis, Ioannis. *Corpus of Dated Illuminated Greek Manuscripts to the Year 1453.* 2 vols. Leiden: Brill, 1981.

Spencer, W. G. See Celsus.

Stadler, Hermann. "Der lateinische Dioscorides der Münchener Hof- und Staatsbibliothek und die Bedeutung dieser Uebersetzung für einen Teil der mittelalterlichen Medizin." *Janus* 4 (1899): 548–550.

———. "Lateinische Pflanzennamen in Dioskorides." *Archiv für lateinische Lexikographie und Grammatik* 2 (1898): 83–114.

———. "Neues zur alten Botanik." *Bayerische Blaetter für das Gymnasialschulwesen* 34 (1898): 609–614.

Stannard, Jerry. "Asclepiades." In *Dictionary of Scientific Biography,* 1:314–315. 1970.

———. "Byzantine Botanical Lexicography." *Episteme* 5 (1971): 168–187.

———. "The Herbal as a Medical Document." *Bulletin of the History of Medicine* 43 (1969): 212–220.

———. "Medicinal Plants and Folk Remedies in Pliny, *Historia Naturalis." History and Philosophy of the Life Sciences* 4 (1982): 3–23.

———. "Squill in the Ancient and Medieval Materia Medica with Special Reference to Its Employment for Dropsy." *Bulletin of the New York Academy of Medicine* 50, 2d ser. (1974): 684–713.

Stearn, William T. "From Theophrastus and Dioscorides to Sibthorp and Smith: The Background and Origin of the *Flora Graeca." Biological Journal of the Linnean Society* 8 (1976): 285–318.

———. "A Synopsis of the Genus Vinca." In *Vinca Alkaloids,* ed. William I. Taylor and Norman Farnsworth, pp. 19–94. New York: M. Dekker, 1973.

Steinbock, R. Ted. "Lead Ingestion in Ancient Times." *Paleopathology Newsletter,* no. 27 (1979): 9–11.

Steinmetz, E. F. "Crude Vegetable Drugs and Their Galenical Preparations versus Active Principles Derived Therefrom." *Quarterly Journal of Crude Drug Research* 1 (1961): 3–10.

Sternberg, Kaspar Maria von. *Catalogus plantarum ad septem varias editiones commentariorum Matthioli in Dioscoridem.* Prague: J. G. Calve, 1821.

Stieb, Ernst W. "Drug Adulteration and Its Detection in the Writings of Theophrastus, Dioscorides and Pliny." *Journal Mondial de Pharmacie* 2 (1958): 117–134.

Stone, W. S. "A Review of the History of Chemical Theory in Cancer." *Medical Record* 90 (1916): 628–634.

Susemihl, Franz. *Geschichte der griechischen Litteratur in der Alexandrinerzeit.* 2 vols. Leipzig: Teubner, 1892.

Swain, Tony, ed. *Plants in the Development of Modern Medicine.* Cambridge, Mass.: Harvard University Press, 1972.

Théodoridès, J. "Intérêt scientifique des miniatures zoologiques d'un manuscrit de Matiere médicale de Dioscuride." *Acta Biologica Debrecina* 7–8 (1969–1970): 265–272.

———. "Remarques sur l'iconographie zoologique dans certains manuscrits médicaux byzantins et étude des miniatures zoologique du Codex Vaticanus Graecus." *Jahrbuch der oesterreiches byzantinische Gesellschaft*, 1961, pp. 24–27.

Thompson, C. J. S. *The Mystic Mandrake.* New York: University Books, 1968.

Thomson, William A. R. *Medicines from the Earth.* New York: McGraw-Hill, 1978.

Thorndike, Lynn. *A History of Magic and Experimental Science.* 8 vols. New York: Columbia University Press, 1923–1958.

———. *The Place of Magic in the Intellectual History of Europe.* New York: Columbia University Press, 1905.

Trease, George Edward. *A Text-book of Pharmacognosy.* 2d ed. Baltimore: W. Wood, 1936.

———, and William C. Evans. *Pharmacognosy.* 11th ed. London: B. Tindall, 1978.

Tschirch, Alexander. *Handbuch der Pharmakognosie.* 3 vols. Leipzig: Tauchnitz, 1909–1925.

Tyler, V. E., L. R. Brady, and J. E. Robbers. *Pharmacognosy.* 7th ed. Philadelphia: Lea and Febiger, 1976; 8th ed. Philadelphia: Lea and Febiger, 1981.

Ullsperger, R. "Die Entwicklung der Crataegusforschung." *Planta Medica* 1 (1953): 43–50.

Usher, George. *Dictionary of Plants Used by Man.* London: Constable, 1974.

Van Gerven, Dennis P. "Nubia's Last Christians: The Cemeteries of Kulubnarti." *Archaeology* 34 (1981): 22–30.

Van Straten, S., Flora de Vrijer, and J. C. de Beauveser, eds. *Lists of Volatile Compounds in Foods.* 3d ed. Zeist: Centraal Institut voor Voedingsonderzoek, 1973.

Von Reis, Siri Altschul. *Drugs and Foods from Little Known Plants.* Cambridge, Mass.: Harvard University Press, 1974.

Waldron, H. A. "Lead Poisoning in the Ancient World." *Medical History* 17 (1973): 391–399.

Waldron, Tony, and Calvin Wells. "Exposure to Lead in Ancient Populations."

Transactions and Studies. College of Physicians of Philadelphia ser. 5, 1 (1979): 102–115.

Walker, R. E. "Roman Veterinary Medicine." In *Animals in Roman Life and Art*, ed. J. M. C. Toynbee, pp. 303–343, 404–414. London: Thames and Hudson; Ithaca: Cornell University Press, 1973.

Watt, John Mitchell, and Maria Gerdina Breyer-Brandwijk. *The Medicinal and Poisonous Plants of Southern and Eastern Africa*. 2d ed. Edinburgh: E. & S. Livingstone, 1962.

Webster, Graham. *The Roman Imperial Army*. London: Black, 1969.

Weitzmann, Kurt. *Ancient Book Illumination*. Cambridge, Mass.: Harvard University Press, 1959.

———. *Die byzantinische Buchmalerei des 9. und 10. Jahrunderts*. Berlin: Gebr. Mann, 1935.

———. *Illustrations in Roll and Codex*. Rev. ed. Princeton: Princeton University Press, 1970.

———. *Late Antique and Early Christian Book Illumination*. New York: G. Braziller, 1977.

———. *Studies in Classical and Byzantine Manuscript Illumination*. Ed. Herbert L. Kessler. Chicago: University of Chicago Press, 1971.

Wellmann, Max. "Athenaios." No. 24, *P.W.* 2 (1896): 2034–2036.

———. "Bassus." No. 122, *P.W.* 10 (1918): 180–181.

———. "Chrysippos." No. 15, *P.W.* 3 (1899): 2509–2510.

———. "Diagoras." No. 3, *P.W.* 5 (1903): 311.

———. *Die Fragmente der sikelischen Ärzte Akron, Philistion und des Diokles von Karystos*. Fragmentsammlung der Griechische Ärzte, vol. 1. Berlin: Weidmann, 1901.

———. "Die Pflanzennamen des Dioskurides." *Hermes* 33 (1898): 360–422.

———. *Die Schrift des Diokurides Περὶ ἁπλῶν φαρμάκων: Ein Beitrag zur Geschichte der Medizin*. Berlin: Weidmann, 1914.

———. "Dioskurides." No. 12, *P.W.* 5 (1903): 1131–1142.

———. "Dorion." No. 4, *P.W.* 5 (1905): 1563.

———. *Krateuas*. Abhandlungen der königlichen Gesellschaft der wissenschaften zu Gottingen, Phil.-Hist. Klasse, Neue Folge, 2: no. 1. Berlin: Weidmann, 1897.

———. "Λεκάνιος Ἄρειος." No. 13, *P.W.* 2 (1895): 626.

———. "Sextius Niger: Eine Quellenuntersuchung zu Dioscorides." *Hermes* 24 (1889): 530–569.

———. "Zur Geschichte der Medizin im Alterthum." *Hermes* 23 (1888): 556–566.

———. See Dioscorides.

White, Lynn, Jr. *Machina ex Deo: Essays in the Dynamism of Western Culture*. Cambridge, Mass.: MIT Press, 1968.

Wilsdorf, Helmut. "Die architektonische Rekonstruktion antiker Produktionsanlagen für Bergbau und Hüttenwesen." *Klio: Beiträge zur alten Geschichte* 59 (1977): 11–24.

Winstedt, E. O. "Some Greek and Latin Papyri in Aberdeen Museum." *Classical Quarterly* 1 (1907): 257–267.

Woodburn, Dixon M., and Edward Fingl. "Analgesic-Antipyretics, Anti-inflammatory Agents, and Drugs Employed in the Therapy of Gout." In *The Pharmacological Basis of Therapeutics*, ed. Louis S. Goodman and Alfred Gilman, pp. 325–358. 5th ed. New York: Macmillan, 1975.

INDEX

There are ten sections: I, Persons; II, Places; III, Plants; IV, Animals and Drugs from Animals; V, Minerals; VI, Drugs; VII, Medical Actions and Therapeutic Procedures; VIII, Diseases and Afflictions; IX, General; X, Greek Terms.

I. PERSONS

II. PLACES

III. PLANTS

IV. ANIMALS AND DRUGS FROM ANIMALS

V. MINERALS

VI. DRUGS

VII. MEDICAL ACTIONS AND THERAPEUTIC PROCEDURES

VIII. DISEASES AND AFFLICTIONS

IX. GENERAL

X. GREEK TERMS

Milton Keynes UK
Ingram Content Group UK Ltd.
UKHW030740040924
447866UK00001B/3